FOUNDATIONS OF THERAPEUTIC INTERVIEWING

FOUNDATIONS OF THERAPEUTIC INTERVIEWING

John Sommers-Flanagan
University of Portland

Rita Sommers-Flanagan
University of Montana

Allyn and Bacon
Boston   London   Toronto   Sydney   Tokyo   Singapore

Series Editor: Ray Short
Production Administrator: Annette Joseph
Production Coordinator: Holly Crawford
Editorial-Production Service: Linda Zuk/WordCrafters Editorial Services, Inc.
Cover Administrator: Linda K. Dickinson
Cover Designer: Suzanne Harbison
Manufacturing Buyer: Louise Richardson

Copyright © 1993 by Allyn and Bacon
A Division of Simon & Schuster, Inc.
160 Gould Street
Needham Heights, MA 02194

Library of Congress Cataloging-in-Publication Data

Sommers-Flanagan, John
    Foundations of Therapeutic Interviewing
  John Sommers-Flanagan, Rita Sommers-Flanagan.
      p.   cm.
    Includes bibliographical references (p.   ) and index.
    ISBN 0-205-14063-7
    1. Interviewing in mental health.   2. Interviewing in psychiatry.
  I. Sommers-Flanagan, Rita   II. Title.
  RC480.7.S66   1993
616.89'023—dc20   92-16647
                                                                    CIP

Printed in the United States of America

10 9 8 7 6 5 4   97 96 95

We wish to dedicate this book to those who shake their heads at us, worry about us, are late to lessons and eat cold pizza because of us, who hug us, love us, put up with us, and believe in us: Grandma Lucy; our parents, Max, Paula, and Mary Lou; and our children, Chelsea and Rylee.

CONTENTS

Preface   xiii

Section I   FUNDAMENTALS OF THERAPEUTIC INTERVIEWING

Chapter 1   Introduction: Philosophy and Organization   1

Teaching Philosophy, 2
>   Quieting Yourself and Listening to Clients, 2
>   Developing Positive Therapeutic Relationships, 3
>   Learning Diagnostic and Assessment Skills, 3
Theoretical Orientations, 4
Basic Requirements for Therapeutic Interviewers, 7
Goals and Objectives of This Book, 8
Total Awareness Interviewing, 8
Textbook Organization, 9
Chapter Summary, 10
Suggested Readings, 11

Chapter 2   Foundations   13

Toward a Definition of Therapeutic Interviewing, 14
Clarifying Initial Assumptions and Issues, 14
>   The Nature of a Professional Relationship, 15
>   Two Functions of Therapeutic Interviews, 17
>   Listening Skills: The Foundation of Therapeutic Interviewing, 18
>   Factors that Guide Therapeutic Interviewing Behavior, 20
Self-Awareness, 21
>   Objective Self-Awareness, 22
>   Forms of Self-Awareness, 23
Interviewing Expectations and Misconceptions, 28

Effective Interviewing: Seven Vocational Perspectives, 28
Chapter Summary, 31
Suggested Readings, 32

Chapter 3   Preparations   33

The Physical Setting, 34
    The Room, 34
    Seating Arrangements, 35
    Note Taking, 38
    Videotape and Audiotape Recording, 40
Professional and Ethical Issues, 41
    Self-Presentation, 41
    Time, 43
    Confidentiality, 45
    Stress Management for Therapeutic Interviewers, 47
Chapter Summary, 48
Suggested Readings, 49

Section II   NONDIRECTIVE LISTENING AND RELATIONSHIP DEVELOPMENT

Chapter 4   Basic Attending Skills   51

Attending Behavior, 52
    Positive Attending Behavior, 53
    Negative Attending Behavior, 56
Individual and Cultural Differences, 59
    Cultural Issues, 59
    Individual Differences, 60
The Relationship between Attending and Listening, 61
    Poor Attending and Good Listening, 61
    Good Attending and Poor Listening, 62
Giving Constructive Feedback, 62
Chapter Summary, 64
Suggested Readings, 64

Chapter 5   Nondirective Listening Responses: A Continuum   67

Nondirective Listening Responses, 70
    Attending Behavior, 71
    Silence, 71
    Paraphrase or Reflection of Content, 72

Clarification, 74
Nondirective Reflection of Feeling, 76
Summarization, 77
Interviewer Development Activities, 80
Brief Nondirective Interviews, 80
Enhancing Your Feeling Capacity and Vocabulary, 81
Silence Desensitization, 81
Generating Sensory-Based and Feeling Words, 82
Chapter Summary, 83
Suggested Readings, 84

Chapter 6   Directives: Listening and Action Responses   85

Directive Listening Responses, 86
Interpretive Reflection of Feeling, 86
Interpretation, 88
Feeling Validation, 90
Questions, 92
Confrontation, 93
Directive Action Responses, 95
Explanation (Providing Information), 97
Suggestion, 100
Giving Advice, 101
Agreement-Disagreement, 103
Urging, 105
Approval-Disapproval, 105
Chapter Summary, 108
Suggested Readings and Professional Recordings, 110

Chapter 7   Relationship Variables and Therapeutic Interviewing   111

Rapport, 112
Common Client Fears, 113
Putting the Client at Ease, 114
Carl Rogers's Core Conditions, 115
Congruence, 116
Unconditional Positive Regard, 119
Accurate Empathy, 121
The Relationship Among Rogers's Core Conditions, 127
Psychoanalytic and Interpersonal Relationship Variables, 127
Transference, 127
Countertransference, 130
Identification and Internalization, 133
Resistance, 135
Working Alliance, 138

Relationship Variables and Behavioral and Social Psychology, 138
    Expertness (Credibility), 139
    Attractiveness, 140
    Trustworthiness, 141
Feminist Relationship Variables, 141
    Mutuality, 142
    Empowerment, 143
Integrating Relationship Variables, 144
Chapter Summary, 144
Suggested Readings, 145

Section III STRUCTURING AND ASSESSMENT

Chapter 8 An Overview of the Interview Process   147

Structural Models, 149
The Introduction, 150
    Telephone Contact, 150
    Initial Face-to-Face Meeting, 152
    Conversation and Small Talk, 155
    Educating Clients and Evaluating Their Expectations, 156
The Opening, 158
    The Interviewer's Opening Statement, 159
    The Client's Opening Response, 160
    Evaluating Client Verbal Behavior During the Opening, 162
The Body, 163
    Sources of Clinical Judgment: Making Inferences, 165
    Defining Psychological and Emotional Disorders, 166
The Closing, 170
    Reassuring and Supporting Your Client, 171
    Summarizing Crucial Themes and Issues, 172
    Instilling Hope, 172
    Guiding and Empowering Your Client, 173
    Tying Up Loose Ends, 174
Termination, 174
    Watching the Clock, 174
    Guiding or Controlling Termination, 175
    Facing Termination, 176
Chapter Summary, 177
Suggested Readings, 179

Chapter 9 The Intake Interview   181

Using Questions, 182
    Types of Questions, 183

Benefits and Liabilities of Questions, 187
Guidelines in Using Questions, 189
Objectives of Intake Interviewing, 192
Identifying, Evaluating, and Exploring Client Problems, 193
Obtaining Background and Historical Information, 199
Evaluating Interpersonal Style, 207
Current Functioning, 211
Identifying Goals and Monitoring Change, 212
Factors Affecting Intake Interview Procedures, 212
Client Registration Forms, 212
Institutional Setting, 213
Theoretical Orientation, 213
Professional Background and Professional Affiliation, 213
Chapter Summary, 213
Suggested Readings, 216

Chapter 10   The Mental Status Examination   217

What Is a Mental Status Exam? 218
A Generic Approach to Mental Status Examination, 219
Appearance, 219
Behavior or Psychomotor Activity, 220
Attitude toward Examiner (Interviewer), 220
Affect and Mood, 221
Speech and Thought, 223
Perceptual Disturbances, 228
Orientation and Consciousness, 230
Memory and Intelligence, 232
Reliability, Judgment, and Insight, 236
When to Use Mental Status Examinations, 240
Chapter Summary, 240
Suggested Readings, 242

Chapter 11   Suicide Assessment   243

Suicide Statistics, 244
Considering Suicide Myths, 246
Risk Factors Associated with Suicide, 246
Conducting a Thorough Suicide Assessment, 250
Assessing Level of Depression, 250
Exploring Suicidal Ideation, 253
Assessing Suicidal Plans, 254
Assessing Client Self-Control, 256
Assessing Intent, 257
Crisis Intervention with Suicidal Clients, 257
Listening and Being Empathic, 257

Establishing a Therapeutic Relationship, 258
Identifying Alternatives to Suicide, 258
Establishing Suicide-Prevention Contracts, 259
Becoming Directive and Responsible, 260
Making Decisions about Hospitalization and Referral, 261
Professional Issues, 263
Can You Work with Suicidal Clients?, 263
Consultation, 264
Documentation, 264
Dealing with Completed Suicides, 265
Chapter Summary, 266
Suggested Readings, 267

Section IV   INTERVIEWING AND DEVELOPMENT

Chapter 12   Facilitating Client *and* Interviewer Development   269

What Is Development?, 270
Client Development, 271
Listening, 271
Intentional Treatment Planning, 271
Interviewer Development, 272
Questions to Ask Yourself, 273
Using Logic and Intuition, 275
Setting Personal Goals, 276
Chapter Summary, 276
Suggested Readings, 277

References   279

Name Index   295

Subject Index   301

PREFACE

This book is designed primarily as an introductory textbook for beginning professional therapeutic interviewers. We have intentionally used the word "therapeutic" in the book's title to describe what has traditionally been referred to as the "clinical" or "counseling" or "helping" interview (Benjamin, 1981; Hutchins & Cole, 1986; Shea, 1988). We chose this word to highlight the multifaceted nature of most initial interview procedures. Specifically, in order to be therapeutic, an interview must involve (a) the development of an alliance or rapport between interviewers and clients; (b) the opportunity for clients to communicate about themselves and their problems to an interested and effective listener; and (c) the elicitation of specific assessment information that allows an individualized and effective treatment plan to be established for each client.

A secondary aim of this book is to emphasize the importance of learning nondirective listening skills prior to more advanced interviewing techniques (i.e., assessment and intervention). Consequently, the first seven chapters are devoted primarily to the goal of developing listening skills and forming effective working relationships with clients. The importance of utilizing interviewing as an assessment procedure is emphasized in Chapters 8 through 11. Chapter 12 is devoted to facilitating the development of both client and interviewer.

Finally, this book is designed so that beginning interviewers are exposed to interviewing perspectives and approaches from a number of theoretical orientations. Current textbooks in this area commonly emphasize cognitive-behavioral, person-centered, or psychoanalytic approaches to interviewing. Because this text is designed for the beginner, it uses a more pan-theoretical approach so that beginners do not feel compelled to prematurely select and adhere to a single theoretical perspective.

Many people have been instrumental in the writing of this text. Perhaps most appropriately, this textbook was made possible because of a senior sales representative of Allyn and Bacon who took the time to effectively listen to a professor's thoughts and ideas about a novel approach to teaching professional interviewing skills. For this, we thank Gerry Bauman of Allyn and Bacon.

Additionally, we wish to thank our supervisors, who helped us in our struggle to quiet ourselves and learn how to listen to clients. We are especially grateful to John Means, H. A. Walters, Philip Bornstein, Janet Wollersheim, David Schuldberg, Bud Orgel, and Brett Steenbarger. Our friends and colleagues Len Burns and Hollie Krueger were continual sources of support; and Susan Davis, Murray Finley, Charlie Hanson of California State University at Northridge, and Scott Meier of State University of New York at Buffalo provided excellent comments in their review of earlier drafts of this book. Finally, we want to express our appreciation to our students and clients, from whom we are privileged to learn by participating in their quest to learn and grow and develop.

1
INTRODUCTION: PHILOSOPHY AND ORGANIZATION

Teaching Philosophy
    Quieting Yourself and Listening to Clients
    Developing Positive Therapeutic Relationships
    Learning Diagnostic and Assessment Skills

Theoretical Orientations

Basic Requirements for Therapeutic Interviews

Goals and Objectives of this Book

Total Awareness Interviewing

Textbook Organization

Chapter Summary

Suggested Readings

There is luxury in self-reproach. When we blame ourselves we feel no one else has a right to blame us.—O. WILDE, Epigrams

Like all other textbooks, this textbook has underlying philosophies. We are not neutral; nor will we feign neutrality. Instead, we will attempt to engage in a bit of self-scrutiny or self-reproach by identifying our biases, explaining them, and allowing you as the reader to weigh them for yourself.

1

We have strong beliefs and feelings about how therapeutic interviewing should be taught. These beliefs are based on our own experiences as students learning to conduct clinical interviews and as instructors teaching interviewing skills to undergraduate and graduate students in psychology and counseling. We cannot present our approach to learning effective therapeutic interviewing skills without at least informing you of our biases. Consequently, this chapter outlines our teaching approach and philosophical orientation. It also describes the book's organization.

Teaching Philosophy

We believe the ability to conduct effective therapeutic interviews is acquired most efficiently when students learn the following interviewing skills and procedures in sequence.

- Quieting oneself and focusing on listening to clients' communication.
- Developing positive working relationships with clients.
- Obtaining diagnostic or assessment information about clients and their problems.
- Searching for and applying individualized and appropriate therapeutic methods and techniques.
- Evaluating client responses to technical interventions.

This text is designed to guide you through the experience of learning the first three skills and processes. We will focus on the process of counseling and psychotherapy within the framework of these three issues; this text does not provide extensive information on implementation and evaluation of therapeutic methods and techniques.

Quieting Yourself and Listening to Clients

Prospective professional interviewers need to quiet themselves and listen nondirectively to what their clients have to say. This task is difficult because when cast into the role of the interviewer many beginning students feel pressure to help clients resolve their problems quickly and efficiently; they try actively and directively to help clients. Our view is that when students (and experienced practitioners) become prematurely active and directive, they run the risk of being insensitive and nontherapeutic. Strupp and Binder (1984) give the following advice to clinicians: "In particular, the therapist should resist the compulsion to do something, especially at those times when he or she feels under pressure from the patient (and himself or herself) to intervene, perform, reassure, and so on (p. 41)."

In a majority of professional interview situations, the best start occurs when clients are allowed to explore their own thoughts, feelings, and behaviors during initial interview sessions. Whenever possible, interviewers should help clients follow their own leads and make their own discoveries (Strupp & Binder, 1984). We consider it the therapeutic interviewer's professional task to encourage clients to express themselves as fully and as completely as possible. We emphasize the term professional because we believe that conducting effective therapeutic interviews is a demanding task requiring professional training.

Developing Positive Therapeutic Relationships

Before developing assessment and intervention skills, interviewers should learn about and experience the process of developing professional and therapeutic relationships with clients. This involves active listening, empathic responding, and other specific behaviors leading to the development and maintenance of positive rapport (Othmer & Othmer, 1989). Counselors and psychotherapists from virtually every theoretical perspective agree on the importance of developing a positive relationship with clients before implementing treatment procedures (Goldfried & Davison, 1976; Luborsky, 1984).

Most clinical interviewers want to be helpful to their clients. They also feel a natural desire to know exactly what to *do* in order to be maximally helpful. These desires sometimes cause interviewers to be impatient, for example, by focusing on what to *do* with clients rather than how to *be* with clients. We recommend focuing first on how to *be* with clients because the practice of being with clients facilitate the development of good working relationships between interviewers and clients (Lambert & Arnold, 1987).

Learning Diagnostic and Assessment Skills

After learning to quiet themselves and develop positive therapeutic relationships with clients, professional interviewers should learn diagnostic and assessment skills and procedures. Although the need for assessment and the validity of diagnosis is controversial along many lines (Szasz, 1961, 1970; Wakefield, 1992), initiating counseling or psychotherapy without adequate assessment is ill-advised, unprofessional, and potentially dangerous (Corey, 1991; Hadley & Strupp, 1976). Think about how you would feel if, after taking your automobile to the local repair shop, the mechanic simply began trying to fix various components of the engine without asking you diagnostic questions designed to identify the problem. Although the profession of therapeutic interviewing is much different than auto mechanics, the analogy reveals the importance of completing assessment and diagnostic procedures before beginning therapeutic interventions. Phares (1988) concludes that the need for diagnosis before intervention is no longer a controversial issue in psychology:

> Intuitively, we all understand the purpose of diagnosis or assessment. Before physicians can prescribe, they must first understand the nature of the illness. Before plumbers begin banging on pipes, they must first determine the character and location of the difficulty. What is true in medicine and plumbing is equally true in clinical psychology. Aside from a few cases involving blind luck, our capacity to solve clinical problems is directly related to our skill in defining them (p. 142).

Our view is that interviewers may begin experimentation with the application of specific therapeutic methods and techniques only after three conditions have been fulfilled. *

1. They have quieted themselves and listened to their clients' communications.
2. They have developed positive relationships with their clients.
3. They have identified their clients' individual needs through a diagnostic and assessment process.

*Additionally, beginning interviewers should obtain professional supervision when experimenting with therapeutic methods.

Theoretical Orientations

We believe advanced interviewers should have some training and experience in conducting therapeutic interviews from each major theoretical perspective. However, as noted previously, we believe therapeutic skills are best developed by focusing first on nondirective interviewing approaches. Because this text is designed primarily for beginning interviewers, approaches and activities throughout this book borrow liberally from person-centered and psychodynamic schools of thought.

Although person-centered and psychodynamic approaches are often considered philosophically quite different from each other, they both teach that interviewers should initially allow clients to freely verbalize their concerns with minimal external structure and direction (Freud, 1940/1949; Luborsky, 1984; Rogers, 1951, 1961). In other words, person-centered and psychodynamically oriented interviewers are alike in that they allow clients a significant amount of freedom to discuss whatever personal issues or concerns they want to discuss. Consequently, these interviewing approaches have been labeled "nondirective" and they heavily emphasize listening techniques (actually, it might be more appropriate to label person-centered and psychodynamic approaches as "less directive," because all interviewers intentionally or unintentionally influence or direct their clients some of the time).

Person-centered and psychodynamic interviewers are nondirective for very different reasons. Briefly, person-centered interviewers believe that by allowing clients to talk freely and openly in an atmosphere characterized by acceptance and empathy, personal growth and change will begin to occur. Carl Rogers (1961), the originator of person-centered therapy, has stated this directly: "If I can provide a certain type of relationship, the other person will discover within himself the capacity to use that relationship for growth, and change and personal development will occur (p. 33)."

For Rogers, an interviewer's expression of unconditional positive regard, congruence, and accurate empathy constitute the necessary and sufficient ingredients for the client's positive personal growth and healing. We will look more closely at how Rogers defines these three ingredients in Chapter 7.

Psychodynamically oriented interviewers advocate nondirective approaches because they believe free association enables clients to communicate unconscious conflicts to their interviewers (Freud, 1940/1949). Eventually, through interpretation of unconscious conflicts, psychodynamic interviewers bring underlying conflicts into awareness so they can be dealt with more directly and consciously.

Similar to person-centered therapists, psychodynamic therapists acknowledge that empathic listening may be a powerful source of healing in its own right: "Frequently underestimated is the degree to which the therapist's presence and empathic listening constitute the most powerful source of help and support one human being can provide another" (Strupp & Binder, 1984, p. 41).

For psychodynamically oriented clinicians, empathic listening constitutes an ingredient that is necessary, but not sufficient, for personal growth and healing to occur (Meissner, 1991).

In contrast to person-centered and psychodynamic interviewers, behavioral or cognitively oriented interviewers are more inclined to take the role of an expert even at the onset of therapy because they believe it is necessary to direct or lead clients to explore specific behaviors or thoughts. This is because cognitive-behavioral clinicians believe that specific thoughts and behaviors cause social and emotional distress (Beck, 1976; Kazdin, 1979).

Cognitive-behavioral clinicians want to identify and then modify or eliminate maladaptive thinking and behavioral patterns and replace them with more adaptive patterns as quickly and efficiently as possible, thereby alleviating the client's social and emotional problems. Kendall and Bemis (1983) clearly state the necessarily directive orientation of the cognitive-behavioral therapist:

> The task of the cognitive-behavioral therapist is to act as a diagnostician, educator, and technical consultant who assesses maladaptive cognitive processes and works with the client to design learning experiences that may remediate these dysfunctional cognitions and the behavioral and affective patterns with which they correlate (p. 566).

Despite this description, most cognitive-behavioral clinicians also recognize the importance of empathic listening as a necessary, albeit not sufficient, factor in adaptive behavior change (Goldfried & Davison, 1976). Moreover, Mahoney (1991) has stated that "a secure and caring relationship" constitutes one of the most basic of all of the "general principles of human helping" (p. 270).

We should clarify that it is not our intent to suggest that person-centered and psychodynamic approaches are more effective than cognitive, behavioral, or other therapeutic approaches. In fact, controlled studies of cognitive and behavioral therapies generally have found them at least as effective as psychodynamic and person-centered approaches (Luborsky, Singer, & Luborsky, 1975; Sloane, Staples, Cristol, Yorkston, & Whipple, 1975; Smith, Glass, & Miller, 1980). Instead, our intent is to assert, as Corsini (1989) has suggested, that nondirective interviewing approaches provide the best foundation of knowledge and skill for beginning therapeutic interviewers. A number of important facts support this assertion (see Box 1-1).

BOX 1-1

Why Be Nondirective?

Many great psychotherapists began with a psychoanalytic orientation, among them Aaron Beck, Albert Ellis, Fritz Perls, and Carl Rogers. These respected theorists and therapists developed their unique approaches after years of listening nondirectively to distressed individuals. An underlying philosophy of this book is that beginning interviewers also need to begin by listening nondirectively to distressed individuals. Although it is natural for beginning interviewers to feel impatient and eager to help their clients, their safest and probably most helpful behavior is effective listening. As Strupp and Binder (1984) note, "Recall an old Maine proverb: 'One can seldom listen his way into trouble'" (p. 44). Many advantages are associated with nondirective interviewing approaches, especially for beginning therapeutic interviewers. Some of these advantages are listed below.

1. It is much easier to begin interviewing someone in a nondirective mode and later shift to a more directive mode than it is to begin interviewing in an active or directive mode and then change to a less directive approach (Luborsky, 1984; Wolberg, 1989).

2. Strategies designed to deliberately influence clients in a particular manner require that the interviewer have extensive knowledge of the psychopathology involved, enabling the interviewer to make sound judgments regarding how a given strategy can help the client change. Most beginning interviewers do not have the training in psychopathology and the supervised psychotherapy experiences needed as a foundation when implementing directive therapeutic strategies.

3. Nondirective interviewing approaches are very effective in helping beginning interviewers enhance their own self-awareness (Sommers-Flanagan & Means, 1987). It is through self-awareness that beginning interviewers become capable of *choosing* a particular theoretical orientation and effective therapeutic interventions.

4. A nondirective listening approach, properly implemented, should help reduce the tension beginning interviewers feel to perform, to help, and to prove something to their initial clients. In short, nondirective approaches help beginning interviewers effectively cope with that urge to 'do something and do it right.'

5. Nondirective approaches have less chance of offending or missing the mark with early clients (Meier, 1989). Although therapeutic interviewers often start out with volunteers, even analogue or role-play clients are real people, with either real or role-played reasons for being interviewed. Nondirective interviewers, who are there only to listen, place more responsibility on the shoulders of the client and can therefore lessen their own fears (as well as the real possibility) of asking the wrong questions or suggesting the wrong course of action. In addition, beginning interviewers tend to feel too responsible for their clients, and a nondirective approach can help prevent interviewers from feeling an inappropriate degree of responsibility.

6. A nondirective listening stance helps clients establish feelings and beliefs of independence and self-direction. This stance also communicates respect for the client's personal attitudes, behaviors, and choices. Such respect is rare, gratifying, and possibly healing (Strupp & Binder, 1984).

Specific helping strategies developed from all major theoretical orientations can be important tools for professional interviewers. Evidence indicating that some forms of psychotherapy may be better than others for particular clients and particular problems is beginning to accumulate (Barlow & Cerny, 1988; Beck, Rush, Shaw, & Emery, 1978; Lazarus, Beutler, & Norcross, 1992). The day when every therapist rigidly adhered to a single psychotherapeutic orientation may be drawing to an end (Goldfried, 1990; Prochaska, 1984). Although we welcome theoretical rapprochement and the identification of specific treatment strategies for specific clinical problems, we believe that, before using any technical therapeutic intervention, therapists require advanced clinical training and supervision. Therapists should receive such training only after they have mastered basic nondirective listening, relationship development, and diagnostic skills.

Basic Requirements for Therapeutic Interviewers

Four basic requirements must be met in order for you to become an effective therapeutic interviewer. First, you must master the technical knowledge associated with therapeutic interviewing. This means you must know the range of interviewing responses available to you and their likely influence on clients; for example, you must know different types of questions and how clients typically respond to them. You must know when the interview situation dictates structured information gathering and when less directive approaches are warranted. You must know ethical guidelines associated with professional therapeutic interviewing. In other words, you must have an intellectual grasp of the basic tools of the trade.

Second, you must be self-aware. You need to know how you affect other people and how you are affected by other people, both those within your own cultural and socioeconomic set and those without. You need to be familiar with the sound of your own voice, body posture, level of interpersonal attractiveness, patterns of eye contact, and interpersonal distance, because all of these variables will influence your clients. Further, you must constantly be willing to learn and grow with regard to blind spots you may have because of your personal and social background.

It is also important that you develop an awareness of how your own culture has shaped your personal values and ways of behaving. You need to become aware that others, both within and outside your culture, may have been taught much different values and behaviors. It is incumbent upon you as interviewer to realize when cultural—and gender—differences may be influencing or hampering effective communication between you and your client. To be a culturally ignorant or biased helping professional is considered unprofessional and unethical (Sue, Arrendo, & McDavis, 1992; Watkins & Francis, 1988; Westermeyer, 1987).

Third, therapeutic interviewing requires you to be able to observe and assess others (to acquire "other-awareness"). This skill requires that you know of and are sensitive to various individual and cultural values, behaviors, and norms. You also must be able to recognize and appreciate the perspectives of others. (This skill is also known as an "empathic way of being"; Rogers, 1961).

Awareness of others is a basic principle underlying interviewing assessment or evaluation. Therapeutic interviewers must be capable of observing objectively client behavior and evaluating for psychopathology. Assessment and evaluation can involve highly structured procedures such as mental status examination, suicide assessment, and diagnostic interviewing. Therapeutic interviewers must be aware not only of client cultural issues, but also of psychological, behavioral, historical, and diagnostic status (Mezzich & Shea, 1990).

Fourth, to be an effective therapeutic interviewer, you need practice and experience. As you begin to learn about interviewing and how you affect others, you must also begin practice interviews. This usually involves extensive role-playing with fellow students or actors or arranged interview experiences with other people you do not know (Balleweg, 1990; Sommers-Flanagan & Means, 1987; Weiss, 1986). Practice interviewing is designed to prepare you for the real thing—the actual therapeutic interview. In order to reduce your anxiety and increase your competence, you should have extensive supervised practice before beginning to conduct actual interviewing or counseling sessions. As you expand your basic skills, you will want to begin reading about and working on understanding people who are culturally, sexually, and socioeconomically different from yourself.

The more culturally diverse your interviewing and supervision experiences, the more likely you are to develop the broad, empathic perspective you need to understand clients. (Vacc, Wittmer, & DeVaney, 1988). In some ways this process is similar to becoming acculturated (Heinrich, Corbine, and Thomas, 1990).

Goals and Objectives of This Book

The basic objectives of this book are to:

1. Guide you through an educational and training experience based on the previously described teaching approach.
2. Provide technical information about therapeutic interviewing.
3. Introduce methods to facilitate your self-awareness and personal growth as an interviewer.
4. Introduce methods of client assessment and evaluation (i.e., facilitate aquisition of diagnostic skills).
5. Provide suggestions for experiential interviewer development activities.

Total Awareness Interviewing

When we set out to write this book we asked ourselves, If we could write the perfect introductory interviewing text, what would our overall goal be? Our ideal would be to teach "total awareness interviewing" (Means, 1981). Interviewers with total awareness interviewing abilities would be able to stop at any point in a given interview and outline what they were doing (based on technical expertise), why they were doing it (based on technical knowledge and assessment or evaluation information), and whether or not any of their personal issues or biases were interfering with the interview process (based on self-awareness).

Put another way, we wish we could teach people to "tune in" to each client and the world of that person so completely that the interviewer would truly "resonate" with the client, as a sensitive violin string begins to move when a matching tone is played in the room (Watkins, 1978). As if that wish were not impossible enough, we also believe that resonating, while necessary, would not be sufficient, so our perfectly trained interviewers would also be able to use this resonance to determine where every interview needed to go. They would have the ability to assess each client's needs from among the full range of potential needs and to carry out the appropriate therapeutic actions to address the client's needs, from initiating a suicide assessment to beginning a behavioral analysis of a troublesome habit—all during the therapeutic interview. One can only imagine the vast array of skills and the depth of wisdom necessary for such interviewing to be possible.

Therapeutic interviewing is a professional endeavor based on scientific research and undergirded by a long history of careful, extensive, and supervised training. As a consequence, it is inappropriate and unprofessional to, as an old supervisor of ours used to say, "fly by the seat of your pants" in an interview session (Bornstein, 1982). Total awareness interviewing should *not* be confused with such a laissez-faire approach. In no way does total awareness interviewing mean playing it by ear. On the contrary, being aware of oneself, one's client, and the best method of providing therapeutic assistance requires objectivity and knowledge of research data pertaining to therapeutic efficacy.

Textbook Organization

This text is divided into four parts. The first, Fundamentals of Therapeutic Interviewing, includes three chapters that cover issues relevant to learning, defining, and practicing therapeutic interviewing. These chapters focus on basic issues such as theoretical orientations, interviewer self-awareness, ethical considerations, and preparation for a therapeutic interview. We recommend that you thoroughly review this material and discuss it in class before initiating role-play interview activities.

The second part, Nondirective Listening and Relationship Development, is most beneficial when accompanied by extensive role-play interview experiences. Its four chapters focus on technical aspects of listening, the range of possible responses and directives available to therapeutic interviewers, and basic relationship issues associated with interviewing and counseling. Chapters 4 to 7 are designed to teach you how to know when you are listening to your clients nondirectively and how specific listening responses influence the formation and development of a helping relationship.

Part 3, Structuring and Assessment, includes four chapters on conducting a structured clinical assessment interview. The length of this section reflects our emphasis on clinical interviewing as an assessment tool. We believe beginning interviewers should avoid conducting interviews with individuals whom they do not know until the material in this section is thoroughly covered through reading and class discussion. Although some interviewing instructors have recommended that students conduct interviews with actors or analogue clients (Sommers-Flanagan & Means, 1987; Weiss, 1986), we suggest that such interviewing assignments are appropriate only after most of the material in Chapters 8 through 11 has been covered. These chapters focus on how and when therapeutic interviewers can and should shift their primary emphasis from listening to evaluation. Topics include an examination of the therapeutic interviewing process, principles of observation, intake interviews, and the handling of potentially suicidal clients.

Part 4, entitled Interviewing and Development, consists of Chapter 12. As implied by the title, we do not view the obtaining of interviewing skills as a process that suddenly ends. Interviewer development is an ongoing and never-ending process. When it comes to interviewer development, there is always room for growth.

As noted previously, this text emphasizes the importance of technical knowledge, self-awareness, other-awareness, and actual interviewing experience as the four central requirements for acquiring clinical interviewing skills. Therefore, although reading the text should provide you with solid technical knowledge on conducting therapeutic interviews, you must also practice using that knowledge in order to bring your skills to life. Because practicing your interviewing skills will also enhance your self-awareness, most chapters contain self-awareness (or other interviewer development) activities, either integrated in the text or set aside from the text in "Boxes."

Generally, Boxes contain supplementary information or activities designed to promote interviewer self-awareness, enhance recall of technical information, or facilitate skill acquisition. Information and activities in the Boxes are considered crucial to optimal interviewer development, so we recommend that you systematically read the Boxes when you read the text.

Chapter Summary

The underlying philosophy of this book is that students should begin learning therapeutic interviewing skills from a nondirective orientation. This is because we believe therapeutic interviewing is most efficiently learned when interviewers have learned the following skills and processes: (a) quieting themselves and listening to their clients, (b) focusing on developing a positive therapeutic relationship with clients, and (c) obtaining diagnostic and assessment information.

Directive interviewing requires advanced skills and should be avoided until a foundation of nondirective listening responses has been developed. For this reason, psychodynamic and person-centered listening techniques are emphasized in the first five chapters of this book. Nondirective approaches for beginning interviewers offer many advantages.

The goal of this book is to *approach* what has been referred to as total awareness interviewing. This means interviewers should know, to the extent possible, how their particular technical responses, self-presentational styles, cultural background, and gender affect each client, taking into account the client's own particular set of problems, biases, cultural background, and gender. In addition, total awareness interviewing includes knowledge of all potential interviewing techniques and their appropriate usage. Of course, total awareness interviewing is impossible, but the ideal emphasizes that interviewers should strive to have a clear rationale underlying their interview behavior.

This book is organized into four parts that seek to move the beginning therapeutic interviewer through a series of stages designed for optimal skill development. Because actual practice is necessary for interviewer skill development, each part offers suggestions for experiential activities to facilitate interviewer self-awareness and development of technical expertise.

Suggested Readings

We recommend that beginning interviewing students have previous knowledge of personality theory and psychopathology. We recognize, however, that not all interviewing and counseling courses have personality theory and psychopathology prerequisites. For those who lack such background, the following textbooks on theories of personality, theories and approaches to counseling and psychotherapy, and psychopathology can provide a worthwhile foundation for professional interviewer skill development.

Corey, G. (1991). *Theory and practice of counseling and psychotherapy* (4th ed.). Monterey, CA: Brooks/Cole. Corey's text is clear and excellent for beginners who have not read about various theoretical approaches to counseling and psychotherapy.

Corsini, R. (1989). *Current psychotherapies* (4th ed.). Itasca, IL: F. E. Peacock. This is an edited volume with specific chapters on many different approaches to psychotherapy.

Hall, C., & Lindzey, G. (1970). *Theories of personality*. New York: John Wiley & Sons. This is a classic text in the area of personality theory.

Kaplan, H., & Saddock, B. (1989). *Comprehensive textbook of psychiatry* (5th ed.). Baltimore: Williams & Wilkins. This huge volume contains extensive descriptions of virtually all aspects of clinical psychiatry.

Lambert, M. J., & Arnold, R. C. (1987). Research and the supervisory process. *Professional Psychology: Research and Practice, 18*, 217–224. This article discusses issues in research and supervision that pertain to interviewer and counselor training.

Miller, P. H. (1983). *Theories of developmental psychology*. San Francisco: W. H. Freeman and Co. Miller provides excellent descriptions of the various theories of psychological development. Her chapters on Piaget and Freud are especially clear and easy to read.

2

FOUNDATIONS

Toward a Definition of Therapeutic Interviewing

Clarifying Initial Assumptions and Issues
    The Nature of a Professional Relationship
    Two Functions of Therapeutic Interviews
    Listening Skills: The Foundation of Therapeutic Interviewing
    Factors that Guide Therapeutic Interviewing Behavior

Self-Awareness
    Objective Self-Awareness
    Forms of Self-Awareness

Interviewing Expectations and Misconceptions

Effective Interviewing: Seven Vocational Perspectives

Chapter Summary

Suggested Readings

*An interview is an interaction between at least two persons. Each participant
contributes to the process, and each influences the responses of the other. But this
characterization falls short of defining the process. Ordinary conversation is
interactional, but surely interviewing goes beyond that.*
                                                    —E. J. PHARES, *Clinical Psychology*

Many factors are associated with therapeutic interviewing. In some ways it is
hard to discern the difference between what is happening in a formal interview
and what happens in usual social relationships. On the other hand, as Phares
suggests, it is obvious that interviews are significantly different than usual
social interactions. This chapter seeks to demystify therapeutic interviewing
and begin you on your developmental journey toward becoming a professional interviewer.

Toward a Definition of Therapeutic Interviewing

Four basic principles define therapeutic interviewing:

- A professional relationship between client and interviewer is established and maintained.
- The interviewer uses active listening skills to communicate with and understand the client.
- The interviewer's intent is either evaluating the client, or helping the client alleviate distress, or some combination of evaluating and helping, with evaluation always preceding helping.
- The specific behaviors the therapeutic interviewer engages in are shaped and guided by objectives that interviewer and client mutually agree upon at the outset of their professional relationship.

Although it will take much more than a memorization of these principles to give you a complete understanding of all a therapeutic interview involves, it is useful to have an intellectual grasp of what defines an interview. To put these principles another way, therapeutic interviewing involves the development and maintenance of a professional relationship in which an interviewer actively listens to a client in an effort to evaluate and understand the nature of the client's problems and concerns. The quality and quantity of interactions between interviewer and client are determined primarily by mutually agreed upon objectives. If appropriate, therapeutic interviewing may require that the interviewer be an instrument of change enabling the client to reduce or eliminate personal distress.

Consistent with the underlying philosophy of this book, evaluation precedes helping (therapy) in this definition of therapeutic interviewing.

Clarifying Initial Assumptions and Issues

When teaching therapeutic interviewing, we commonly encounter two misleading assumptions. The less common of the two is for students to assume they know about interviewing simply because they can define the word interview or because they have conducted or experienced a few interviews. Students who are initially confident are usually disappointed to find that effective therapeutic interviewing is an art and science at which they must work to improve throughout their careers. To approach a complete understanding of all that a therapeutic interview entails requires extensive reading and experience, while acquiring skills to conduct effective therapeutic interviews takes much effort and practice. Partial knowledge of interviewing techniques combined with an overestimation of one's own skills can be very dangerous. Therapeutic interviewing is a potent activity that can produce negative outcomes and painful experiences as well as positive and healing experiences (Strupp & Hadley, 1979). A friend of ours who is an emergency room physician once claimed, "I know just enough psychology to be a little dangerous" (Wolff, 1989).

Unfortunately, this is sometimes the case for overconfident interviewing students. Often such students must begin by unlearning their neat, tight definition of interviewing in order to let a deeper and more comprehensive definition guide their learning.

The second and more common student assumption is that good therapeutic interviewing requires mysterious or magical skills that, once acquired, will enable them to see into the very heart or psyche of the client. Further, students often believe they know nothing already about this mysterious process, and they enroll ready to be apprenticed into the order by the master. By definition, beginning therapeutic interviewers are usually those who have never seen a client or conducted a therapeutic interview and therefore have good reason to be intimidated by what appears to be a mysterious process. It comes as a surprise to these students that most of them, naturally, in their own personal relationships, have engaged in activities basic to good therapeutic interviewing. They may also be disappointed to realize that there is no magic; therapeutic interviewing is a skill that is sometimes harder to learn than throwing touchdown passes or executing a perfect backhand in tennis.

You may recognize in yourself the first assumption, or the second, or even a blend of the two. You may also be wincing at our emphasis on the hard work and difficulty involved in learning good interviewing. Whether or not you hold one of these false assumptions, remember this important fact: although you may be a novice, your social relationships have provided you with a foundation of interpersonal experience to draw upon as you learn therapeutic interviewing skills.

Therapeutic interviewing involves a systematic modification of normal social interactions. Unfortunately, these modifications often serve to increase the social discomfort and self-consciousness of beginning interviewers. We usually tell our students that therapeutic interviewing requires socially inappropriate behavior. This is because social rules in a professional counselor-client or clinician-client relationship are much different than social rules to which we all conform in casual social relationships.

The Nature of a Professional Relationship
Most clients come to helping professionals because at some level they have one or all of the following characteristics:

- They are experiencing personal distress (Frank, 1973, 1982).
- They feel demoralized or unable to cope with their distress (Frank, 1973, 1982).
- They hope a professional can help them reduce or eliminate their distress (Frank, 1973, 1982; Korchin & Sands, 1982).

Usually professional relationships are characterized by the fact that the client or another funding source is paying for the services of the professional. For you as a professional counselor, this will be true whether you receive payment directly (as in private practice) or indirectly (as when you receive a paycheck from a department of family services, local mental health center, psychiatric hospital, or other institution). As a professional interviewer you are providing a service to someone in need—a service that should be worth its cost (see Box 2-1).

At its very essence, a professional relationship involves the purchase of services. Some have labeled psychotherapy "the purchase of friendship" (Korchin, 1976, p. 285), but clearly there are many differences between a therapy relationship and a friendship. Your friends do not meet formally with you in an office or schedule appointments. They do not regard your self-expression, personal growth, and the resolution of problems as their sole objective each time you meet. Therefore, although there are social and friendly aspects to a professional relationship, it is much different than a typical social relationship. Professional interviewers must learn to understand and control the extent of their friendliness; in fact, in order to be professional and therapeutic, interviewers must sometimes ignore and reject customary social behavior. This may sound extreme, but keep in mind that it is much easier to begin a relationship with a client very cautiously and to gradually introduce social, friendly compo-

---

BOX 2-1 ━━━

Just How Much is Your Professional Help Worth?

In 1991, when this text was being written, private mental health practitioners' fees ranged from $60 to $120 or more for a 50-minute session. Psychiatrists' fees were usually at the upper end of this range, while counselors with a master's degree charged rates nearer the lower end. Clinical and counseling psychologists charged in the middle range, between $75 and $100 for fifty minutes of therapy. Most psychology and counseling students begin seeing clients at training clinics designed specifically to provide services while at the same time allowing beginning therapists to practice doing therapy under supervision. Such clinics ordinarily provide services for a fee that is considerably lower than the going professional rate, and clients are aware they are receiving services from psychologists- or counselors-in-training. Nonetheless, many beginning therapeutic interviewers react strongly to their first experiences of charging a fee, no matter how small, for their services. For example, as a graduate student, author John Sommers-Flanagan can recall commenting to several fellow students that he felt he should be paying clients a small fee because they had graciously volunteered to allow him to practice his therapeutic interviewing skills on them!

Think for a moment about how you will feel charging someone who receives your professional services. How will you react to introducing financial reward and obligation into the therapy situation? How much will you feel comfortable charging? If the training clinic where you were employed required you to obtain at least $25 from each client, how might receiving such a fee influence how you handle yourself during the session? Consider the possibility that the client may wish to obtain the service for less than you are allowed to charge. You may find it helpful to write a list of potential effects that charging a fee for your services might have on your actual behavior in the therapeutic interviewing room.

---

nents than it is to retract overly social gestures or overly friendly messages. Part of becoming a mature professional is learning to be warm, interactive, and open with clients while not violating the constraints of the professional relationship. If how to achieve this balance is not entirely clear, not to worry, it is a theme to which we return many times in this book (see, for example, chapter 3).

Two Functions of Therapeutic Interviews

Therapeutic interviewing has two essential functions: evaluating prospective clients and helping those clients. To maximize your chances of effectively helping clients, it is necessary for you to thoroughly evaluate each client's presenting problems and personality style. As noted previously, a common behavioral tendency of beginning interviewers is to rush into helping strategies before they have conducted an adequate assessment. Mahoney (1991) states, "We yearn to learn technique because we desire the power of enacted knowledge, which is the heart of praxis ('doing,' the existential basis of 'Being')" (pp. 286–287).

Rather than succumb to the yearning Mahoney speaks of, interviewers need to obtain clear knowledge of their clients' presenting problems, expectations for therapy, previous efforts at solving their problems, general personality style, and other information before they use directive helping interventions (see chapters 5, 6, and 9). Impulses to quickly and efficiently help one's clients are normal and natural for all interviewers, both beginning and experienced. The problem for beginning interviewers is unique in that they often hold unrealistic expectations regarding how quickly therapeutic progress should occur and they may feel pressure to "prove their worth" because they are being paid for their services for the first time.

While the impulse to offer advice or try to help is understandable, it is important to realize that learning to quiet this impulse is a major step in your development as an effective interviewer. All too often, the interviewer does not fully grasp or appropriately respond to the thoughts, feelings, and situation presented by the client because the interviewer is too busy thinking of solutions instead of listening.

When a premature intervention is offered, a number of negative outcomes might occur, including, but not limited to, the following:

- The interviewer may choose an inappropriate therapeutic approach or technique that is potentially damaging to the client's condition (e.g., one that increases rather than decreases anxiety).
- The client may feel misunderstood and rushed, and may conclude either that the problem is too awful for even a professional interviewer to understand or that the interviewer is not very bright or competent.
- The client may follow the therapist's incorrect or inappropriate guidance and become frustrated with therapy. As a result, the client's openness to subsequent therapy interventions, and possibly subsequent therapists, will be significantly diminished.

- The therapist may not have taken time to listen to what the client has already done to try to solve the problem and may suggest a "remedy" that the client has already tried without success. The therapist's credibility is thereby diminished.

Clearly a therapeutic interview may produce effects that are less than positive. Negative effects often result from misguided, inappropriate, or premature efforts to help clients. Moreover, clinical research indicates that negative therapy outcomes are frequently associated with inadequate assessment or evaluation procedures (Hadley & Strupp, 1976). Therefore, it is crucial for interviewers to learn how to evaluate clients so they may help them effectively.

In some situations the helping and evaluative functions of therapeutic interviewing are kept almost completely distinct; one interview might be strictly a helping interview while another is solely an evaluation or assessment interview. However, most therapeutic interviews combine the helping and evaluative functions.

The clinical skills required for insightful evaluation are also required for effective helping. Good evaluators closely observe clients in order to objectively assess their psychological condition, but they also listen well and sometimes integrate potentially therapeutic responses into their interviews. On the other hand, good helpers seek to influence the client in a positive manner, but they also listen thoughtfully and constantly evaluate whether or not their therapeutic interventions are effective and appropriate. They need to have adequate evaluative skills in order to judge in which areas they might be able to help at once and which may be best left for later. Helping therapists also need to know how to ascertain whether the help a client is seeking or needs is the product of an acute problem requiring swift intervention, such as in the case of clients who are potentially suicidal, homicidal, or delusional.

The common element underlying both types of interviewing is sensitive and effective listening. Good evaluators and good therapists are similar in that they are sensitive listeners and can actively demonstrate to their clients that they are hearing accurately the central messages each client communicates during the session.

Listening Skills: The Foundation of Therapeutic Interviewing

To conduct an effective evaluation or therapeutic interview, interviewers must first listen to clients' stories about themselves and the reasons they have come for an interview. People who seek a professional counselor or therapist do so for their own unique reasons. Consequently, therapeutic interviewers must learn quickly how to stay out of their clients' way so the clients may freely tell their stories (Gustafson, 1986; Luborsky, 1984; Strupp & Binder, 1984).

Although it is commonly assumed that one of the best ways to listen to clients' stories is to ask questions liberally, thereby demonstrating skill and interest as an interviewer, we must state unequivocally that this assumption is incorrect. Asking questions is a directive interviewing activity that does not allow clients to freely express themselves. Each question guides and restricts client verbalizations so that the material produced is that which the interviewer thinks the client should produce. It may or may not actually represent what clients would say if left to their own whims, associations, and verbal patterns. Because questions are an advanced and directive technique, interviewers need to first focus on how to listen without interfering with their clients' verbal flow by asking questions (we will discuss the advantages and disadvantages of questions in detail in chapter 9). This is not to suggest that questions should be excluded from all interviews. Rather, a pattern of listening first and asking questions later assists interviewers in accomplishing both tasks of therapeutic interviewing: evaluating and helping.

Skillful interviewers listen, evaluate, and help in a manner that makes these three activities seem simultaneous. Beginning interviewers, on the other hand, usually should restrain themselves from using helping techniques until they have adequately listened (nonjudgmentally) and evaluated (clinically). Therefore, the following guideline is useful for most beginning interviewers (and for some advanced interviewers seeking to improve their skills): No matter how backward it might seem, you should begin training sessions by *not* trying to help the client. Instead, try only to listen to the client. Doing so will probably help the client more than if you actually *tried* to help (Rogers, 1961; Strupp & Binder, 1984). This fact may seem paradoxical, but it is nonetheless true.

Jerry Fest, a therapist who works with street youth in Portland, Oregon, wrote of the following encounter in a manual for persons working with street youth (Boyer, 1988). One night he was working in a drop-in counseling center. A young woman came in obviously agitated and in distress. Jerry knew her from other visits, so he greeted her by name. She said, "Hey, man, do I ever need someone to listen to me." He showed her to an office and listened for five or six minutes to a moving tale of difficulties. He then made what he thought was an understanding, supportive statement. The young woman immediately stopped talking. When she began again a few moments later, she stated again that she needed someone to listen to her. The same sequence of events played itself out. After her second stop and start, however, Jerry decided to take her literally, and he sat absolutely silent for the next ninety minutes. The woman poured out her heart, finally winding down and regaining control. As she prepared to leave, she looked at Jerry and said, "That's what I like about you. You don't get it right right away, but you finally catch on." The young woman's need that day is a basic need shared by all human beings: to have someone listen. Interviewers cannot go wrong by listening well, but as we pointed out earlier, they can get in trouble by rushing into premature action. The moral of this story should be obvious. Restrain the impulse to directively help solve clients' problems in early interviews; plenty of opportunities for directive helping will arise later (see chapters 5 and 6 for distinctions between listening and directive interviewer responses). Your interviewing policy should be "listen first and ask questions later . . . maybe." Only by establishing yourself as an effective listener can you facilitate open, nondefensive expression by the client (see Box 2-2).

Factors that Guide Therapeutic Interviewing Behavior

We have recommended very clearly that you adopt a goal of nondirective listening during your initial therapeutic interviews because nondirective listening skills provide an excellent foundation for all forms of therapeutic interviewing. However, it is not always appropriate to follow this suggestion. There is a time and a place for directive interviewing. To help you determine the best time and place for directive interviewing, we offer the following basic principle of therapeutic interviewing: Your specific interviewing behaviors will be strongly influenced by the purpose or objective of your interview.

Each interview you conduct should have clear and specific objectives; these objectives will guide your interviewing behavior. For example, evaluation or diagnostic interviews are much more likely to be characterized by a series of specific questions than are helping interviews (Hersen & Turner, 1985). You should begin determining and identifying interview objectives before starting an interview, and you should modify them as the session proceeds so they are consistent, or at least compatible, with the expectations of the client being interviewed.

The objectives you have during interview sessions will be influenced by the particular policies and functions of the agency where you are employed as well as the time available to you and the client. Most clinics and private practices ask clients to complete registration forms describing their background, ability to pay, and reasons for coming to the clinic. Reading over these forms carefully is one important step in beginning to understand your client's expectations. Often, too, the institution's setting and the services it offers determine the types of clients and problems you are most likely to encounter. You should be very familiar with the public's understanding of what your agency or clinic offers. Author Rita Sommers-Flanagan once had the experience of beginning an interview with a noticeably overweight man who indicated on his paperwork he had come in to lose weight.

BOX 2-2

Self-Statement for Beginning Therapeutic Interviewers

Listening should be your primary function as a therapeutic interviewer. If you do not listen adequately, you have no right to suggest helping strategies to a client. If you do listen adequately, you may not need to offer suggestions because your clients may tell you themselves which strategies would be most helpful. In fact, our position on suggestions and directive questions is that they should be avoided entirely by the beginning interviewer and remain minimized even as the interviewer develops in skill. Questions tend to reduce the clients' freedom of expression. We often have students use the following cognitive self-statement to keep this first learning goal firmly in mind before and during their initial therapeutic interviews: "The goal of my initial interviews is simply to listen well. If I do this, I will be providing an essential service to the client and learning what I need to learn."

She began the session with one of the classic open-ended statements we will later describe (see chapter 8), something like "Tell me what brings you here today." He told a story about a friend of his who had lost weight and how encouraged it made him feel. He went on to talk about his wife's pressuring him to lose weight and their vacation plans next summer. After a while he stopped and asked, "So what does the program cost with your fancy food and all?" At this point Rita could have remained nondirective by replying, "Seems like the cost is a concern for you." However, the mention of "fancy food" alerted her that perhaps, just perhaps, the man was harboring a slight misconception about the services the clinic offered.

Across campus another agency administered a weight-loss program. Carefully, in case she was mistaken, Rita said, "I think there are many ways for people to change their eating behavior, change their exercise behavior, and lose weight. We *do* work with people along those lines here, but over at the ABC agency, they have a more specific program that involves purchasing food from them. Your question about the cost of the service and the food makes me wonder if you wanted to get some help there instead of here." That was indeed the case—he had the agencies confused. Not wanting him to feel embarrassed for having come to the wrong place and begun talking about his problems, Rita phrased her interruption as casually as she could. The man left for the other agency, feeling fine, if a little awkward. Months later, he stopped by to say that his program there was going well.

Except when an interviewer handles cases with couples or families, there are exactly two people involved in the process of therapeutic interviewing. Although most of this book addresses the skills interviewers need in order to effectively focus on clients, interviewers also need to focus on themselves. We now turn our attention to an issue that further complicates the process of therapeutic interviewing.

Self-Awareness

> There is no more fascinating sight than your own image looking back at you in a mirror. You are drawn to it in a half embarrassed way, excited and intensely involved. Do you remember the last time someone showed you a picture of yourself? Wasn't there a surge of feeling and a deep curiosity about "How do I look?" (Fisher, 1973)

We believe competent therapeutic interviewing is one of the most complex and difficult activities in which an individual can engage. Of course, everyone believes their particular profession requires special talent and skill. Physicians, sculptors, computer programmers, and even used-car salespeople take pride in the art and science of their trade. Author John can recall an old college baseball coach who would discuss with pride the difficulty associated with the act of hitting a baseball. He claimed the task of making solid contact with a round ball and a round bat left virtually no room for miscalculation. Hitting a baseball required that player's body be an instrument that could constantly respond and adjust to a small, round, spinning object traveling at varying but always high speeds.

The process of becoming a good hitter requires knowledge, practice, and excellent body awareness and hand-eye coordination. Therapeutic interviewing also requires knowledge, practice, and self-awareness, and it involves a strikingly similar process. As a professional therapeutic interviewer, you must consistently make solid psychological, social, and emotional contact with a large number of individuals you have never before met. You are ordinarily required to accomplish this task in the short span of fifty minutes. To make such contact you must be very sensitive to and tolerant of the limitless number of ways people can present themselves *and* be just as sensitive to and aware of your own physical, psychological, social, cultural, and emotional presence. (Now which of these processes seems more difficult, hitting a baseball or consistently conducting effective therapeutic interviews? Author Rita points out that, depressing—or perhaps encouraging—as it may be, after a certain point efficiency at hitting a baseball rapidly decreases with age, while effective therapeutic interviewing enjoys a much longer efficiency curve.)

A high level of self-awareness is considered a positive personality trait, and it can be an especially important attribute for therapeutic interviewers. Self-awareness helps interviewers know how their personal biases or emotional states influence and potentially distort their understanding of clients. Self-awareness also aids interviewers in recognizing and understanding positive and negative aspects within given interviewer-client relationships. Working with therapy clients on a regular basis can produce emotional reactions within interviewers (e.g., anxiety, depression, or euphoria). An ability to recognize quickly their own emotional reactions toward specific clients and toward practicing psychotherapy in general is obviously an advantage to interviewers. We therefore recommend that interviewers strive to understand themselves and their own interpersonal relationships before entering into professional interviewer-client relationships (Clark, 1986; Greenberg & Staller, 1981; MacDevitt, 1987; Strupp, 1955). Just as the superior athlete must possess a high level of body awareness in order to perform effectively, the effective interviewer must possess superior psychological, emotional, and social self-awareness in order to perform at optimum levels.

Objective Self-Awareness

Many components of learning to conduct therapeutic interviews will increase your level of self-awareness. We recommend that you audio- or videotape as many of your practice interviews as possible. As you listen to your voice and speech patterns and as you watch your facial expressions and physical mannerisms during the interview, you will become more keenly aware of how others are likely to respond to you. This increased awareness of how you are perceived by others can be very valuable both personally and professionally. On the other hand, you may also become exceptionally uncomfortable, distressed, and self-conscious as a function of listening to and watching yourself.

Research has confirmed that most people initially experience personal discomfort, inhibition, and self-consciousness when they are made to feel more self-aware (Carver & Scheier, 1978; Fenigstein, 1979; Fenigstein, Scheier, & Buss, 1975). Therefore, the problem for interviewers in the process of training is increasing self-awareness without simultaneously producing discomfort and a paralyzing sense of self-consciousness. One potential solution to this dilemma is for you to embrace the self-consciousness and view it as a positive step toward enhancing your clinical skills. This task can be challenging.

Many people choose to avoid examining themselves closely through video or other feedback mechanisms because of the high levels of discomfort associated with such a process (although other people feel attracted to recordings of themselves). Despite the discomfort caused, training programs almost universally require videotaped presentations as a portion of practicum or interviewing courses. We strongly endorse this practice. We believe the self-awareness gained from video and audio feedback is so crucial that it should be used in all training programs. After initial discomfort, most students find they can videotape themselves, survive, and even use the knowledge they gain from the tape to their benefit. Perhaps you will be reassured to know that the discomfort associated with audio and video recording is normal, natural, and nearly universal (Yalom, 1985). It may also help to know that over time you will become more comfortable with yourself, and this feeling, in turn, will improve your therapeutic interviewing skills.

Forms of Self-Awareness

There are several aspects of self-awareness to be explored prior to conducting therapeutic interviews: physical self-awareness, psychosocial self-awareness, developmental self-awareness, cultural self-awareness, and awareness of one's expectations and misconceptions about therapeutic interviewing.

Physical Self-Awareness Physical self-awareness involves becoming conscious of your voice quality, body language, and other physical aspects of self. It is particularly important to be conscious of how your individual physical presentation affects others in an interpersonal setting. Some people have especially soft, warm, and comforting voices, while others come across as authoritative in their oral presentation. Take time to listen to yourself on an audiotape, or ask others to listen to your voice as you speak and give you feedback on what they think of your voice. We once had a foreign student in an interviewing class who indicated privately that he believed others were uncomfortable with his accent. We asked the class to give him feedback about his voice after he presented an audiotaped interview. His classmates were uniformly positive about the warm and pleasant aspects of his voice, and this feedback proved to be a very positive step for the young interviewer. The point is that because others hear us differently than we hear ourselves, we need direct feedback from others to find out how they perceive us.

Clients' perceptions of their interviewers are sometimes influenced by the interviewer's sex. For example, male interviewers are commonly described as more rational and authoritarian and females as more warm and compassionate (Basow, 1980). This stereotyping is inaccurate and usually has more to do with a client's history of male-female relationships than with the interviewer's actual presentation style. Nevertheless, as sensitive and self-conscious interviewers you must remain aware of these common reactions. Clients come to an interview because of negative interpersonal experiences; these experiences strongly shape how they perceive other people. As a result, interviewers may be quickly judged as cold, rational, sensitive, warm, or even abusive simply because of their gender (similarly, interviewers may stereotype their clients based on whether their clients are female or male (Morshead, 1990).

Closely exploring your own physical presentation through self-awareness activities will help you avoid taking a client's inaccurate evaluation of you at face value. For example, author John Sommers-Flanagan recalls a client who used to periodically accuse him of being as unemotional as a robot. She would say, "You're so cold. . . . I bet if I were to cut open your arms I'd find wires, not veins." It helped for John to know already that he was not a cold and unemotional interviewer. At the same time he was seeing another female client who consistently accused him of "being out of control emotionally," complaining that he overreacted to what she told him. Both of these clients were extremely disturbed (both were inpatients on a psychiatric unit) and their perceptions of their therapist were distorted by their own personal problems. However, even less disturbed clients can have significantly distorted perceptions of your physical, social, and emotional presentation; this can disconcerting if you have not received other feedback from peers and supervisors about your interpersonal style.

We will discuss this process in greater detail in chapter 7, when we focus on transference and the distorting qualities of defense mechanisms. For the time being, Box 2-3 outlines a method for obtaining greater physical self-awareness and for coping with the discomfort associated with examining yourself closely.

Psychosocial Self-Awareness   Psychosocial self-awareness refers to how you view yourself as relating to others. As suggested by Bennett (1984), it is an elusive concept: "The social self is more elusive. There is no mirror in which we may actually examine interpersonal relations. Most of the feedback, most of the self-percepts come from others"(p. 276).

Not only does psychosocial self-awareness involve our perceptions of and feedback about how others view us, it also involves psychological, social, and emotional needs and how they influence your interpersonal life. In his oft-cited hierarchy of needs, Maslow (1970) contended that all humans have basic physiological needs; safety needs; self-esteem needs; self-actualization needs; and needs for love, acceptance, and interpersonal belongingness. Good therapeutic interviewers are aware of their own particular psychological and interpersonal needs and how such needs can affect their interviewing and counseling behavior. One way of enhancing your psychosocial self-awareness

BOX 2-3 ━━

Desensitization and Objective Self-Awareness

Objective self-awareness is the term coined by researchers to describe feelings of discomfort associated with listening to or viewing yourself on audio- or videotapes (Fenigstein, 1979). The discomfort usually has to do with your appraisal of physical aspects of yourself (e.g., voice quality, physical appearance, or idiosyncratic mannerisms). To watch or listen to yourself produces increased self-awareness, but also increased levels of self-consciousness and inhibition. You should expect to experience at least moderate levels of objective self-awareness as you playback and review recordings of your interviews. Another way to produce high levels of objective self-awareness is to conduct therapeutic interviews while facing a mirror. We recommend that you take advantage of every opportunity to observe yourself doing interviews on tape. Viewing yourself will help you identify specific aspects of your physical presentation you do not like and want to modify, and, over time, you will become more comfortable with yourself and perhaps be able to identify attractive aspects of your physical presentation that you wish to keep and even showcase. The following advice is provided to help you through the initial stages of objective self-awareness.

1. Video- or audiotape your interviewing sessions as often as possible.
2. Keep a personal library of both your positive and negative taped sessions.
3. Watch or listen to the tapes by yourself first, if you prefer. This can help you feel more comfortable (or unfortunately, less comfortable) when you present your work to a group.
4. Admit to someone, perhaps to the whole group who will listen to or watch your recorded session, your feelings of discomfort. You will probably find many in the group who acknowledge their own discomfort and who support you for the brave act of presenting your tape to the class. Also, simply talking about your feelings to people you trust is a good coping strategy.
5. Be open to positive or negative feedback from others, but if you don't want feedback, feel free to request there be no feedback.
6. If someone gives you feedback you don't completely understand, ask for clarification.
7. Be sure to thank people who have given you feedback, even if you did not like or agree with some of the feedback. It is rare in our culture to have the opportunity to receive direct feedback about how we come across to others. Take advantage of the opportunity and use it for personal growth.
8. As Rogers (1961) and Maslow (1970) suggested, the self-actualized or fully functioning person is "open to experience" (Rogers, 1961, p. 173). We believe the healthy interviewer possesses similar qualities. There is nothing to be gained by defensiveness. Try your best to adopt an open and nondefensive attitude toward feedback. If this is too difficult or overwhelming for you, look for support from people you trust.
9. If you cannot identify anyone in your class or group whom you trust you have several choices. First, keep trying to build trust with your classmates. Sometimes persistence pays off in interpersonal relationships. Second, find someone outside the group (a friend, colleague, or therapist) in whom you can confide, with the eventual goal of also identifying someone in the group. Third, find a new group or individual whom you can trust. Sometimes pathological groups or classes form that do not provide empathy or support for their members. If you are sure this is the case, then move on to more healthy

(continued)

BOX 2-3 *Continued* ━━━

surroundings. On the other hand, always examine yourself and your role in the process before leaving a group. You may be able to modify some of your own attitudes in order to stay with the group successfully.

10. Learn a relaxation technique. Many methods of physical and mental relaxation can help you manage the stress and anxiety that accompany self-awareness (see Borysenko, 1986; Charlesworth & Nathan, 1985; and Siegel, 1986).

━━━

is to examine yourself and your life and career goals through self-reflection. Some questions you should ask yourself include:

- How do I define myself?
- What are my life goals? What do I really want out of life, and why? Does my everyday behavior help me move toward my life goals?
- What are my career goals? If I want to become a counselor or psychotherapist, how do I envision myself achieving this goal? Why do I want to be a counselor or psychotherapist?
- How would I describe myself in only a few words? How would I describe myself to a stranger? What do I particularly like and what do I especially dislike about myself?

Another method for evaluating your psychosocial self involves traditional psychological testing. Many tests are available that can provide you with insight regarding your psychosocial needs and tendencies. Some tests commonly used by therapeutic interviewers in training to become more familiar with their psychosocial selves include the Minnesota Multiphasic Personality Inventory (Hathaway & McKinley, 1943), California Psychological Inventory (Gough, 1957), and Personality Adjective Inventory (Retzlauff, Gibertini, Scolatti, Laughna, & Sommers, 1986).

Developmental Self-Awareness   Although developmental self-awareness is closely associated with the concept of psychosocial self-awareness, we believe it to be of great enough significance to merit separate discussion and attention. Developmental self-awareness refers to a consciousness of one's personal history, that is, of specific events that significantly influenced personal development. Everyone has at least a few vivid memories that characterize and capture very personal aspects of self. These memories usually mark personal struggles, victories, or traumas that occurred during particular developmental transitions (e.g., adolescence). In the tradition of the object relations movement in psychoanalytic thinking, it is suggested that you explore your own history of interpersonal relationships, beginning with childhood. Reviewing and perhaps uncovering consistencies in your patterns of relating to others can provide you with insight regarding ways you will react to clients during therapeutic interviews. One way to begin this exploration is to sit quietly and recall all the people and events in your life that made a pivotal difference in where you are today. Go back as far as you can, picturing each person or scenario in as much detail as possible. You may even want to list them chronologically and fashion a psychosocial developmental map of your history. Another way of exploring your developmental history is through psychoanalytic psychotherapy (Clark, 1986; Greenberg & Staller, 1981).

Cultural Self-Awareness The belief in the innate superiority of one's own tribe to neighboring tribes, or one's own nation or 'race' to other nations or races, is probably as old as our species. (Zuckerman, 1990, p. 1297)

In the past, geographical isolation and consequent inbreeding resulted in similarities among the members of inbred human groups that laypeople have referred to as characteristics of race. As Zuckerman (1990) points out, these characteristics lie along a continuum, and constitute only surface differences with regard to species distinction. Commonality between the races overrides the distinctions, just as commonalities among cultures are more numerous than are differences among them. So why do we advocate caution when you deal with clients whose background is different from yours? Why the admonitions to know yourself culturally? Why the belief that to be effective interviewers, therapists must pursue knowledge of other cultures and backgrounds to the extent that they strive to be multicultural? Slowly we are beginning to awaken to the truth that our ideas about what is proper and improper, right and wrong, appropriate and inappropriate—even abnormal and normal—are highly influenced by our particular cultural, religious, political, and gender-typed upbringing. Whether two people can understand each other depends not so much on racial or cultural backgrounds, but on how strongly each of them believes in the correctness or even the superiority of that which is personally familiar. Truly understanding someone from another culture begins with acceptance of differences as normal, interesting aspects of being human.

Social scientists have explored the phenomenon we refer to as stereotyping from a number of perspectives. One important finding for the interviewer to consider is that, in general, the frequency with which people stereotype others varies inversely with the extent of their personal experience with individual members of other groups. Certainly, simple exposure is not sufficient to end stereotyping, but it is an important first step.

We suggest you and your classmates take time to consider your own cultural, religious, and political biases. It is helpful to explore these, even among yourselves. How many in your class were raised to believe in a God referred to as masculine? How many were raised to believe that to care for the poor is a high calling in life? How many were raised to believe that being on time and standing in line are signs of weakness? The list of varying beliefs and values is endless. And to further complicate matters, it is not only how we were raised or even what we believe now that we need to explore, but also the interaction of the two. How have we matured? How do we now respond to those who believe as we once did? There is no easy way to become culturally self-aware, but we recommend exposure, introspection, discussion, reading, and even personal therapy to uncover these biases and blind spots and to begin work on increased effectiveness with and sensitivity to people of different cultures (Jones & Thorne, 1987; Sue & Sue, 1987).

Interviewing Expectations and Misconceptions

We began this chapter by suggesting that interviewing students often begin their training with erroneous expectations. Before you conduct therapeutic interviews, we suggest you explore this area of your professional development in more depth. Specifically, think about the expectations you hold for yourself as a therapeutic interviewer. Do you expect you will be effective and successful or that you will fail miserably? What thoughts or images come to mind when you think of therapeutic interviewing? What preconceived ideas do you have about how you should act in an interview? Do you believe that in order to be a good clinician you must be a certain type of person? As you examine these questions, you may want to write down your thoughts, feelings, and expectations. You may also want to respond to the sentence completion items in Box 2-4.

Effective Interviewing: Seven Vocational Perspectives

As noted throughout this chapter, there are many factors that make becoming an effective therapeutic interviewer a complicated and difficult process. Despite our emphasis on the complex and difficult aspects of learning therapeutic interviewing, we remain convinced that learning effective interviewing is possible—and can even be fun. We encourage you to consider the following similarities between therapeutic interviewing and other human activities.

First, you must know what famous philosophers know: the importance of knowing thyself (Bennett, 1984). Because you are the instrument through which you hear and respond to clients, you must be keenly aware of your physical presentation, personality style, and individual biases. In other scientific enterprises scientists always calibrate their instruments prior to using them for research or practice. Checking in with your most central instrument, your self, is one of your essential duties as an interviewer.

Second, you must know what good landscapers know: the terrain. You must learn about how to set up an environment that is maximally conducive to your objective. Obviously, a number of situational factors can make clients more (or less) willing to discuss their personal concerns with you. It is your job to establish an environment that allows clients to feel comfortable and open with you about their thoughts, feelings, and concerns.

Third, you must have what successful music teachers have: a good ear. You must know how to listen with every one of your senses in order to quickly evaluate how the client is relating to you. You must have knowledge of which behaviors effective listeners use and which they avoid. Good therapeutic interviewers engage in specific listening behaviors that enhance listening accuracy and that demonstrate to clients that their message has been heard.

BOX 2-4 *Continued* ━━

A Sentence Completion Test for Beginning Therapeutic Interviewers

1. I expect that as a therapeutic interviewer I will

    _____.

2. All therapeutic interviewers should

    _____.

3. My first interview will be

    _____.

4. The biggest fear I have about interviewing is

    _____.

5. Clients are always

    _____.

6. The type of person who makes a good interviewer is

    _____.

7. If the person I was interviewing was suicidal, I would

    _____.

8. The way I most want to be perceived by my clients is

    _____.

9. Counseling or psychotherapy is needed when

    _____.

10. If I become a professional therapist, my parents will think

    _____.

11. If I become a professional therapist, my friends will think

    _____.

(continued)

BOX 2-4 *Continued*

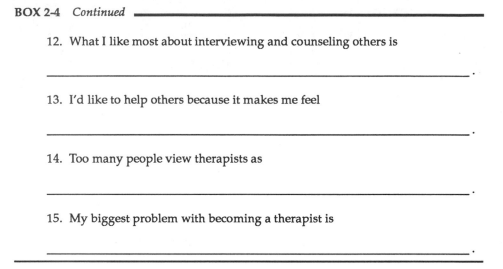

12. What I like most about interviewing and counseling others is

_____ .

13. I'd like to help others because it makes me feel

_____ .

14. Too many people view therapists as

_____ .

15. My biggest problem with becoming a therapist is

_____ .

Fourth, you must do what the successful athlete does: practice. It takes dedicated practice to move skills from brain to body, or from theory to practice. Without an accumulation of interviewing experiences, the knowledge you obtain about therapeutic interviewing and sixty cents will buy you a cup of coffee. It is only through the experience of conducting interviews that you will begin to become more self-aware and truly learn how to apply the principles discussed within this text.

Fifth, you must know what good office managers know: how to prioritize information. As an interviewer you must be able to quickly sort through the huge amount of verbal and nonverbal messages given to you by clients so you can focus on important clinical material.

Some information given to you by clients may require immediate attention and possibly action. For example, if you are interviewing someone whom you discover has been thinking about suicide, you will need to consider this issue as top priority. Furthermore, you may suddenly need to determine whether or not your client needs further evaluation by a licensed professional or hospitalization. On the other hand, some information produced by your client requires a much different kind of attention. It is very important that as a novice interviewer you begin to develop prioritization and evaluation skills as soon as possible, simply because it is difficult to predict when and where you will face your first major clinical decision. You will probably have to make your first difficult clinical decision before you feel prepared or experienced.

Sixth, you must know what good wardrobe managers know: how to mix and match. Good therapeutic interviewers must learn how to apply their evaluation and listening skills to a variety of situations. Conducting intake interviews, suicide assessments, and mental status exams in preparation for choosing therapeutic techniques and assisting clients with referrals all constitute applications of the interviewer's evaluation and listening skills.

Seventh, you must know what good car mechanics know: how to trouble-shoot. Just as car mechanics know the various sounds and symptoms indicative of bad wheel bearings or troubled fuel injectors, you need to know the signs and symptoms of depression, anxiety, paranoia, and more. Even beginning therapeutic interviewers need to have a rudimentary knowledge of psychopathology so that they can judge whether clients have come in for their regular tune-up or are in need of something closer to a major overhaul.

Chapter Summary

Beginning interviewers often hold one of two mistaken assumptions. Some may be overconfident and believe they know more about interviewing than they actually do, while others believe they know virtually nothing about this mystical process through which they can instantly analyze people and lead them toward therapeutic solutions. Neither of these initial assumptions is accurate, because therapeutic interviewing involves a systematic modification of normal social interactions. All therapeutic interviewers must learn a new set of social rules associated with interviewing.

The client-interviewer relationship is a professional one wherein the client usually pays a fee for the clinician's services. These services are designed to help clients alleviate their personal distress. Although the relationship established between interviewer and client is a friendly one, it is much different than friendship. It is a challenge for beginning interviewers to sort out the differences between professional and friend relationships. Some aspects of professional relationships may be initially difficult and uncomfortable (e.g., fee setting and collection).

Therapeutic interviews serve a dual function: to evaluate and to help clients. A common tendency for beginners is to rush in and try to help clients before an adequate evaluation has been conducted. This tendency should be avoided because it may result in a number of negative side effects. Because all therapeutic interviews emphasize active listening techniques, it is sometimes difficult to distinguish between evaluative and therapeutic activities.

Effective listening skills constitute the foundation of therapeutic interviewing. Although many people believe one of the best ways to listen effectively is to ask questions liberally, this is simply not the case. Questions are a directive interviewing technique associated with interrogation rather than listening. It is recommended that therapeutic interviewers listen first and ask questions later.

Many factors determine the specific behaviors clinicians use during an interview. Perhaps the most important of these factors is the objective of the interview. For example, if the objective is particularly evaluative (e.g., diagnosis), it is likely that the interviewer will be engaging in more frequent question-asking behavior. Other variables, such as the amount of time available to interviewers and clients and the particular agency's policies or functions, also influence interviewer behavior greatly. Interviewers and clients need to agree explicitly on mutual, or at least compatible, interviewing objectives.

Therapeutic interviewing is generally defined as the development and maintenance of a professional relationship in which a professional interviewer actively listens to a client in an effort to evaluate and understand the nature of the client's problems and concerns and, if appropriate, be an instrument of change that enables the client to reduce or eliminate personal distress. The quality and quantity of interactions between interviewer and client are influenced primarily by mutually agreed upon objectives.

It is important for therapeutic interviewers to have a high level of self-awareness and insight. Although the development of self-awareness is encouraged, self-awareness also can increase interviewer discomfort and inhibition. It is natural for interviewers to experience the discomfort of objective self-awareness when they receive feedback based on an audiotpae or videotape of their interviews.

There are many forms of self-awareness, including physical, psychosocial, developmental and cultural. Cultural self-awareness, means awareness of the influence of one's own culture, religion, gender, and political beliefs. Interviewers also should be aware of their preconceived biases and beliefs about themselves and others during the therapeutic interviewing process. Several methods for enhancing awareness in each of these areas have been discussed and offered in this chapter.

Suggested Readings

Arkoff, A. (Ed.). (1980). *Psychology and personal growth* (2nd ed.). Boston: Allyn & Bacon. This is an edited text with many stimulating readings on personal growth. Chapter 2, which focuses on body image, is especially interesting.

Bennett, C. C. (1984). "Know thyself." *Professional Psychology, 15*, 271–283. This article explores the many dimensions of self.

Borysenko, J. (1986). *Minding the body, mending the mind.* New York; Simon & Schuster. Borysenko's book is written for the general reader but contains many practical cognitive and behavioral approaches to stress management.

Charlesworth, E. A. & Nathan, R. G. (1985). *Stress management: A comprehensive guide to wellness.* New York: Ballantine Books. An excellent resource, this book takes a more technical and lengthy approach to describing stress-management procedures.

Zuckerman, M. (1990). Some dubious premises in research and theory on racial differences: Scientific, social, and ethical issues. *American Psychologist, 45*, 1297-1303. This article provides a good analysis of current theory and research on racial differences.

_3_

PREPARATIONS

The Physical Setting
    The Room
    Seating Arrangements
    Note Taking
    Videotape and Audiotape Recording

Professional and Ethical Issues
    Self-Presentation
    Time
    Confidentiality
    Stress Management for Therapeutic Interviewers

Chapter Summary

Suggested Readings

Farmers . . . need good land for their work to prosper.
          — _RICHARD BACH, Illusions_

Farmers also need good weather, adequate machinery, methods of pest and weed management, and a work ethic to be productive. They need to invest time, money, and effort in planning and preparation or else their farming enterprise is destined to failure. Like farming, therapeutic interviewing requires certain basic ingredients to ensure a maximally productive outcome.

Before you meet with your first client, there are practical issues to consider and settle so you can begin the session feeling prepared and professional. Once these preparations are complete, you can focus all your skill and energy on accomplishing your task, although, like the farmer, sometimes you will find there are variables beyond your control and you end up simply hoping for good weather. This chapter examines two general aspects of presession preparation: the physical setting and professional and ethical issues.

The Physical Setting

> The environment not only prods or lashes, it *selects*. Its role is similar to that in natural selection, though on a very different time scale, and was overlooked for the same reason. It is now clear that we must take into account what the environment does to an organism not only before but after it responds. Behavior is shaped and maintained by its consequences. Once this fact is recognized, we can formulate the interaction between organism and environment in a much more comprehensive way. (Skinner, 1972, p.18)

When interviewer and client sit down together to talk, a multitude of environmental factors may influence their behavior. Although the interviewer is probably the most important environmental stimulus affecting client behavior, many other physical or external variables also can significantly influence the process and outcome of therapeutic interviews. Interviewers should be conscious of these variables and consider them carefully before conducting therapeutic interviews.

The Room

What kind of room is most appropriate for therapeutic interviewing? First, we should note that circumstances beyond your control can determine what kind of room you have available for interviewing. Many undergraduate programs and some graduate programs do not provide clinical facilities with rooms for practice interviews. In fact, interviewers do not have a room at all; Benjamin (1981) once reported conducting interviews in a tent in a desert. Most readers of this book will have slightly better facilities available to them than Dr. Benjamin did, but no matter what the circumstances, there are certain features to which you should pay attention.

Most counseling and psychotherapy interviews take place within a room, but there are some exceptions. Behavioral therapists sometimes take clients to a scene that produces anxiety in order to implement anxiety-reduction or response-prevention techniques (Marks, 1981). Other counseling and psychotherapy activities have been reported as taking place while interviewer and client were outside jogging, walking, dancing, or sitting in a comfortable setting, such as under a tree on a pleasant day (Abt & Stuart, 1982). We take a fairly rigid and conservative approach for students in clinical training. We require a room, especially for the beginning interviewer.

The minimum requirements for the room are that it provide privacy and a reduced likelihood of interruptions and other distractions. Privacy and freedom from interruption are minimim requirements because most therapeutic interviews involve very personal communication; the room should help facilitate such communication. Some practitioners are very particular about room specifications, believing that for optimal communication to occur a soundproof room with covered windows is required (Langs, 1986). While we are not as narrow in our beliefs about requirements, we want to emphasize that you should not underestimate the importance of physical surroundings.

People are not inclined to reveal their deepest fears or secrets at the student union building over coffee, at least not to someone whom they have just met. Privacy and comfort are as central to a good interview as the interviewer. On the other hand, in attempting to present oneself professionally, it is not necessary to hide behind a massive oak desk with a backdrop of velvet curtains and twenty-seven professional degrees. As is true regarding many variables associated with interviewing, when choosing a room it is useful to strike a balance between professional formality and casual comfort. Consider the room an extension of your professional self. In an initial interview, your major purpose is to foster rapport, trust, and hope in your client in an effort to help the client talk openly. Your choice of room should reflect that purpose.

As illustrated in Box 3-1, control is a central issue in setting up and planning the atmosphere in which the interview will take place. The client may certainly be given small choices, such as in which chair to sit, but overall the interviewer should be in control of the surroundings. A pleasant, well-lit, comfortable room, free from outside noise and distraction, is a basic necessity. Beyond this, each interviewer must consider the purpose of the interview and the type of setting most conducive to that purpose.

As we mentioned in chapter 2, a number of elements distinguish the therapeutic interview from other social encounters. One such distinction is that the time devoted to the interview is to be set aside and its exclusive purpose respected. Whereas interruptions during a business or social encounter may be permissible or even welcome, this is not true in interviewing or therapy. In our view, interruptions of interviews are nearly intolerable. In our own training clinic, everyone from the janitor to our supervisors realizes that while interviewers are in session, they are not to be disturbed. The secretary would never dream of interrupting, and in fact, guards the students' client hours with a fierce loyalty to both student and client. Apparently after he moved out of his tent, Benjamin wrote the following comment on the issue of interruptions:

> Outside interruptions can only hinder. Phone calls, knocks on the door, people who want "just a word" with you, secretaries who must have you sign this document "at once," may well destroy in seconds what you and the interviewee have tried hard to build over a considerable time span. (1981, p.4)

This statement would hold true even if Benjamin were speaking about interviews held in his tent. A place and time set aside to do therapeutic interviewing should be just that—set aside. If you do not have access to rooms in which privacy is assured, you may want to place a "Do not disturb" or "Session in progress" sign on the door to reduce the probability of interruptions.

Seating Arrangements

When teaching therapeutic interviewing, we routinely ask students how two people should sit during an interview. The variety of student responses to this

BOX 3-1 ━━━━━━━━━━━━━━━━━━━━━━━━━━━━━━━━━━━━━━

Stay in Control of the Interview Setting

Picture this: An interviewing student calls a volunteer interviewee.

"Hello, is Sally Sanders there?"

"Yes, this is she."

"Sally, my name is Beth McNeece and I'm taking Interviewing 443. I believe you signed up to be interviewed for extra credit in your Psychology 101 class. I got your name, so I'm calling to set up a time."

"Oh sure. No problem . . . but it *is* almost finals time. I'm pretty busy."

"Uh, yeah. I had hoped to do this sooner in the term, but uh, well, let's see if we can find a time"

After much searching they find a time. Unfortunately, Beth forgot to check the room availability schedule, and finds no rooms are available at the time chosen. She calls Sally back.

"Sally, this is Beth McNeece again. I'm sorry, but there are no rooms available at the time we decided . . . " Sally is a bit irritated, and it shows in her voice. Beth is feeling apologetic, indebted, and a little desperate. There is only one week left in the term. They discuss their limited options. Beth suggests:

"Maybe I should call someone else."

Sally counters with, "Hey, look, I really want to do this. I need the extra credit. Why don't you just come to my room? I live in University Hall, right here on campus."

Knowing she is violating the rules, Beth reluctantly agrees to do the interview in the dorm room. After all, it's just a class assignment, right? What's wrong with a nice, quiet dorm room? Who will ever know where the interview was conducted? Besides, it's better than inviting Sally to her house, isn't it? Beth asks Sally to make sure they will have the room to themselves. "No problem," says Sally, sounding distracted.

The next day Beth arrives. It is late afternoon. It just happens to be the one hour designated as the time when residents can make as much noise as they please to compensate for quiet hours and finals stress. The Grateful Dead, Madonna, and U2 compete for air space. Sally's friend from across the hall is getting her hair permed, which, except for the odor, should not be all that relevant, but somehow, Sally's digital clock is being used to time the perm. No one besides Beth and Sally are actually in the room, but there are numerous interruptions and the phone rings six times, twice with calls for Sally.

Unfortunately, this is a true story. "Beth" had the courage to report her rule violation and "horrible" experience. She shared with us her dismal failure in establishing any kind of meaningful communication with the young woman she interviewed and admitted feeling totally out of control. Although this example is extreme, it illustrates the importance of controlling the interview setting. Loss of such control can happen all too easily.

question is surprising. Some students suggest a face-to-face seating arrangement, others report liking the feeling of having a desk between themselves and the client, and still others note that sitting at about a 90- 120-degree angle provides clients and interviewers the option of looking away from one another without discomfort. Also, a few students usually point out, correctly, that many professional psychotherapists still use a couch for the client, with the therapist seated behind the client and out of view.

In the interviewing rooms of many training clinics, the seating provided includes a single, soft reclining chair along with two or three more austere wooden chairs. Theoretically, the soft recliner provides clients with a comfortable and relaxing place from which they can freely express themselves. The recliner is also an excellent seat to use for hypnotic induction, for learning of progressive relaxation, and even for free association. Unfortunately, our experiences with having a designated seat for clients is that it produces discomfort, especially during early sessions. In the training facilities that use such an arrangement, clients are notorious for avoiding the selected seat or complaining that they feel they're on the throne or hot seat.

Several factors are associated with individual interviewers' choices of seating arrangements. Interviewer theoretical orientation is one factor. Psychoanalysts often choose couches, behaviorists often choose recliners, and person-centered therapists usually emphasize the importance of having chairs of equal status and comfort. In classes, we have consistently noticed a connection between students' suggestions for seating arrangements and their personality styles. More assertive students tend to suggest and choose the face-to-face arrangement, while students with needs for control more frequently choose to put their clients on the couch or recliner. We recommend you try out a number of different seating arrangements in order to get a sense for what feels best for you. This doesn't mean you should then choose whatever arrangement feels best for you, but you may be enlightened to discover your preference. We also suggest you remain sensitive to your clients' preferences, as there will be certain arrangements that feel better and worse to each of them too.

We usually recommend seating the interviewer and client at somewhere between a 90- and 150-degree angle to one another during initial interviews. Benjamin (1981) states the rationale for such a seating arrangement quite nicely:

> [I] prefer two equally comfortable chairs placed close to each other at a 90-degree angle with a small table nearby. This arrangement works best for me. The interviewee can face me when he wishes to do so, and at other times he can look straight ahead without my getting in his way. I am equally unhampered. The table close by fulfills its normal functions and, if not needed, disturbs no one (p. 3).

The 90-degree angle arrangement is safe and conservative. It is doubtful that using it will offend anyone. Nonetheless, many interviewers (and clients) prefer a less extreme angle so they can look at the client more directly but not quite face to face (perhaps at a 120-degree angle). In some cases clients may

BOX 3-2 ━━

Watch Where Your Client Sits

In some cases the therapeutic interviewer will want to lead the client into a room and allow the client free choice in choosing a chair. Family therapists are careful to observe seating arrangements to give them clues as to potential coalitions or discordant relationships within the family. With individuals, allowing the client to choose a seat may provide the clinician with clues about client personality style or, in extreme cases, diagnostic category.

Uncle Herman's Guide to Armchair Diagnosis

The following exaggerated and stereotypic statements are provided as humorous anecdotal information rather than a serious or valid diagnostic approach.

- The paranoid client chooses the seat farthest away from you with his back to the corner of the room (where no one can sneak up on him).
- The agoraphobic client will seat herself in the hall supply closet (that is, if she makes it to your office building).
- The dependent client asks you where to sit, when to sit, and if he can hang up his coat.
- The schizotypal client usually sits behind you or anywhere that allows her to avoid direct eye contact.
- The anxious client moves from seat to seat, or just paces and chews his nails.
- The depressed client always sits in the most uncomfortable seat available.
- The sexually inadequate client usually covers his privates with a book or strategically crosses his legs.
- The alcoholic usually sits far away from you so you can't smell her breath.
- The narcissistic client will move her chair so she sees herself clearly in the one-way mirror. She will make more eye contact with her image than with you.
- The oppositional client asks which chair you prefer he sit in and then sits in another.
- The antisocial client always takes your chair, and sometimes sips your coffee as well.

Uncle Herman points out that this same schema may serve as a diagnostic guide for colleagues, blind dates, faculty, and even yourself, if you are brave enough to admit it.

━━

disrupt your prearranged setting by moving their chair to a different position. We recommend that the interviewer avoid insistence on any given seating arrangement. If a client appears more comfortable with an unplanned or unusual seating arrangement, simply allow the client to choose, make a mental note of this behavior, and proceed with the interview.

Note Taking

The question of whether or not a clinical interviewer should take notes has been taken up by many therapists and writers (Benjamin, 1981 see Box 3-3; Pipes & Davenport, 1990). Although some experts have recommended that

BOX 3-3 ───

Some Rules for Note Taking

1. Never let note taking interfere with the flow of the interview or with the development of rapport.

2. Always explain the purpose of your note-taking behavior to your clients. Some clients will be disappointed if you don't take notes; you will need to explain to them why you have chosen not to take notes.

3. Never hide or cover your notes or act in any manner that might suggest to clients that they are not supposed to see your notes.

4. Never write anything on your notepad that you would not want the client to read. If you note certain personal observations you intended to keep to yourself, rest assured that your client will want to read what you've written. Clients who tend to be a bit paranoid will always be suspicious about what you've written and may ask to read your notes or, in extreme cases, simply stand up and take your notes (or read the notepad over your shoulder).

5. If your clients ask to see what you've written, explore their concerns with them and then offer to let them read through your notes. Rarely do clients accept such an offer. However, in the unusual case when a client does read through your notes, you had better have followed rule #4.

───

interviewers take notes only after a session has ended, others accurately point out that interviewers do not have perfect memories and thus some ongoing record of the session is desirable (Benjamin, 1981; Pipes & Davenport, 1990; Shea, 1988). The bottom line is that note taking may in some cases offend clients while in other cases it may enhance rapport and interviewer credibility. Clients' reactions to note taking are usually a function of their intrapsychic issues, interpersonal dynamics, previous experiences with note taking behavior, and of how much tact the interviewer utilizes in introducing note taking. Because you cannot predict a client's reaction to note taking in advance, you should explain the activity at the time you begin to take notes in a session. Shea (1988) recommends the following approach:

> I frequently do not even pick up a clipboard until well into the interview. When I do begin to write, as a sign of respect, I often say to the patient, "I'm going to jot down a few notes to make sure I'm remembering everything correctly. Is that alright with you?" Patients seem to respond very nicely to this simple sign of courtesy. This statement of purpose also tends to decrease the paranoia that patients sometimes project onto note taking, as they wonder if the clinician is madly analyzing their every thought and action. (p. 169-170)

We agree that whenever interviewers take notes they should introduce the note taking in a courteous manner and proceed with tact (i.e., the interviewer should always pay more attention to the client than to the notes). However, we recommend that beginning interviewers practice conducting interviews both with and without taking notes. It is important for beginning interviewers to explore how it feels to take notes and to not take notes during a session.

Videotape and Audiotape Recording
If you choose or are required to record the session with either video or audio equipment, make it as unobtrusive as possible. As discussed in chapter 2, virtually everyone is initially uncomfortable with tape recording. In general, the more comfortable and matter-of-fact you are in your presentation of the recording equipment, the more quickly the client will become comfortable being recorded. This is a classic "easier said than done" statement, since the purpose of recording the session is probably for later viewing with a supervisor or your fellow students. Even though you are the interviewer, you will be the one most closely observed on the subsequent review of the tape, so you may be as nervous as, or even more nervous than, your client. Some students find it easier to explain that the purpose of recording the session is for the student's own growth, and that recording the interview ensures the best service possible for the client. This explanation takes the focus away from the performance aspects of being taped, from the client's perspective.

When planning to audiotape or videotape a session, you must always obtain the client's permission to do so before actually starting the recording. Usually permission is obtained on a written consent form. This is important for a number of reasons. Recording clients without their knowledge seriously invades clients' privacy, which is a basic violation of trust. It is also important for ethical and legal reasons to explain the potential future uses of the recording and how it will be stored, handled, and eventually destroyed.

We are aware of a number of awkward, embarrassing, and even destructive situations that occurred because interviewers failed to inform their clients about recording sessions. In one case, in an effort to obtain a recording of initial interactions he was about to have with a new client, a doctoral intern decided he should start his audiotape recorder before the client came into the interviewing room. He assumed that after preserving the important initial material on tape, he could then discuss the issue of recording the sessions with the client. Unfortunately, he was unable to convince the client to return to therapy because she considered his actions to be a violation of her privacy. Furthermore, she delivered to the young intern a punishing tirade against which he had no defense (and, of course, he recorded this tirade for himself loud and clear). The intern had unwittingly pinpointed one of the best ways of destroying trust and rapport early in the interview: he failed to ask the client ahead of time whether he could record the interview on tape.

We should note one final observation about taping we have made over the years. It seems that whenever you have recorded your best session ever, you subsequently discover there was some minor problem with the equipment and consequently your session was not recorded or not recorded properly. On the other hand, when you have conducted a session poorly and wish you could quickly forget it ever happened, the audio or video equipment always works perfectly and the session turns out to be the one your supervisor wants to listen to or watch. We recommend you closely examine the equipment prior to recording the session and take time to test the audio and video quality.

Professional and Ethical Issues

Interviewers must also consider various professional and ethical issues before conducting practice therapeutic interviews. Beginning interviewers often struggle with how to dress professionally, how to present themselves and their lack of credentials, how to handle time boundaries, and what to say about confidentiality. Below we provide some guidelines for dealing with these issues effectively.

Self-Presentation
As stressed in chapter 2, you are your own primary instrument for a successful therapeutic interview. Your appearance and how you present yourself to new clients is an important component in the process of professional and effective therapeutic interviewing.

Grooming and Attire   Students often have difficulty deciding how to dress for the therapeutic interview. Some ignore the issue and some overdo it, which makes the question of how to dress seem a symptom of a larger developmental issue: how seriously you take yourself as a professional. Is it time to take off the Salvation Army sweats, or stop trying to capture the title of Most Likely to Be on the Cover of *Seventeen*? Is it time to don the dreaded three-piece suit and come out to do battle with mature reality, as perhaps some of your parents or friends have suggested? Don't worry. We are not leading up to a point where we say "yes" to these questions, but then, neither are we saying "no." Our point again involves self-awareness. You need to be aware of how your clothes may affect others. Even if you ignore this issue, your clients—and your supervisor—will not. Your choice of dress communicates a great deal to your clients and can be a source of conflict between you and your supervisor.

We knew a student whose distinctive style included closely cropped, multicolored hair; earrings that seemed likely to prominently elongate his earlobes over time; and an odd assortment of scarves, vests, sweaters, runners' tights, and sandals. He easily stood out in most crowds. Imagine his effect on, say, a middle-aged dairy farmer referred to the clinic for depression or on a mother-son dyad having trouble with discipline, or on the daughter of the mayor. No matter what effect you imagined, the point is that, it is easy to imagine *some* kind of effect. Dress is not neutral, it always provokes a reaction. The issue of interviewer dress can certainly be worked through by interviewers and clients, but it may use up time and energy better devoted to other issues.

Physical self-presentation issues that have become increasingly controversial include whether male interviewers should wear earrings or ponytails. Whether it is appropriate for female interviewers to wear pants will probably always be an issue for some. Regardless of where you stand on these issues of self-presentation, at least take the time to ask yourself why you have chosen your particular style of dress and grooming and how your dress and grooming might be interpreted by a wide range of potential clients. Although it is unfortunate that people quickly form first impressions and that these impressions may be inaccurate, your clients will judge you by the way you look and dress (Lennon & Davis, 1990). The first impression often takes the form of a vague positive or negative emotional reaction: "Typically, a first impression of a stranger . . . is poorly differentiated and hard to put into words; yet it often yields a distinct emotional flavor of liking or dislike. This affective reaction may be a source of both useful information and error" (Holt, 1969, p. 20).

Your goal as a therapeutic interviewer is to present yourself in a manner that takes advantage of first impressions. Dress and grooming should be a useful source of information for the client that fosters the development of rapport, trust, and interviewer credibility (Strong, 1968). If anything, it may be best to err on the conservative side until you have a firm understanding of the effects of your presentation. This is sometimes a good practicum or supervision topic as well.

Presenting Your Credentials Students notoriously have difficulty introducing themselves to clients. Referring to yourself as a student may bring forth spoken or imagined derogatory comments such as, "So I'm your guinea pig?" Our advice to the beginning interviewer is to clearly and firmly state your full name and an accurate description of your training status to your clients. For example: "My name is Holly Johnson and I'm in the graduate training program in clinical psychology," or "I'm working on my master's degree," or "I'm enrolled in an advanced interviewing course." You should pause after this description in order to provide the client a chance to ask questions regarding your credentials. If the client asks questions, try to answer them directly and nondefensively.

It is important to practice even these simple introductory portions of the therapeutic interview. Before reading further, formulate exactly how you want to introduce yourself in the clinical setting. You may want to write out your introduction or state it into a tape recorder. We also recommend practicing introductions during role plays with fellow students. These practice techniques may help you to avoid introducing yourself by stating: "Well, I'm just a student and I'm taking this interviewing course, and I have to practice, so . . . uh, here we are."

There is nothing wrong with being a student and there is no need to behave apologetically for being inexperienced. An apologetic action or attitude will quickly erode your credibility and rapport. If you have a tendency to feel guilty about "practicing" your interviewing skills, we suggest a small dose of cognitive therapy (i.e., "reframing"). Remind yourself that people usually enjoy a chance to talk about themselves. It is rare for most people in our culture to be listened to and attended to as completely as you will listen to your client. You can provide a positive experience for clients and learn more about the interviewing process at the same time.

With regard to introducing yourself, always be honest and straightfor-ward with your clients, whether analogue or actual. It is an ethical violation to misrepresent yourself by overstating your credentials. No matter how inexpe-rienced or inadequate you feel inside, you should not attempt to compensate by pretense or fraudulent misrepresentation.

Student interviewers are normally supervised. You should mention this fact at the beginning of an interview by saying something like, "As I've noted, I haven't completed my degree, so my work here at the clinic is being super-vised by Dr. Bornstein. What this means is that I will be reviewing your case occasionally with Dr. Bornstein to ensure that you are receiving high-quality professional services. Dr. Bornstein is a licensed clinical psychologist, and we will maintain the highest professional and ethical standards possible in our discussion of your case."

Time

Time is of the essence. Or, perhaps when it comes to therapeutic interviewing it would be more accurate to say: Time is the essence. Time is what you are providing the client. If the client is paying a fee, the fee is based on your time. Although therapeutic interviewing is a rich, involved, and complicated pro-cess, time is the commodity you are selling. Therefore, you should always attend to and be respectful of time boundaries.

It is typical for a therapeutic interview to last 50 minutes. This time period, while somewhat arbitrary, is convenient; it allows the interviewer to meet with clients on an hourly basis, with a few minutes at the end and beginning of each session to write notes and read files. Despite this usual and customary time period, some situations warrant briefer contacts while other situations require longer sessions. For example, initial (intake) or assessment interviews are sometimes longer than the classic psychotherapy hour because of the difficulty of obtaining all of the information needed to begin conceptual-izing a case and establishing treatment goals. Depending upon the setting, up to ninety minutes, or even two hours, may be provided for an initial clinical interview. On the other hand, some crisis situations require extreme flexibility and deviation from scheduled time limits (Wollersheim, 1974).

Start the Session on Time The guiding principle for starting sessions is to be punctual as often as possible and to briefly explain any lateness directly to the client at the beginning of the session. If you are late, you should apologize to the client and offer to extend the session or somehow "pay back" the client for the lost time. You may want to state something like, "I apologize for being late today; I had an appointment at another building that lasted longer than was expected. Because we have missed ten minutes of our session, perhaps we can extend this session or our next session an additional ten minutes to make up for the lost time."

Although most students are not faced with fee collection, another option professional interviewers use for repaying clients for lost time is to offer to prorate the fee for whatever portion of the usual interview hour remains.

You should also avoid beginning sessions early in cases in which the client arrives before her scheduled time and no one else is in your office. Pipes and Davenport (1990) state this position succinctly: "Clients will show up early and may ask if you are free. The answer is no, unless there is a crisis" (p. 18).

It may seem that we are being overly rigid regarding time boundaries. Our intent is to point out how your punctuality can communicate respect to your clients. Clients appreciate interviewers who begin sessions at the scheduled time. Many times our classes have discussed the contrast between the attitudes of psychotherapists and physicians (excluding psychiatrists) when it comes to punctuality. Physicians are notoriously late for patient appointments and such lateness communicates plenty about the nature of typical physician-patient relationships (Siegel, 1986). One student of ours commented in class, "It doesn't matter if physicians offend you by being late because they would never take the time to talk about it with you afterward anyway" (Hayes, 1990). This comment captures an important value that good therapeutic interviewers uphold: respect for the feelings and reactions (even irrational reactions) of their clients.

In cases when clients are late for a session, an interviewer may have an impulse to extend the length of the session or to punish the client by canceling the session entirely. Neither of these alternatives is desirable. Clients should be held responsible for their lateness and thus must suffer the natural consequences of their behavior, an abbreviated session. This is true regardless of the reasons for the client's tardiness. In some cases the client may sincerely regret his lateness and will ask you for additional time. Be empathic but firm in such situations. You might want to state something like, "I'm also sorry this session has to be brief, but I believe strongly in the importance of us sticking with our scheduled appointment time." If you have an appointment scheduled for the next hour, you may want to mention that you have previous commitments you must uphold.

One option professional interviewers use in cases of client lateness is to offer to schedule an additional appointment at another time you have available during the week so the client doesn't feel she is falling behind, or being cheated, in terms of therapy or assessment progress. For example: "If you feel you'd like to make up the time we've lost today, perhaps we can arrange to meet for an additional session sometime this week."

It is not unusual for therapeutic interviewers to have feelings of anger or irritation in response to a client who is late for a session. As is the case with many emotional reactions interviewers have toward clients, it is important for you to notice and examine them, but you should refrain from acting on them. For example, even though you would like to leave the office if a client is twenty minutes late, you should not do so unless you have previously made it perfectly clear that you only wait a certain length of time (such as fifteen to twenty minutes) for late clients. You should clarify your policy on lateness and no-shows in each client's initial session. If your agency or clinic has a policy of charging clients for a full hour if they do not call in and cancel, then you must inform your clients of this policy. Similarly, you should inform volunteer clients of the consequences of "missing" their scheduled appointments (e.g., loss of extra credit).

End the Session on Time   Interviewers should end therapeutic sessions in a timely manner. We have heard many excellent excuses why clinicians consciously let sessions run overtime, but rarely have these excuses constituted an adequate rationale for breaking prearranged time agreements. Some reasons we have heard from our students:

- We were on the verge of a breakthrough.
- She brought up a clinically important issue with only five minutes to go.
- He just kept talking at the end of the hour, and I felt uncomfortable cutting in (i.e., he seemed to need to talk some more).
- I thought I hadn't been very effective during the hour and felt the client deserved more time.
- I forgot my watch and couldn't see the clock from my chair.

For most of these situations, our advice is for the interviewer to calmly and tactfully point out that time is up for the day, but that if the client wishes, the session can continue along similar lines next time. We also recommend that you sit in a position that affords you direct visual contact with a clock. It is rude and distracting to glance repeatedly at your watch or to look over your shoulder at the clock during an interview.

There are very few situations in which it is acceptable for an interviewer to extend the therapeutic hour. These situations are usually considered emergencies—for example when the client is suicidal, homicidal, or floridly psychotic. (Recently, a close friend of ours was held at gunpoint by one of his clients for about forty minutes [Clucas, 1990]. This is certainly a situation when time boundaries become irrelevant.)

Confidentiality

A major challenge of therapeutic interviewing is to help clients talk with you about very personal information. This not only a difficult task (people are usually uncomfortable disclosing personal information to someone they hardly know), but a heavy burden as well. It is a burden because clients entrust interviewers with a wide range of very private information, some of which they may have never told anyone before. In this sense the therapeutic interviewer becomes a "confidant," which is by definition someone who is entrusted with "private" or "secret" information (*Webster's Ninth New Collegiate Dictionary*, 1985, p. 275). If you have ever had someone tell you a special secret, you know about the burden associated with being a confidant.

When it comes to being a confidant, therapeutic interviewers are in a unique situation. There are legal and ethical limits of confidentiality. In other words, although you want every client to be as open and honest with you as possible, there are some specific types of information that you simply cannot keep secret. For example, a client could come to you and say, "I'm very depressed and am sick and tired of life. I've decided to quit dragging my family through this miserable time with me . . . so I'm going to kill myself. I have a gun and ammunition at home and I plan to blow myself away this weekend." In this case you are legally and ethically obligated to break confidentiality and report your client's suicidal plans to the proper authorities (e.g., police, county mental health professional, or admission personnel at a psychiatric hospital).

The central statement regarding the confidentiality policy of the American Psychological Association (APA) (1990) is provided below:

> Psychologists have a primary obligation to respect the confidentiality of information obtained from persons in the course of their work as psychologists. They reveal such information to others only with the consent of the person or the person's legal representative, except in those unusual circumstances in which not to do so would result in clear danger to the person or to others. Where appropriate, psychologists inform their clients of the legal limits of confidentiality (pp. 392-392).

Unfortunately, the APA statement is necessarily general and leaves room for different interpretations. To better clarify the standard, Box 3-4 provides you with a summary of APA guidelines concerning confidentiality and some examples of situations in which therapeutic interviewers are obligated to break confidentiality.

Confidentiality constitutes an ethical, legal, and clinical issue in professional therapeutic interviewing. Additional discussion of this crucial issue is provided intermittently throughout this book.

One final point should be made regarding the APA ethical standards of confidentiality. The APA specifically states: "Where appropriate, psychologists

---

BOX 3-4

Confidentiality and Its Limits

1. You must respect the private, personal, and confidential nature of communications from your client.

2. You may disclose information (or break confidentiality) in the following situations:

- You have the client's (or the client's legal representative's) permission.
- The client is suicidal and you determine there is a clear danger of suicide.
- The client is homicidal or is threatening to engage in behaviors where significant danger to others is likely. For example, your client tells you of her plans to sabotage a local nuclear plant and you determine there is significant danger to others' lives if she carries out such an activity.
- The client is a child, and you have evidence to suggest he is being sexually abused.
- You have evidence to suggest the client is sexually abusing a minor.

3. If appropriate, tell your client about the legal limits of confidentiality.

inform their clients of the legal limits of confidentiality" (APA, 1990, pp. 392-393). Concerning this standard, Pipes and Davenport (1990) wrote:

> Although it has been argued that clients deserve information about the legal limits of confidentiality and privileged communication, in actual practice the majority of psychotherapists probably give limited information until specifically asked by the client. (p. 14)

We strongly believe that it is *always* appropriate to inform clients of the legal limits of confidentiality. This should be done both orally and in writing. It is important for clients to understand very clearly the ground rules of the professional relationship.

Imagine a scenario wherein a client who has not been informed of the legal limits of confidentiality begins talking about suicide. At that point the therapeutic interviewer should begin to consider whether or not the client's suicidal thoughts are serious enough to warrant breaking confidentiality. As a result, the interviewer may suddenly feel compelled (and rightly so) to inform the client that the interviewer is obligated to break confidentiality under certain circumstances. To inform a client *after* the client has begun talking about secret information that the information may not be held in confidence is like changing the rules of a game as you go along. Clients deserve to know up front the rules and ethics that guide your interactions. It may be that the result of informing your clients of the limits of confidentiality is that the clients choose to be more selective in what they disclose to you. This is an unfortunate but natural side effect of the limits of confidentiality.

Stress Management for Therapeutic Interviewers

Therapeutic interviewing is stressful, particularly for beginning interviewers. In fact, all mental health workers are consistently exposed to high levels of stress (Rodolfa, Kraft, & Reilley, 1988) and the stress is always especially acute for those in the early learning stages.

Therapeutic interviewing is not something one can learn about in the abstract and then apply perfectly. The fact is you will make mistakes. The trick is to learn to use the mistakes for learning and for growth. Sometimes an interviewer's mistakes can even serve to humanize the process for the client, because the client sees that even the interviewer is not perfect.

We knew one student interviewer who reported high levels of anxiety accompanied by a tendency to pick at skin around the edges of his fingers. During his first session he picked at his fingers until he began feeling some moisture, which prompted him to conclude he was so nervous his fingers were sweating. He looked down and discovered one finger had begun to bleed. He spent the rest of the session trying to cover up the blood and worrying over whether or not the client had seen his bleeding finger. While this example is an extreme one, it illustrates how nervousness and anxiety can interfere with therapeutic interviewing. We believe that managing stress effectively so that it does not interfere with therapeutic interviewing is a professional issue.

Interviewers may be affected by stress before, during, or after the interview. Stress reactions may result in physical, mental, emotional, social, and spiritual symptoms. It is important for interviewers who are strongly affected by stress to seek out resources specifically designed to help individuals develop stress-coping responses. Readings that may help you manage your stress effectively are included in the suggested readings at the end of this chapter and of chapter 2.

Chapter Summary

This chapter describes and discusses practical and abstract factors therapeutic interviewers need to consider before conducting interviews. These factors include the physical setting and professional and ethical issues.

Generally, clinicians need to conduct their interviews in rooms that afford maximum privacy and minimal potential for interruption. The room is the safe place where clients begin disclosing personal and private information about themselves. Consequently, even during practice interviews, care should be taken to provide a room that facilitates client openness.

Although there is no hard and fast rule about how therapeutic interviewers and their clients should sit during a session, interviewers should be aware of how different seating arrangements may affect clients. Choices of seating arrangements may reflect underlying personality traits of the interviewer and the client. The most unobtrusive seating arrangement is probably one in which the interviewer and client sit in equally comfortable chairs at a 90- to 150-degree angle to one another with a small table nearby.

Experts on interviewing disagree as to whether it is appropriate for the interviewer to take notes during a session. Note taking is important because it can enhance the interviewer's memory of the session, but it can also offend some clients. If interviewers choose to take notes, it is recommended that they do so tactfully by explaining their purpose to the client and taking care to pay more attention to the client than the notes. Also, interviewers should never write anything in their notes that they would not want the client to read.

Video- and audiotape equipment affords interviewers another method of recording sessions, but the presence of such equipment sometimes produces discomfort and inhibition in both interviewers and clients. Interviewers should always obtain prior written and oral permission from clients when using audio or video recording equipment. The equipment should also be tested and made as unobtrusive as possible before initiating recording.

Professional and ethical issues include interviewer self-presentation, time boundary maintenance, confidentiality, and interviewer stress management.

Interviewers' dress and grooming can have a strong effect on clients. Interviewers generally should dress comfortably but conservatively. First impressions can strongly influence whether clients return for additional counseling; therefore, interviewers should dress and groom themselves in a manner unlikely to offend clients.

Another aspect of self-presentation is how therapeutic interviewers describe themselves and their credentials to clients. Interviewers should be honest and straightforward in their self-descriptions and should avoid introducing themselves in a demeaning manner, such as, "I'm just a student."

Time is the commodity therapeutic interviewers are selling to their clients. Therefore, interviewers need to be very careful in their management of time. Interviewers should start and end the session on time whenever possible. The primary exception to this rule is when there is an emergency. If interviewers are late for a session, they may offer to repay the client for lost time.

Confidentiality is a central ethical issue in therapeutic interviewing. Interviewers are obligated to maintain their clients' confidence unless the clients clearly present a danger to themselves or others. Interviewers should inform their clients of the limits of confidentiality before clients begin disclosing personal information, even though this may cause clients to be less open during sessions.

Because therapeutic interviewing is a stressful activity, stress management can be a professional issue for interviewers. It is recommended that interviewers who are having stress reactions seek methods of coping with their stress more effectively. The suggested readings at the end of this chapter and of Chapter 2 provide useful information regarding stress management for therapeutic interviewers.

Suggested Readings

Benjamin, A. (1981). *The helping interview* (3rd ed.). Boston: Houghton Mifflin Co. Chapter 1, on physical conditions, such as the room, and Chapter 4, on recording interviews, of Benjamin's classic text include information related to the content of this chapter.

Pipes, R. B., & Davenport, D. S. (1990). *Introduction to psychotherapy: Common clinical wisdom*. Englewood Cliffs, NJ: Prentice Hall. Chapter 2 of this text consists of "questions beginning therapists ask." Many of the questions address the physical interview setting, as well as professional and ethical interviewing issues.

Rodolfa, E. R., Kraft, W. A., & Reilley, R. R. (1988). Stressors of professionals and trainees at APA-approved counseling and VA medical center internship sites. *Professional Psychologist: Research and Practice, 19,* 43-49. This article discusses common stressors experienced by counselors and psychologists in training.

Wolberg, B. (1989). *The technique of psychotherapy*. (4th ed.). New York: Grune & Stratton. Chapter 62 of this huge text provides extended answers to common questions asked by beginning counselors and therapists.

4

BASIC ATTENDING SKILLS

Attending Behavior
    Positive Attending Behavior
    Negative Attending Behavior

Individual and Cultural Differences
    Cultural Issues
    Individual Differences

The Relationship Between Attending and Listening
    Poor Attending and Good Listening
    Good Attending and Poor Listening

Giving Constructive Feedback

Chapter Summary

Suggested Readings

He started going into this nodding routine. You never saw anybody nod as much in your life as old Spencer did. You never knew if he was nodding a lot because he was thinking and all, or just because he was a nice old guy that didn't know his ass from his elbow.—J. D. SALINGER, The Catcher in the Rye

When you pay attention to someone who is speaking, your intent is to receive information from that other person. It is a truism, however, that during an interview session it is impossible for the interviewer to only pay attention or listen. As Cormier and Cormier write, "Communication is ever two-way" (1985, p. 89). In the excerpt above, Salinger's fictional narrator Holden Caulfield nicely illustrates the "ever two-way" nature of communication. The person speaking is almost always simultaneously paying attention to the listener, receiving and judging important information. Just as while Holden speaks he evaluates old Spencer's nodding behavior, your clients will evaluate you on the basis of your attending behavior.

Although old Spencer's intent was to listen, he simultaneously communicated important information to Holden. As a clinical interviewer, your attending behavior is a message to your client—a message that should be interpreted as an invitation to speak openly and freely. You need to avoid potentially distracting mannerisms, such as old Spencer's nodding. Put another way, your job is to stay out of the way and not interfere with client disclosure. You do this by sounding, looking, and acting interested. It may seem ingenuine or phony to suggest that interviewers consciously try to appear to their clients as interested. Nonetheless, it is a fact that effective clinical interviewers consciously and deliberately engage in specific behaviors that clients interpret as a sign of interest and concern. These behaviors are referred to in the interviewing and counseling literature as "attending behaviors" (Ivey, 1988, p. 13).

In the ideal, interviewers are always genuinely interested and concerned about their clients' problems and welfare. In reality, there are always times, at least moments, when even the best interviewers become uninterested and unconcerned about their clients. Exploring why interviewers become interested or uninterested in their clients and how they should handle such feelings is very important. We will focus on these topics later (see the sections on congruence and countertransference in chapter 7).

Many people who enter the counseling field have a natural tendency to obtain satisfaction and enjoyment from listening to other people. In addition, they usually want to be more than just a naturally caring and compassionate person (although that is praiseworthy in itself); they also want to know the specific methods and techniques associated with effective counseling. This chapter's purpose is to explore the technical aspects of listening. Reading this chapter and practicing behaviors associated with effective listening will enable you to behave in ways that facilitate client verbal behavior and self-disclosure. This chapter also examines behaviors associated with poor listening. You can use these techniques to reduce or inhibit client expression or verbal behavior when you want the client to talk less, rather than more.

Attending Behavior

Ivey (1988) refers to "attending behavior" as the "foundation" of interviewing (p. 13). He goes on to define attending behavior as "culturally and individually appropriate eye contact, body language, vocal qualities, and verbal tracking" (p. 13). It is obviously important for interviewers to pay attention to their clients in culturally and individually appropriate ways, simply because if interviewers don't sound, look, and act like they're paying attention to their clients, they won't have any clients; clients will stop coming because of the interviewer's poor attending skills.

It is refreshing to find a concrete principle in the fields of psychology and counseling upon which virtually everyone agrees. Ivey's attending behavior, and in a more general sense, the importance of the art of listening well, is spectacularly uncontroversial (Cormier & Cormier, 1991; Egan, 1986; Goldfried & Davison, 1976; Strupp & Binder, 1984). Perhaps the only group of helping professionals who minimize the importance of eye contact and body language are staunch psychoanalysts who continue to use the couch in psychotherapy. Still, even psychoanalysts pay very close attention to their own vocal qualities, to tracking client verbal behavior, and to the general principle of listening well.

Attending behavior is primarily nonverbal. Edward T. Hall claimed that communication is 10 percent verbal and 90 percent a "hidden cultural grammar" (1966, p. 12). Others have similarly suggested that 65 percent or more of a message's meaning is conveyed through nonverbal channels (Birdwhistell, 1970). With respect to interviewing and counseling, Gazda, Asbury, Balzer, Childer, and Walters (1977) have noted that "when verbal and nonverbal messages are in contradiction, the helpee will usually believe the nonverbal message" (p. 93). Consequently, as an interviewer, you must utilize these powerful nonverbal channels in your communications with clients.

Positive Attending Behavior

Positive and negative attending behaviors have been identified by many authors (Cormier & Cormier, 1991; Ivey, 1988; Pipes and Davenport, 1990; Shea, 1988). Positive attending behaviors are usually those which open up communication and encourage free expression. In contrast, attending behaviors labeled "negative" tend to close down communication or inhibit expression. When it comes to identifying positive and negative attending behaviors, there are few universals because clients' cultural background and learning experiences may affect whether they view a particular attending behavior as positive or negative. Although there are some basic fundamentals, what works with one client will not always work with the next. Therefore, the manner in which you pay attention to clients must vary to some degree depending upon each client's individual needs, personality style, and family and cultural background. In other words, you need to be flexible; in some cases you must be very attentive, while in others you need to be less attentive— to "turn down the heat."

Ivey (1988) has identified four dimensions of attending behavior. Ivey's dimensions are simple and useful and have been studied cross-culturally to some degree:

- Eye contact
- Body language
- Vocal qualities
- Verbal tracking

Eye Contact The eyes have been said to be the windows of the soul. Cultures vary greatly in what they regard as appropriate eye contact behavior, and there is also a great deal of individual variation. For some interviewers, sustaining eye contact during an interview is easy and natural. For others, it can be difficult and painful; they may have a tendency to look down or away from the client's eyes because of shyness or inhibition. The same is true for clients; some prefer more intense and direct eye contact, while others would just as soon look at the floor, the wall, or anywhere but into your eyes.

Generally, for white American clients, interviewers should maintain about 70 to 90 percent eye contact. In contrast, Native and Black American clients prefer less direct eye contact. Some interviewers naturally look at the client's mouth or face rather than into the eyes; you may want to observe yourself to determine your own visual style with clients. For most clients it is appropriate to maintain more constant eye contact when they are speaking and less constant eye contact when you are speaking. Some research suggests that clients' pupils tend to dilate when they're emotionally aroused or interested and constrict when they're bored or uncomfortable (Hess, 1975; Ivey, 1988). While it is likely that the same process is true for interviewers, it is not likely that clients will be examining your pupils closely in an effort to determine whether you're interested in what they're saying. In fact, we have rarely met interviewers who are consistently able to pay close attention to their clients' pupil size. For most people eye contact is a simple method of making personal contact with someone else. It usually does not involve intense scrutiny of the other person's physical characteristics.

Body Language Aspects of communication that involve what most people, including Ivey (1988), refer to as body language are known technically as kinesics and proxemics (Birdwhistell, 1952; Hall, 1966; Knapp, 1972). Kinesics denotes variables associated with physical features and physical movement of any body part, such as eyes, face, head, hands, legs, or shoulders. Proxemics refers to personal space and environmental variables such as the distance between two people and whether any objects are between them. As most people know from personal experience, a great deal is communicated to others through simple, and sometimes subtle, movements. When we discussed client-interviewer seating arrangements in chapter 3, we analyzed proxemic variables and their potential effect on the interview.

Positive interviewer body language entails the following behaviors (derived from Walters, 1980):

- Lean slightly toward the client.
- Maintain a relaxed but attentive posture.
- Place your feet and legs in an unobtrusive position.
- Keep your hand gestures unobtrusive and smooth.
- Minimize the number of other movements.
- Make your facial expressions match your feelings or the client's feelings.
- Seat yourself at approximately one arm's length from the client.
- Arrange the furniture to draw you and the client together, not to erect a barrier.

One aspect of body language that receives attention in the interviewing field has been termed synchrony, or mirroring. Mirroring refers to efforts by the interviewer to be consistent or synchronous with clients' movements and verbal activity. When mirroring occurs, the interviewer's physical and verbal activity is "in sync with" the physical and verbal activity of the client. Mirroring is an advanced nonverbal interviewing technique that, when effective, enhances rapport and empathy (Banaka, 1971 [see Box 4-1]; Maurer & Tindal, 1983), but when ineffective, can be disastrous. Specifically, when mirroring is too obvious it may be perceived by clients as mimicking, which in turn is interpreted as mocking. Therefore, we recommend that mirroring be used only in moderation. Its potential benefits are small, while its potential costs are great.

Vocal Qualities   If your friends described your voice, what do you think they would say? Vocal quality is referred to as paralinguistics in the field of communication and consists of loudness, pitch, rate, and fluency. Think about the potential effects of these vocal variables on clients. Often, interpersonal influence is determined not so much by what you say but by how you say it.

Effective interviewers use their vocal qualities to enhance rapport, communicate interest and empathy, and emphasize specific issues or conflicts. In

---

BOX 4-1 ───

Mirroring: The Rubber Band Exercise

In this exercise, you select a partner, stand face to face, and raise both hands as if you were facing yourself in a mirror (your partner serves as your reflection. You then pretend your hands are attached to one another's with rubber bands, although you keep your hands about two inches apart). For the next two or three minutes partners are not allowed to speak to one another and are not allowed to touch one another's hands. Both partners can move their hands in any manner they desire, but the hands must stay together, as if connected by rubber bands.

The point of this exercise is to explore pacing and feelings of control. Pacing refers to "staying with" someone, as opposed to leading someone. After the exercise, ask one another the following questions: Who led and why? How was leadership initially determined? What was it like to lead, and what was it like to follow? Did leadership change at any point in the exercise, and if so, how did the transition occur?

In a variation of this exercise, partners sit with one another as in an interviewing setting. It is best to have a group of three so that each person can play the role of interviewer, client, and observer in turn. Choose a topic of discussion and assign roles. The client will be the leader, that is, the person the interviewer will mirror. Proceed to talk, with the interviewer practicing mirroring the leader as subtly as possible. The leader should occasionally change positions as a client might shift around during an interview session (e.g., cross and uncross legs, grimace, or fold hands). The purpose of this mirroring exercise is to experience how it feels to mirror a client, as well as how it feels to be mirrored. You may discover that you're comfortable mirroring particular types of behavior (e.g., leg crossing), but very uncomfortable mirroring other types of nonverbal behavior (e.g., grimacing). After all three partners have played every role, discuss how it felt to be mirrored, how it felt to mirror, and what it looked like from an outside observer's perspective.
Source: Banaka, 1971.

───

general, interviewers' voices should be soft yet firm, indicating both sensitivity and strength. As with body language, it is often useful to follow the client's lead, speaking in a volume and tone similar to the client's. Meier (1989) refers to this practice as "pacing the client" (p. 6).

On the other hand, interviewers can utilize voice tone, as with all interviewer responses and directives, to lead clients toward particular content or feelings. For example, speaking in a tone that is soft and gentle can sometimes encourage clients to explore their feelings more thoroughly, while speaking with increased rate and volume may help convince them of your credibility or expertise (Myers, 1989).

Although people perceive emotions through all sensory modalities, some research suggests people are better at discerning emotion from auditory input than visual input (Levitt, 1964; Snyder, 1974). This finding indicates the importance of vocal qualities in emotional expression and perception. Actors use their entire bodies, including their voices, when portraying various emotions. As an interviewer you should understand the impact of your own voice qualities and exercise control over your vocal emotional expression.

Verbal Tracking It is very important that interviewers accurately track the content of what clients communicate to them. In most cases, clients are not accustomed to being attended to (and listened to) as thoroughly as they are during an interview session. Although eye contact, body language, and vocal quality are important, they will not suffice by themselves. As an interviewer you must demonstrate your ability to track the content of your clients' speech by stating aloud some of the key words and phrases they have used. In most cases, clients do not know if you are really tracking what they're saying unless you prove it to them through accurate verbal tracking.

To use Meier's (1989) terminology again, the purpose of verbal tracking is to "pace" the client by staying with the content of the client's speech (as well as speech volume and tone, as mentioned previously). You need only reflect on the content of what the client has said; it is not important to evaluate the information or to add to it. Let us caution you: this is much easier said than done. At times clients talk about so many topics, it is very difficult to track them coherently. At other times you may become distracted by the content of what the client is saying and drift into your own thoughts or evaluations. For example, a client may mention something about New York City, abortion, drugs, AIDs, divorce, or some other topic about which you may have personal opinions or emotional reactions. In order to verbally track a client effectively, your personal reactions must be minimized; your focus must remain on the client, not yourself. This rule also holds true when it comes to more advanced verbal tracking techniques, such as clarification and paraphrasing, which we will discuss in chapter 5.

Negative Attending Behavior
It has been said that familiarity breeds contempt. In the case of attending skills, it might be more accurate to say that overuse breeds contempt. The chapter's

BOX 4-2 ───

Enhancing Your Emotional Expression and Perception

Researchers have identified seven to ten basic emotions that infants and children across many different cultures express and perceive as they develop (Izard, 1977; 1982; Levitt, 1964; Plutchik, 1980). Plutchik has identified eight specific emotions: anger, sadness, joy, acceptance, anticipation, disgust, fear, and surprise. This exercise involves practicing the expression and perception of Plutchik's eight basic emotions through visual and auditory modalities.

Visual expression of emotion requires the use of a partner or some form of visual feedback system (i.e., mirror, camera, or videotape recorder). Once you have set up a system, practice facial expression of each of the eight emotions listed above, one at a time. In order to adequately express the emotions through your face, you may need to reflect on previous experiences during which you felt those emotions. If you haven't experienced such feelings recently, or if you prefer not to reflect upon a negative experience, you may simply imagine situations that would make you react with the emotions you need to portray. If you use a video camera to record your emotional expressions, be sure to code the exact sequence of your emotional expressions. Then you can later show the tape to students working on emotional perception and let them evaluate the accuracy of your expressions by trying to identify them. You can also watch the video yourself later and attempt to identify the emotions you tried to express.

Auditory emotional expression is best practiced with an audiotape recorder. Emotions are expressed auditorily through one of two modes:

- Word content, (that is, whether or not emotionally laden words are used (see chapters 5 and 6 and Hutchins & Cole, 1986, p. 31).
- Vocal qualities or paralinguistics, including loudness, pitch, rate, and fluency (see Knapp, 1978; Cormier & Cormier, 1991).

Because the goal of this procedure is to produce a particular emotional expression based solely on vocal quality rather than word content, a standard script is required. The script we prefer, after having tried several, is "I am going out now, I won't be back all afternoon. If anyone calls, just say I'm not here" (Levitt, 1964; Snyder, 1974). You should have a written copy of the script so you can focus on utilizing your vocal qualities to express each of Plutchik's eight basic emotions. As with the visual emotional expression and perception task, you can subsequently seek partners to evaluate your accuracy or conduct your own self-analysis.

In some ways it is more efficient to complete these exercises within an interviewing class, where group feedback and appraisal is possible. When we use this exercise in class, we write the script on the chalkboard and hand out three-by-five inch cards, each with one of the eight emotions written on it, to eight randomly selected students. The students then try to express the emotion written on their card while the rest of the class listens with their eyes closed. The class tries to identify which of the eight emotions each person was expressing. Class discussion focuses on what factors contributed to the accurate, or inaccurate, expression and perception of each of the emotions. Source: Izard, 1982; Levitt, 1964.

opening example from *The Catcher in the Rye* is a great illustration of this. Most positive attending behaviors, when overused, become at best ineffective and at worst obnoxious. Interviewers should monitor the following attending behaviors to determine whether they are being overused.

1. Head nods. Interviewers can bother clients with excessive head nods. After a short while clients sometimes break eye contact with such interviewers in order to stop watching their heads bob. The most negative comment (outside of Holden Caulfield's) we have ever heard about head nods was "I couldn't stand it, it gave me a sore neck just to look at her."

2. Saying "uh huh." This is one of the most overused interviewer attending behaviors. Some novices and professionals fall into this pattern. When listening to someone for two minutes they sometimes utter as many as twenty "uh huhs." Our response (and the response of many clients) is to simply stop talking in order to force the person to say something besides "Uh huh."

3. Eye contact. Some interviewers worry too much about the importance of adequate eye contact. For example, some professionals believe that during group therapy each participant should receive approximately the same amount of eye contact from the group leader. Consequently, they slowly rotate their heads around the group throughout the session. Group members (patients in a psychiatric hospital) are often offended and sarcastic regarding such "mechanical and robotic" patterns of eye contact.

4. Repeating the client's last word. Some interviewers are very adept at selecting a single key word, often the last word, that the client had used. Unfortunately, they sometimes tended to overuse this attending technique, partly because they are so good at it and partly because they may not know what else to say. One result of this pattern is that clients sometimes feel overanalyzed, because interviewers reduce their thirty-second statement into a single-word response.

5. Mirroring. As suggested previously, excessive or awkward attempts at mirroring can be disastrous. We recall a psychiatrist who used this technique with rather disturbed, nearly nonverbal psychiatric inpatients. At times his results were astoundingly successful; at other times the patients became angry and aggressive because they perceived him as mocking them. A related concern is that often clients worry that counselors may know and use subtle techniques to exert special control over them. They may notice that you're trying to get into a physical position similar to theirs and wonder if you're using a psychological ploy to manipulate them. The result is usually resistance and pursuit. Clients begin moving into new positions, the interviewer notices and changes position to establish synchrony, and the client moves again. It is especially interesting to watch this process using the fast forward button on your VCR.

Several other nonverbal interviewer behaviors have been identified by researchers as negative, that is, they are perceived by clients as potentially indicating deception and they produce increased interpersonal distance. "Negative nonverbal messages" (Cormier & Cormier, 1985, p. 83; Graves & Robinson, 1976; Smith-Hanen, 1977) are conveyed by the following interviewer behaviors:

- Making infrequent eye contact
- Turning 45 degrees or more away from the client
- Leaning back from the waist up
- Crossing one's legs away from the client
- Folding one's arms across the chest

As noted, although it is certainly helpful to know these basic guidelines regarding positive and negative attending behaviors, there are some cases when individual clients do not respond to your attending in ways that you expect. Perhaps the best examples result from interviews of individuals from cultures other than the interviewer's own.

Individual and Cultural Differences

Many individual and cultural differences can potentially affect the clinical interview. It is advisable for clinical interviewers to be aware of and sensitive to gender differences, as well as other divergent social and cultural issues particular to each individual client (Gilligan, 1982; Miller, 1986; Vacc, Wittmer, & DeVaney, 1988). Remember every client is part of a distinct subculture with associated behavior patterns and social norms. Obviously, the way interviewers attend to clients who are young gang members is somewhat different than the way they deal with geriatric patients. Working knowledge of a wide range of social and cultural norms will help interviewers attend more effectively. Individual, social, and cultural differences are discussed briefly here and intermittently in other chapters. Suggestions for additional reading regarding this important facet of clinical interviewing are provided at the end of this chapter.

Cultural Issues

It is important to be sensitive to cultural differences when it comes to attending behavior, whether with regard to eye contact, body language, vocal qualities, or verbal tracking. Although most of the white population of the United States interpret eye contact as a positive sign of interest, people from many other cultures (e.g., Asian and Native American) tend to prefer less direct eye contact and may view excessive eye contact as disrespectful or invasive.

During a recent visit to Europe and North Africa, we became acutely aware of cultural differences in body language. We had only limited ability to speak other languages, and therefore our experience of different cultures was based largely on nonverbal perceptions. Our trip began in central Germany and northern Switzerland, where we hardly noticed any body language differences among the German, Swiss, and our own dominant culture. However, as we proceeded south to southern Switzerland and Italy, the average amount of personal space and distance between people shrank. We found ourselves observing much more of what could be described as nose-to-nose communication. In addition, hand gestures were much more vigorous and emphatic. Perhaps our greatest discovery occurred while we were lining up for tickets at railway stations. In Germany and most of Switzerland, the lines were organized and polite, with little cutting or verbal exchanges between those waiting to be served. In southern Italy and Tunisia, lines were extremely disorganized, chaotic, and characterized by intense rubbing together of masses of bodies near the entrance or destination. We discovered that waiting patiently in a line was viewed as passive and low-class. People were respected for being pushy and aggressive in their approach to obtaining services or reaching their destination.

It is generally useful to assume clients from cultures other than yours may have different social habits than your own. This does not mean they necessarily require different interviewing methods or attending behaviors, but it is safer to explore their cultural differences rather than assume they are comfortable with the same degree of eye contact as are the clients who share your culture. It is acceptable to discuss directly with clients what types of attending behaviors are comfortable for them. You are more likely to offend clients from other cultures by assuming they have adopted your values and norms than you are by exploring types of attending behavior with which they are uncomfortable. We also recommend you read about and experience other cultural systems before attempting to conduct clinical interviews with someone from a different cultural background than your own.

Individual Differences

If you were to invite twenty people, one by one, into your office for a clinical interview, you would probably discover that each person was optimally comfortable with slightly different amounts of eye contact, personal space, mirroring, and other attending behaviors. The guidelines we have given above are based on averages and probabilities. For example, if you were to interview Italian-American clients, you might find them, on average, comfortable with closer seating arrangements than clients with roots in Scandinavia. This is not the whole story. There also will be times when a particular Italian-American prefers greater interpersonal distance than a particular Scandinavian. If you expect all Italian-Americans, all Scandinavians, all African-Americans, all women, and so on to be similar simply because of average group likenesses, you are stereotyping in a manner that may result in prejudicial behavior. This is because differences between particular individuals is often greater than the average difference between particular groups, cultural or otherwise. Therefore, you should be aware of the potential differences between members of various groups, but you should suspend judgment until you have explored the issue with each individual. Interviewers can explore their clients' individual differences and levels of comfort with specific attending behaviors through observation and by directly discussing personal comfort and attending behavior with clients.

The Relationship between Attending and Listening

Ivey's (1988) "attending behavior" is the most basic and fundamental of what he has described and popularized as "microskills" (p. 13). Interviewers and counselors must learn how to attend well to the clients' talk before moving on to more advanced skill development.

Ivey's attending behaviors are usually considered the basic ingredients required for effective listening. This does not mean that attending and listening are synonymous processes or even that they are causally related. Their relationship consists in the fact that because attending behavior is *associated* with listening, it is often interpreted by clients as evidence of listening.

People are inclined to incorrectly assume that attentive eye contact, body language, vocal qualities, and verbal tracking constitute "effective listening." Although good attending behavior is generally associated with good listening and poor attending behavior is associated with poor listening, the fact is that people can attend very poorly and listen very well or attend very well yet listen very poorly.

Poor Attending and Good Listening

You probably all know a few people who can look like they are not listening while, in fact, they are absorbing everything going on around them. Children are especially good at playing while at the same time monitoring their parents' interactions in case they, the children, are being left out of something fun or in case there is trouble on the horizon. Sometimes these nonattending quirks can be endearing, such as the kindly professor who always straightens her pens when she is really interested in what you are saying, or a grandparent who knits and fusses around the house, all the while listening to the grandchild's tall tales.

We all have our own style of listening and have individualized ways of signaling to those around us that we are listening—our own personalized attending ritual. Those who know us well and trust us tolerate these attending variations, but sometimes ignoring the basic attending behaviors can cause misunderstanding and feelings of being ignored, even among those who know us well. In interviewing situations the risk is much higher because initially you are trying to communicate effectively with a virtual stranger. Thus, your personal style may need to be more carefully monitored in order to communicate that you are, indeed, listening.

Author Rita Sommers-Flanagan is a doodler. Her concentration is actually enhanced when she is free to sketch, make lists, and generally let her pen wander as it likes. In graduate school this habit had many opportunities for expression and, in fact, she attained a certain notoriety for writing letters, lists, and single-line poems and for drawing pictures during class or group discussions. As you may guess, this activity was not well received by professors and fellow students. She was called to task on several occasions by professors, who, suspecting she was not listening to lectures, directly questioned her knowledge of the lecture material during discussion periods. The truth of the matter was,

Rita really was listening and contemplating the material at hand, so she could usually answer appropriately. Finally, during an end-of-the-year evaluation, her advisor said, "Rita, if you can't stop it entirely, then the faculty would like you to try to disguise your doodling. They realize you are listening, but you are still a distraction to your fellow students. Cool it." Doodling less has not been easy, and Rita's preferred style of listening is still with pen in hand, happily spreading ink around while the verbal interactions go on. However, in an interview or therapy situation, it is extremely rare that she feels free to doodle in any form, with one exception: she has found that sometimes she can enhance what is being said by a list or diagram that comes to mind; she jots it down and shares it with the client in the process of their work together.

Good Attending and Poor Listening

Although most of us are reluctant to admit it, many interviewers or psychotherapists fall into this category. Having been effectively trained in Ivey's microskills, author John Sommers-Flanagan confesses to being a good attender but poor listener. During lectures, and even during counseling situations, he can automatically make good eye contact, nod his head sincerely, speak in appropriately sensitive tones, and even verbally track to some degree by repeating occasional key words and phrases, and yet not actually hear and retain the message the other person is communicating. All too often his mind is somewhere else, while his body is automatically performing the skills he so thoroughly learned from family, friends, teachers, students, and clients. At one point when John and Rita were dating, John was startled into full attention when Rita said, rather emphatically, "OK, I am done talking to Carl Rogers. Is John Sommers around?"

It is important for you to note what causes you to go into this "automatic-pilot" sort of attending. You may be tired, bored, upset, or preoccupied on occasion, and simply need to conserve energy in this way. However, except for short periods or extreme situations, it is not advisable to allow yourself to appear to be listening more keenly than you actually are. By doing so, you rob the interaction between you and the client of authenticity and of the opportunity for deeper, more meaningful interactions. If you find yourself attending better than you listen on a regular basis, take time to find out why and take steps to address the problem.

Giving Constructive Feedback

Repeated practice is required to master the skills of attending. Throughout this chapter we have included various attending activities in order to facilitate your improvement. We recommend engaging in extensive role-playing and obtaining feedback about yourself as a supplement to this chapter. The following discussion regarding how to cope with and give constructive feedback is provided to help you get started.

Individual and group feedback regarding the efficacy of your attending skills is useful to your development as an interviewer. You can solicit feedback through in-class activities, demonstrations, role-plays, and audio- or videotape presentations. We recommend that students receive specific and concrete feedback regarding their eye contact, body language, vocal qualities, and verbal tracking. For example: "You looked into your client's eyes with only two or three breaks and although you fidgeted somewhat with your pencil, it didn't appear to interfere with the interview." Generally positive comments such as "Good job!" are encouraging and useful, but should be used in combination with more specific feedback; it is nice to know what was "good" about your "job."

Sometimes class activities or role-plays do not proceed smoothly, and negative feedback is appropriate. Of course, we recommend that negative feedback be worded constructively (i.e., recipients of feedback are given clear examples of more positive behavior patterns they could adopt). This issue is sensitive because it can be very painful for people to hear that others view their performances as imperfect. In contrast to positive feedback, general negative comments such as "Terrible job!" that are not constructive should always be avoided. In order to be constructive, negative feedback should always be specific and concrete. Several other guidelines are useful when giving negative feedback:

- The class should be reminded occasionally of the disappointing fact that no one performs perfectly, including the teacher or professor.
- Remember that the purpose of being in an interviewing class is to improve your interviewing skills. Though hard to hear sometimes, constructive feedback is useful for skill development.
- Feedback should never be uniformly negative. Everyone engages in positive and negative attending behaviors. If you happen to be the type who easily sees what is wrong but has more trouble offering praise, you may want to impose the following rule for yourself: If you cannot think of something positive to say about an interviewer's performance, don't say anything at all.
- Negative feedback usually can be stated in a positive manner. For example, "your body posture was stiff and rigid" can be rephrased as "you might be more effective if you relaxed your arms and shoulders more thoroughly."
- Role-players can be asked to evaluate themselves. Usually students are more negative regarding their own interviewing behavior than others who observe them.
- Students should be asked directly after a class interviewing activity whether or not they would like feedback. If they say "no," then no feedback should be given.
- Feedback that is strongly negative is the responsibility of the instructor and should be given during the privacy of an individual supervision session.

Chapter Summary

This chapter focuses on basic attending skills that interviewers can learn to facilitate client disclosure. Because communication is a two-way process, interviewers must strive to behave in ways clients are likely to interpret as indicative of interest and concern. Positive attending behavior serves as the foundation of effective listening.

Attending behavior is primarily nonverbal and consists of appropriate eye contact, body language, vocal qualities, and verbal tracking. Most white American clients feel comfortable with the following interviewer behaviors: approximately 70 to 90 percent eye contact, a slight lean forward, minimal to moderate unobtrusive gestures, facial expressions that match the client's or that match the interviewer's inner feelings, occasional head nods, occasional "uh huhs," and short phrases or words capturing the essence of what the client said. Clients and interviewers from other cultures may have different preferences when it comes to nonverbal behavior.

Negative attending behavior may consist of any positive attending behavior taken to the extreme. Inattentive or distracting verbal or nonverbal behavior is also generally viewed as nonfacilitative.

Considerable differences may exist among clients regarding the amount and type of eye contact, body language, vocal qualities, and verbal tracking they prefer. For example, Italians tend to require less interpersonal distance than northern Europeans, while Native Americans prefer less direct eye contact than European-Americans. However, it is important to remember there are great individual differences, even within cultures. Therefore, to avoid stereotyping and prejudice the interviewer should consider and explore these issues with each individual client.

Many people mistakenly believe that attending skills are synonymous with listening. Simply because someone sounds, looks, and acts as if they're listening doesn't mean they are effective listeners. Some people listen very effectively, yet appear as if they're not paying attention. Attending is a skill that can facilitate listening and serve the purpose of communicating to clients that you're trying to listen.

Practice is crucial to the development of positive attending behavior. Therefore, exercises that promote attending skill development are given throughout the chapter. Guidelines are provided for giving positive and constructive feedback to students trying to improve their skills.

Suggested Readings

Several textbooks and workbooks offer additional information and exercises on basic attending skills. As noted in this chapter, knowledge of and sensitivity to various social and cultural groups is important.

Brodsky, A.M. (1982). Sex, race, and class issues in psychotherapy research. In J.H. Harvey & M.M. Parks (Eds.), *The Master Lecture series: Vol. I. Psychotherapy research and behavior change.* Washington, DC: American Psychological Association. This is a good general overview of issues associated with race, class, and sex issues in psychotherapy.

Brody, C.M. (Ed.). (1984). *Women therapists working with women: New theory and process of feminist therapy.* New York: Springer. This edited volume of general and specific concerns regarding feminist therapy is also a very good reference for other works related to feminist therapy.

Cormier, W.H., & Cormier, L.S. (1991). *Interviewing strategies for helpers: Fundamental skills and cognitive behavioral interventions* (3rd ed.). Monterey, CA: Brooks/Cole. Chapter 4 in particular (pp. 63–86) of this text provides extensive and in-depth information regarding nonverbal behavior.

Egan, G. (1985). *Exercises in helping skills: A training manual to accompany the skilled helper* (3rd ed.). Monterey, CA: Brooks/Cole. Egan's manual provides attending skill exercises that can be very useful for beginning students.

Gilligan, C. (1982). *In a different voice: Psychological theory and women's development.* Cambridge, MA: Harvard University Press. Gilligan clarifies female and male differences and discusses how the field of psychology has persistently viewed women inaccurately.

LeVine, S., & LeVine, R.A. (1985). Age, gender, and the demographic transition: The life course in agrarian societies. In A.S. Rossi (Ed.), *Gender and the life course.* pp. 29–42. New York: Aldine. This book discusses patterns of age and sex subordination within the families of agricultural societies.

Miller, J.B. (1986). *Toward a new psychology of women* (2nd ed.). Boston: Beacon Press. This book is about women (and men) and the issues they deal with in contemporary society. It helps articulate the depth and meaning of some difficulties traditionally associated with being female.

Pederson, P.B. (1988). *A handbook for developing multicultural awareness.* Alexandria, VA: American Association for Counseling and Development. This handbook is already a classic with regard to multicultural sensitivity training.

Scheflin, A.E., & Scheflin, A. (1972). *Body language and social order.* Englewood Cliffs, NJ: Prentice-Hall. This classic book focuses on the various ways in which body movement and the use of space influence human interaction.

Sue, D.S. Arredondo, P., & McDavis, R.J. (1992). Multicultural counseling competencies and standards: A call to the profession. *Journal of Counseling and Development, 70,* 477–486. Standards and competencies in the area of multicultural issues are outlined for the counseling profession.

Vacc, N.A., Wittmer, J., & DeVaney, S.B. (1988). *Experiencing and counseling multicultural and diverse populations.* Muncie, IN: Accelerated Development Inc. This book presents an overview of thirteen diverse ethnic subgroups within American society. It includes chapters on experiencing and counseling gay and lesbian populations, Native Americans, Southeast Asian refugees, and others.

5
NONDIRECTIVE LISTENING RESPONSES: A CONTINUUM

Nondirective Listening Responses
    Attending Behavior
    Silence
    Paraphrase or Reflection of Content
    Clarification
    Nondirective Reflection of Feeling
    Summarization

Interviewer Development Activities
    Brief Nondirective Interviews
    Enhancing Your Feeling Capacity and Vocabulary
    Silence Desensitization
    Generating Sensory-Based and Feeling Words

Chapter Summary

Suggested Readings

. . . Hurriedly, he raised his head from his hand, and stood forth upon the rock and listened. But there was no voice throughout the vast illimitable desert, and the characters upon the rock were SILENCE. And the man shuddered and turned his face away, and fled afar off, in haste, so that I beheld him no more.
        —EDGAR ALLAN POE, *Silence: A Fable*

Many interviewers are uncomfortable with silence. There is pressure associated with responsibility and usually the person designated as interviewer is viewed as having most of the responsibility for producing a "good" interview. As a consequence, when silence occurs, it is often the interviewer who feels pressure, responsibility, and possibly discomfort. This is natural and normal, especially for beginning interviewers. A common response of beginning interviewers is to exclaim, "I don't know what to say!" And they are usually correct in their appraisal. Not knowing what to say can be a dilemma for *all* clinical interviewers, both beginning and experienced. Both of us authoring this book have learned to readily admit that at times we don't know exactly what to say either.

In some ways, it would be nice if we could launch into an authoritative guide to interviewer responses with a structured format for determining which interviewer response should be used at each specific point in the interview. Unfortunately, or perhaps, fortunately, individual clients are so different and unique that it is impossible to develop a standard procedure to tell you which interviewing response to use at a given point in an interview. Differences among clients make it impossible to reliably predict their reactions to various interviewing responses. Some clients react very positively to responses that we judge as poor or awkward, while others react negatively to what might otherwise be considered a perfect paraphrase. Although this chapter systematically and scientifically breaks down nondirective interviewing responses into rather distinct categories, it provides only general guidelines in the use of these responses. Knowing when and how to apply particular interviewing responses constitutes the artistic side of interviewing and requires sensitivity and experience as well as other intangibles you cannot absorb from a book. Although this is not the kind of confident approach to interviewing we wish we could provide, it is honest; no one should pretend to know all the right things to say in an interview.

Experienced and effective interviewers have developed the patience required to appreciate, or at least endure, silence. Then, when they decide to speak, they say something they intended to say. We would like to echo Meier's (1989) recommendation: "When you don't know what to say, say nothing" (p. 10). In other words, there will be times when even the best interviewers do not know what to say and when that occurs, the best advice is to stay with basic attending skills (introduced in the previous chapter). Luborsky (1984) also emphasizes the importance of keeping quiet: "Listen . . . with an open receptiveness to what the patient is saying. If you are not sure of what is happening and what your next response should be, listen more and it will come to you" (p. 91).

Experienced and effective interviewers have the confidence required to wait; they know they will eventually think of something useful to say, or they will know that the most useful thing to do is to say nothing.

You may find yourself feeling a bit suspicious about our claims that often even experienced professionals truly don't know what to say. Margaret Gibbs explores her feelings along these lines in her chapter The Therapist as Imposter in Claire Brody's book *Women Therapists Working with Women*. Gibbs states:

> Once I began my work as a therapist . . . I began to have . . . doubts. Certainly my supervisors seemed to approve of my work, and my patients improved as much as anybody else's did. But what was I actually supposed to be DOING? I knew the dynamic, client-centered and behavioral theories, but I continued to read and search for answers. I felt there was something I should know, something my instructors had neglected to tell me, much as cooks are said to withhold one important ingredient of their recipes when they relinquish them. (1984, p. 22)

As Gibbs suggests, experience and hard work will help take the edge off the feeling of not knowing what to say. It also will help interviewers have more confidence in their skills. Nonetheless, part of being an honest professional is to admit and tolerate the fact that sometimes you don't know what to say. Gibbs ends her chapter with the following statements (and we heartily concur):

> Strategies can cover up, but not resolve, the ambiguities of clinical judgments and interventions. Imposter doubts need to be shared, not suppressed, in the classroom as elsewhere. Arkes (1981) cites evidence to support the idea that uncertainty and humility about the accuracy of our clinical inferences is an aid to increased accuracy. I find this notion enormously comforting. (p. 32)

We are spending a great deal of time on the issue of knowing what to say, when to say it, and when to be quiet, because this is the heart of the interview. Knowing what to say and when to say it is central to the process of clinical interviewing, and saying the wrong thing is the most common fear stated by our students (Sommers-Flanagan, 1990). Therefore, the purpose of this chapter is to outline and describe the range of nondirective listening responses available to clinical interviewers.

We have followed Robinson's (1950) and Benjamin's (1981) organizational format in this and the next chapter. We begin with responses that are considered, for the most part, nondirective or "client-centered," and proceed along a continuum toward increasingly directive or "therapist centered" responses. Although Robinson and Benjamin distinguish in their writing between interviewer "responses and leads" (Benjamin, 1981, p. 114), we refer to all possible interviewer behavior as responses. This is because even very directive or "leading" interviewer statements are usually in "response" to client communications. Potential interviewer responses are categorized into three groups.

- Nondirective listening responses (e.g., silence; see Table 5-1)
- Directive listening responses (e.g., interpretation; see Table 6-1)
- Directive action responses (e.g., advice; see Table 6-2)

Nondirective listening responses are the focus of the remainder of the chapter.

Nondirective Listening Responses

Nondirective listening responses are designed to encourage clients to talk freely and openly about whatever issues come to mind. These techniques are not designed to direct or lead clients into a particular topic area. Nondirective listening responses track central client messages by reflecting back to clients what they have already said.

On the other hand, because of the potentially powerful influence interviewers have, even nondirective responses may be used to direct and lead clients into disclosing particular information. This is true despite the fact that most interviewers intend to use such responses in a nondirective manner. There are two major reasons why nondirective responses become directive responses. First, interviewers may inadvertently, or purposefully, pay closer attention to clients when they discuss certain issues. For example, perhaps an interviewer wants a client to talk about his relationship with his mother. Through eye contact, head nodding, and positive and interested facial responses whenever the client talks about his mother, the interviewer is likely to direct the client toward "mother talk." Conversely, the interviewer can look uninterested whenever the client shifts topics and discusses something other than his mother. Technically, such an interviewer is using social reinforcement to influence the client's verbal behavior. Unfortunately, this type of selective attending probably occurs fairly frequently in clinical practice. After all, psychoanalytic interviewers are theoretically more interested in mother talk, person-centered interviewers are more interested in feeling talk, and behaviorists are more interested in specific, concrete behavioral talk.

Second, clients talk about such a wide range of topics in interviews that it is impossible for interviewers to pay equal attention to every issue a client brings up; some selection is necessary. For example, imagine a case in which a female client begins a session with: "We didn't have much money when I was growing up, and I suppose that was one thing that frustrated my father. . . . He beat us five kids on a regular basis. Now that I'm grown and have kids of my own I'm doing OK, but sometimes I feel I need to discipline my kids more . . . harder . . . you know what I mean?" Now as an interviewer, what do you say and how do you act in response to what the client has just said? This woman brought up many important and significant issues in the first twenty seconds of the session—being beaten by her father, being poor, doing OK now, and feeling like disciplining her children more severely. Which do you focus on? To focus on any single aspect of this woman's message, to select only one of these topics to paraphrase or nod your head to, would be, in essence, to use a directive listening response. In order to be truly nondirective, an interviewer would need to respond equally to the entire message, which is unrealistic and inappropriate. Therefore, you must be aware of the powerful influence even theoretically nondirective responses can have on what clients choose to talk about.

Despite these cautions, nondirective responses are still the least influential of interviewer responses and provide the greatest opportunity to encourage clients to freely express themselves (Table 5.1).

Attending Behavior

Attending behavior was described in the previous chapter and will be only briefly discussed here. The primary purpose of attending behavior is to facilitate client talk. Ideally, positive attending behavior allows clients freedom to speak about whatever topics they would like; the interviewer paces or tracks what clients say. However, as noted above, attending behavior also may be utilized in a directive or leading manner. Eye contact, head nods, facial expressions, and other attending behaviors may be used to encourage, or discourage, a client talking about a particular topic.

Silence

Silence is perhaps the most nondirective of all responses. It is also one of the most powerful of all responses. It takes time for both interviewers and clients to adjust to silence. As the excerpt from Edgar Allan Poe's writing at the beginning of this chapter suggests, silence can be frightening. On the other hand, when used appropriately, silence can be quite soothing.

Silence doesn't just frighten beginning interviewers, it frightens clients as well. Most people feel awkward about silence in social settings and strive to keep conversations alive. Interviewers often feel a heavy burden of responsibility during their initial practice sessions; they feel they must keep the session going smoothly.

The primary function of silence as an interviewer response is to encourage client talk. Silence may also serve to allow clients to recover from or reflect upon difficult material they have just discussed. However, a word of caution is needed here. Interviewers who begin their sessions with silence and continue using silence liberally, without explaining the purpose of their silence to their clients, run the risk of scaring clients away. This is because when interviewers are nonexpressive, great pressure is placed on the clients to speak. Any silence that occurs is then viewed as caused by clients, who then may feel anxiety or a great burden of responsibility for the silence.

Silence is a major tool used by psychoanalytic psychotherapists to facilitate free association. Effective psychoanalytic therapists, however, explain the concept of free association to their clients in advance. They explain that this type of therapy will primarily involve the client's free expression accompanied by occasional comments or interpretations by the psychotherapist. Explaining the therapy or interviewing process to clients is always important, but especially so when the interviewer is using potentially threatening techniques, such as silence (Luborsky, 1984; Meier, 1989).

We think it useful for beginning interviewers to experiment with silence. We recommend you try letting some periods of silence pass by during role-plays. Keep the following guidelines in mind:

- When a role-play client pauses after making a statement or after hearing your paraphrase, let a few seconds pass rather than immediately jumping in with further verbal interaction. Given the opportunity, clients often flow naturally into very significant material *without* your guidance or urging. Give them a chance to associate to new material.

- As you're sitting silently and waiting for your client to resume speaking, try to tell yourself that this is the client's time to express herself, not your time to prove you can be useful. If you assume the role of an "expert" interviewer, you will probably feel greater responsibility (i.e., as if you need to say the right thing or ask the right question).
- Try not to get into a rut regarding your use of silence. When silence comes, sometimes you should wait for the client to speak next and other times you should break the silence yourself.
- Avoid using silence if you believe your client is confused, experiencing an acute emotional crisis, or psychotic. Excessive silence, and the anxiety it provokes, tends to exacerbate these conditions.
- If you feel uncomfortable during silent periods, try your best to relax. Use your attending skills to look expectantly toward clients. This will help them understand that it's their turn to talk.
- If clients appear uncomfortable with silence, you may give them instructions to free associate (i.e., tell them "just say whatever comes to mind."). Or you may want to use an empathic reflection of content or feeling (say something like, "it's hard to decide what to say next.")
- Remember, sometimes silence is the most therapeutic response available.
- Read the published interview by Carl Rogers (Meador & Rogers, 1984) listed at the end of this chapter. The interview includes excellent examples of how to handle silence from a person-centered perspective.

Paraphrase or Reflection of Content

The paraphrase or reflection of content is a cornerstone of effective communication. The primary purpose of the paraphrase is to assure clients that you have accurately heard the central meaning of their messages. Secondarily, paraphrases are designed to allow clients to hear how someone else perceives them (a clarification function), which usually facilitates further expression. In addition, paraphrases may be used in an effort to keep clients focusing on a particular content area.

Paraphrasing is defined as "giving the meaning in another form" (Webster's Ninth New Collegiate Dictionary, 1985, p. 854). In clinical interviewing a paraphrase has also has been referred to as a "reflection of content." A paraphrase or reflection of content refers to a statement accurately reflecting or rephrasing the essence of what the client has said. Paraphrasing does not give license to change, modify, or add to what the client has said. A paraphrase must be accurate; it is usually brief.

Interviewers often feel awkward when making their first paraphrases. They feel like they're restating the obvious. They often simply parrot back to clients what has just been said in a manner that is rigid, stilted, and at times offensive. This is unfortunate because the paraphrase, properly used, is a flexible and creative technique that enhances rapport and empathy. There are several types of paraphrases.

The Generic Paraphrase The generic paraphrase simply rephrases, rewords, and reflects what the client just said. Some examples:

- C: "Yesterday was my day off. I just sat around the house doing nothing. I had some errands to run, but I couldn't seem to make myself get up off the couch and do them."

- I: "So you had trouble getting going on your day off."

- C: "I do the same thing with every assignment. I wait till the last minute and then I whip together the paper. I end up doing all-nighters and I don't think the final product is as good as it could be."

- I: "You see this as a pattern for yourself. It sounds like your procrastination makes it so you don't do as well as you could on your assignments."

Each of these examples of the generic paraphrase is simple and straightforward. The generic paraphrase does not retain everything that was originally said; it only rephrases the essence of the client's message. It also does not include any evaluative components (i.e., interviewer opinion, reactions, and commentary are excluded, whether positive or negative).

The Sensory-Based Paraphrase Most people have preferred sensory systems through which they obtain most of their information about their environment. The neurolinguistic programming (NLP) movement in counseling recently popularized a concept referred to as "representational systems" (Bandler & Grinder, 1975; Grinder & Bandler, 1976). Representational systems refer to the sensory system—usually visual, auditory, or kinesthetic—that clients prefer to use to experience the world.

If you listen closely to words your clients use to describe their experiences, you will notice that some clients rely primarily on visually oriented words (e.g., "I see" or "it looks like"), others on auditory words (e.g., "I hear" or "it sounded like"), and others on kinesthetic words (e.g., "I feel" or "it moved me"). According to NLP theory, interviewers establish greater rapport and trust with their clients if they use each client's preferred representational system in their responses. In fact, some research suggests that when interviewers speak through their client's representational system, empathy, trust, and desire to see the interviewer again are all increased (Brockman, 1980; Hammer, 1983; Sharpley, 1984).

Listening closely for your client's sensory-related words is the key to using sensory-based paraphrases. To sensitize yourself to the three representational systems, we recommend doing an individual or in-class activity in which you generate as many visual, auditory, and kinesthetic words as you can. (Although clients occasionally refer to olfactory and taste experiences, it is rare that clients utilize these systems as their primary representational modality.) Some examples of sensory-based paraphrases follow with the sensory words italicized:

- C: "My goal in therapy is to get to know myself better. I think of therapy as kind of a *mirror* through which I can *see* myself, my strengths and my weaknesses more *clearly*."

- I: "You're here because you want to *see* yourself more *clearly* and believe therapy can really help you with that."

- C: "I just got laid off from my *job* and I don't know what to *do*. My *job* is so important to me. I *feel lost*."

- I: "*Doing* your *job* has been so important to you, you *feel adrift* without it."

There are other methods available for evaluating a client's primary representational system. However, thus far, analyzing the client's spontaneous use of sensory words appears to be the most reliable method (Sharpley, 1984).

The Metaphorical Paraphrase   Many times interviewers can use metaphor or analogy to capture the central message within a client's communication. For instance, often clients come to a professional interviewer because they're feeling stuck; they're not making any progress in terms of personal growth or problem resolution. In such a case an interviewer might reflect back, "So it seems like you're spinning your wheels" or "Dealing with this particular problem has been a real uphill battle." Although this type of paraphrase is probably best suited to the kinesthetically oriented client, we have found that most clients respond well to it, perhaps because it captures so much of an experience in so few words. Following are some additional examples:

- C: "My sister is so picky. We share a room and she's always bugging me about picking up my clothes, straightening up my dresser, and everything else too. She has this watchful eye that scrutinizes every move I make and criticizes me every chance she gets."

- I: "It's like you're in the army and she's your drill sergeant."

- C: "I'm prepared for some breakdowns along the way."

- I: "You don't expect it will be smooth sailing." (From Rogers, 1961, p. 102)

Clarification

There are several forms of clarification interviewers can use during a session, all with the same purpose: to make clear for yourself, and for the client, the precise nature of what has been said. Clarifications may also be used to ascertain whether you are hearing and understanding the client accurately.

The first form of clarification consists of a restatement of what the client has said and a closed question, in either order. Rogers was a master at clarification: "If I'm getting it right . . . what makes it hurt most of all is that when he tells you you're no good, well shucks, that's what you've always felt about yourself. Is that—the meaning of what you're saying?" (from Meador & Rogers, 1984, p. 167).

The second form of clarification is slightly more probing. It consists of a restatement imbedded in a double question. A double question is defined as an either/or question that includes two or more possible choices of response for the client. For example:

- "Are you feeling anger . . . or is it something else?"
- "Did you get in the argument with your husband before or after you went to the movie?"

As you can see, using clarification along with a double question requires interviewers to take more responsibility for trying to discover what clients are saying. In a sense, interviewers try to guess a client's potential response by providing possible choices, similar to the multiple-choice test format.

The third form of clarification is perhaps the most basic. It is used when a client has stated something barely audible and you're checking to see if you heard the statement correctly.

- "I'm sorry, I didn't quite hear that. Could you repeat what you said?"
- "I couldn't make out what you said. Did you say you'll be going home after the session?"

There will be times during interviews when you do not clearly understand what your clients are saying. There also will be times when your clients won't be sure what they are saying or why they are saying it. The worst possible scenario is when neither of you has a clue as to what the other, or yourselves, are saying. Sometimes the appropriate response is to wait, as Luborsky (1984) suggests, for the understanding to come. However, at other times it is necessary to clarify precisely what clients are talking about. There will also be times when clients will make efforts to clarify something that you've said.

Brammer (1979) provides two general guidelines for clarifying. First, "admit" your "confusion" over what the client has said. Second, "try a restatement or ask for clarification, repetition, or illustration" (p. 73). Asking for a specific illustration or example can be especially useful, because it encourages clients to be concrete and specific rather than abstract and vague.

From the clinical interviewer's perspective, there are two primary factors to consider when deciding whether or not to clarify what a client has said. First, if the information appears trivial and unrelated to therapeutic issues, it may be best to simply wait for the client to move on to a more productive area. It can be a waste of valuable session time to try to clarify minor details that are only remotely related to interview goals. For example, suppose a client says, "My stepdaughter's grandfather on my wife's side of the family usually has little or no contact with my parents." This presents an excellent opportunity for the interviewer to listen quietly and unenthusiastically. To attempt a clarification response might result in a five-minute (or longer) entanglement with distant family relationships. Spontaneous rambling toward discussion of distant familial relationships is often a sign that your client is avoiding pertinent personal issues. You should not use a clarification response, or any response, that might reinforce this avoidance pattern.

Second, if the information your client is discussing seems important but is not being articulated clearly enough for you to understand, you have two choices:

- Wait briefly to see if the client can independently express himself more clearly.
- Immediately seek to clarify the precise nature of what the client is saying.

For example, a client may state, "I don't know, she was different. She looked at me differently than other women. Others were missing . . . something, you know, the eyes, usually you can tell by the way a woman looks at you, can't you? Then again, maybe it was something else, something about me that I'll understand someday." An appropriate interviewer clarification might be, "So she seemed different; it may have been how she looked at you, or it may have been something about you that you don't understand. Is that what you're saying?"

Nondirective Reflection of Feeling

The primary purpose of nondirective reflection of feeling is to let clients know, through an emotionally oriented paraphrase, that you have heard their emotional expressions. Other purposes of nondirective feeling reflections may include enhancing clients' sense of being understood by their interviewer and encouraging further emotional expression.

Consider the following example of a fifteen-year-old male talking with an interviewer about his junior high school teacher:

C: "That teacher pissed me off big time when she accused me of stealing her watch . . . I wanted to punch her lights out."

I: "So you were pretty pissed off."

C: "Damn right."

Notice the interviewer's feeling reflection focuses only on what the client had clearly articulated. This is the basic rule when it comes to nondirective feeling reflections: Restate or reflect *only* what you have clearly heard the client say. Do not probe or interpret or speculate. Although we might guess that there were other underlying emotions causing this boy's fury, we do not address these possibilities with a nondirective reflection of feeling.

Feelings are, by their very nature, personal. This means that any attempt at reflecting clients' feelings should be considered a move toward interpersonal closeness or intimacy. Some clients who are not wanting, or not ready, for the intimacy associated with a counseling relationship will react to feeling reflections by becoming more distant and quiet. Others will deny their feelings even if they have clearly and obviously expressed them. You will minimize potential negative reactions to feeling reflections if you begin with nondirective reflections. Nondirective feeling reflections are the least threatening and least intimate of all feeling responses. You are not trying to teach, guide, or direct with this type of response. Similarly, You are not trying to validate clients' emotional experiences (although clients may experience a sense of emotional validation when an interviewer accurately recognizes their emotional state). Nondirective feeling reflections are designed primarily to take note of clients' descriptions of their feelings and no more.

When giving feeling reflections, interviewers should make every effort to be accurate in terms of feeling content and intensity. If you are unsure of what a client is feeling, it may be appropriate to venture forth with a tentatively expressed reflection. Rogers (1951, 1961) would sometimes check with clients after giving a feeling reflection to see if the reflection fit well. As noted above, feelings are personal, and therefore interviewers should not barge into a client's personal world by forcing a particular emotion onto a client. If you have a good relationship with your clients and are tentative in your feeling reflection, your clients may quickly correct you. For example:

> C: "That teacher pissed me off big time when she accused me of stealing her watch . . . I wanted to punch her lights out."
>
> I: "Seems like you were a little irritated about that. Is that right?"
>
> C: "Irritated, hell, I was pissed."

In this example it would be more appropriate to use the stronger emotional descriptor ("pissed"), because the client clearly expressed the fact that he was more than just "irritated." Empathy may be adversely affected because the interviewer failed to reflect the intensity of the client's feeling. On the other hand, the adverse effect may be minimized because the interviewer phrased the reflection in a tentative manner.

Summarization

The purposes of summarization include demonstrating accurate listening, enhancing client and interviewer recall of major themes, helping clients focus on particularly important issues, and extracting or refining the meaning behind client messages.

After listening to a client for twenty or thirty minutes, or even after an entire session, it may be useful to summarize some of what has been discussed. For example:

> I: "You've said quite a lot in these first fifteen minutes, so I thought I should make sure I'm keeping track of your main concerns. You talked about the conflicts between you and your parents, about how

you've felt angry over their neglecting you, and about how it was a relief, but also a big adjustment, to be placed in a foster home. Does that seem to cover the main points of what you've talked about so far?"

C: "Yeah. I think that about covers it."

Although the concept of summarization is simple, the process of coming up with a summary can be difficult. First, we are all only too human and consequently our memories may fail us at times; we may not remember all of the significant issues discussed during a session. Sometimes because of a desire to be thorough and precise in summarizing the content of a session, interviewers bite off more than they can chew. For example:

"Now I would like to summarize the four main issues or concerns you've discussed today. First, you've noted that your childhood was difficult due to the fact that your father was very authoritarian. Second, in your current marriage you find yourself being overly critical of your wife's approaches to rearing your son. Third, you described yourself as controlling and perfectionistic, which you think contributes to some of the ongoing conflict in your marriage. And fourth, uh, fourth, [long pause], uh, I think I forgot what was fourth . . . but I'm sure it will come to me."

Many interviewers who make this type of summarizing mistake are outstanding clinicians, but such a meticulous and comprehensive style is not always necessary or appropriate when summarizing what clients have discussed. And even with a meticulous approach, it is doubtful that an interviewer can catch all of what has been said.

This brings us to the second difficulty in summarizing. Often a session is full of a variety of topics and themes. There may not be a readily apparent underlying pattern that lends itself to summary. This is especially true at the beginning stages of therapy. To provide a concise summary that captures the essence of what was said without being overly redundant and without leaving out a central segment is difficult. Therefore we usually recommend an informal and collaborative approach to summarization. At certain points in a session it is useful to stop and review what has been discussed. But it is not solely the interviewer's responsibility to recall important topics.

There are several advantages to reviewing or summarizing what your clients have said in an informal, interactive, and supportive manner (see Box 5-1). First, doing so takes pressure off you and your memory for details during the interview. Second, it places some responsibility on clients to recall what

BOX 5-1 ━━

Guidelines for Summarizing

We stated in the text that summarizations should be informal, interactive, and supportive. Below we have defined more precisely what we mean by an informal, interactive, and supportive summary.

Informal

- Instead of saying, "Here is my summary of what you've said," you should say something like, "Let me make sure I'm keeping up with the main things you've been talking about."
- Instead of numbering your points, simply state them one by one. That way if you inadvertently forget a point, you won't feel as awkward and uncomfortable as you would if you forgot your fourth point.

Interactive

- As you state the issues you are summarizing, pause so that your client has an opportunity to agree, disagree, or elaborate.
- At the end of a summary, ask the client if what you've said seems accurate.
- In the initial interview, have the client summarize what has been most important to *her*. This way you obtain the client's view first, without tainting it with your opinion on what's been important. You can always add what you thought was important afterward. We find ourselves consistently surprised at what seems important to our clients. If we did not occasionally ask them to summarize, we might never know which issues they believe are important.

Supportive

- In some cases you should openly acknowledge that your client has disclosed a large amount of material. For example: "You've said a lot" or "You've covered quite a bit in a short period of time." These statements are supportive and help clients feel good about what they've produced. Of course, as an interviewer you should remain genuine and make these supportive statements only when they are truthful.
- The manner in which you ask a client for a summary can be supportive. Specifically: "Of course, I'm interested in what *you* feel has been most important out of all you've covered today." Similarly, you might say, "You're the best expert on yourself; how would you summarize the most important things you've talked about today?"

━━━

they think is important. This step will help clients recall what they said in a session and help you to know what they believe is significant. Third, an interactive summarizing approach models a collaborative relationship. In counseling, the counselor is not solely responsible for change or success. Interviewing and counseling are team processes, and allowing clients help decide what is considered important in an interview provides a good demonstration of such teamwork.

TABLE 5-1 Summary of Nondirective Listening Responses and Their Usual Effects

Nondirective Listening Response	Description	Primary Intent / Effect
Attending Behavior	Eye contact, leaning forward, head nods, facial expressions, etc.	Facilitates or inhibits spontaneous client talk
Silence	Absence of verbal activity	Places pressure on clients to talk
Clarification	Attempted restating of a client's message, preceded or followed by a closed question (e.g., "Do I have that right?")	Clarifies unclear client statements and verifies the accuracy of what the interviewer heard
Paraphrase	Reflection or rephrasing of the content of what the client said	Assures clients you hear them accurately and allows them to hear what they said
Sensory-Based Paraphrase	Paraphrase that uses the client's clearly expressed sensory modalities	Enhances rapport and empathy
Nondirective Reflection of Feeling	Restatement or rephrasing of a clearly stated emotion	Enhances clients' experience of empathy and encourages their further emotional expression
Summarization	Brief review of several topics covered during a session	Enhances recall of session content and ties together or integrates themes covered in a session

Interviewer Development Activities

Brief Nondirective Interviews

A good initial assignment for beginning interviewers is the brief nondirective interview. Divide students into groups of three or four. In each group, designate one person as interviewer, another as client, and the others as observers. The interviewer's goal is to conduct a 10-minute minisession using *only* nondirective listening responses. In other words, no questions, no advice, and no directing are permitted. Designated clients are encouraged to talk openly with their interviewers; they should not play the role of a difficult client. Observers take notes on the types of responses used by the interviewer, and if possible, the reactions they appear to produce within the client. After the interview, discussion focuses on the following questions:

1. How did it feel to the interviewer to avoid directive interviewing responses?
2. What kind of responses did the interviewer want to use?
3. What types of responses did the interviewer rely on?
4. Did the interviewer "break the rules" by asking occasional questions or using other directive responses?
5. How did the client feel during the interview (e.g., was any increased sense of responsibility or pressure to talk perceived)?
6. What interaction patterns did the observers notice?

Enhancing Your Feeling Capacity and Vocabulary

There are many approaches to exploring and potentially enhancing your feeling capacity and vocabulary. Carkhuff (1987) and Egan (1985) recommend the following activity.

Identify a basic emotion, such as anger, fear, happiness, or sadness, and then simply begin associating to other feelings you often have in response to that emotion. For instance, state, "When I feel sad . . ." and then finish the thought by associating to another feeling and stating it, for example, "I feel cheated.") An extended example of this process is provided below:

- When I feel joy, I feel fulfilled.
- When I feel fulfilled, I feel content.
- When I feel content, I feel comfortable.
- When I feel comfortable, I feel safe.
- When I feel safe, I feel calm.
- When I feel calm, I feel relaxed.

This feeling association process can help interviewers discover more about their inner emotional lives as well as help them come up with a wide range of feeling words that have meaning for them. We suggest that interviewers conduct this exercise individually, or in dyads, using each of the ten primary emotions identified by Izard (1977):

1. Interest-excitement	6. Disgust
2. Joy	7. Comtempt
3. Surprise	8. Fear
4. Distress	9. Shame
5. Anger	10. Guilt

Silence Desensitization

Most students enjoy playing the client but not the interviewer during the next interviewing activity. The purpose of the activity is to help interviewers adjust to and become more comfortable with silence during an interview. Before beginning, all students should write on cards or small pieces of paper how they think they'll feel and react in response to silent periods during an interview. They also should estimate how long (in seconds) of a silence they think they will be comfortable with. Students should then divide into groups of three or four and designate an interviewer, a client, and one or two observers. The interviewer opens the session with a nondirective statement (e.g., "This is our first interview and so maybe you could just begin by telling me some things about yourself that you think are important for me to know."). The designated client plays the role of a person who is quiet and rather resistant to letting the interviewer know much. Consequently, frequent silences occur. The observers record the length of silences and note who breaks the silence. The interview should last about ten or fifteen minutes.

After the interview, participants discuss how the silence felt to them and the interviewers and clients make estimates regarding the lengths of the longest silent periods. If they report feeling different about the silences than they anticipated feeling, this is explored. Students may feel less uncomfortable than they anticipated because of the artificial nature of this activity. If so, the professor or instructor should help the students identify thoughts they had as they interviewed that decreased their anxiety or discomfort. Perhaps similar thoughts can be used in actual interviews to help manage discomfort with silence. Also, students who are uncomfortable with silence tend to grossly overestimate the length of silent periods. For example, ten to fifteen seconds can feel like thirty seconds or even a full minute.

Generating Sensory-Based and Feeling Words

A simple in-class activity for expanding awareness of sensory-based words can stimulate discussion and class participation. This activity works best with class sizes of between ten and twenty students, although it can be modified for smaller or larger classes.

The instructor identifies one of the three major sensory modalities (i.e., auditory, kinesthetic, or visual). Each student is then asked to come up with one word, experience, or activity that relates primarily to that particular sensory modality. For instance, if "auditory" is chosen, students begin naming words associated with auditory experiences: music, loud, talk, listen, sound, say, and so on. The class is encouraged to generate a list of common (and sometimes not so common) words that might suggest a particular sensory orientation. Students should also be encouraged to discuss their own sensory modality preferences.

A variation of this activity can be used to explore feeling words and expand emotional vocabularies. The instructor simply goes around the room and asks each student to "name a feeling, any feeling." Obviously, larger classes generate larger lists of feeling words. In small classes the instructor may go around the room several times until the class has exhausted itself of feeling words (or until they tire of the activity). Discussion should focus on questions such as: Why do we usually come up with more negative than positive feeling words? How can we compare feeling words in intensity? What interpersonal situations tend to be associated with the different feeling content areas?

Chapter Summary

Much of the time beginning interviewers are unsure as to what they should say during a clinical interview. This occurs despite the fact that many potential nondirective interviewing responses are available to clinical interviewers. Beginning interviewers are more likely than experienced interviewers to speak even when they are unsure of what they should say; experienced interviewers usually have the patience to wait until they can think of something potentially useful to say before speaking. However, even experienced interviewers sometimes feel indecisive about what they should and shouldn't say during interviews. Admitting openly and honestly that one doesn't know what to say is more productive than feigning competence or hiding insecure feelings.

Nondirective interviewing responses generally are designed to facilitate open and free expression by clients, but they may also be used to direct clients to discuss some topics more than others.

Silence is perhaps the most nondirective response available to clinical interviewers. However, because silence can be threatening to clients (and interviewers), the purpose of its use should be discussed with clients in advance. Silence can be used to pull or pressure clients into free associating and thus disclosing information they had not consciously intended to disclose. Silence can also give clients time to reflect, pull things together, and relax with the interviewer.

A restatement or reflection of the content of what a client has said is referred to as a paraphrase. The paraphrase constitutes a cornerstone of effective communication and is used liberally by most clinical interviewers. Used properly, paraphrases are flexible and creative technical responses that enhance rapport and empathy because they communicate to the client that the interviewer is listening closely. Paraphrases can be categorized into generic, sensory, and metaphorical subtypes.

The purpose of a clarification is to make clear to both interviewer and client precisely what has been said. The most basic type of clarification consists of a paraphrase preceded or followed by a closed question. Other forms of clarification include the double question and the simple question directed toward something inaudible or incomprehensible that the client has said. If particular information seems trivial or if an interviewer is waiting to see if a client can notice and clarify his own unclear communication, clarification may be unnecessary.

Nondirective reflection of feeling is a basic restatement of a client's clearly articulated feelings. Effective nondirective feeling reflections enhance empathy and encourage further emotional expression. Because feelings are so personal, caution should be used when reflecting feelings. Good feeling reflections are usually tentatively worded explorations into a client's personal world.

The process of summarization, although conceptually simple, may be difficult to enact. The interviewer may find it hard to recall all that a client has said during a given period of time. Sometimes it may be more useful to let clients summarize, because this can let you know what they believe is important. Summaries are most effective if they are informal, interactive, and supportive.

Three interviewer skill development and personal growth activities are described at the end of this chapter: brief nondirective interviews, an exercise to enhance interviewer feeling capacity and vocabulary, and an activity to help interviewers generate sensory-based and feeling words.

Suggested Readings

Many sources are available to help you explore the issues discussed in this chapter in greater depth. Some of the more useful are briefly described below.

Bandler, R., & Grinder, J. (1979). *Frogs into princes.* Moab, UT: Real People Press. This is one of the early books on NLP. It discusses the concept of representational systems.

Benjamin, A. (1981). *The helping interview* (3rd ed.). Boston: Houghton Mifflin Co. Benjamin provides an excellent discussion of a variety of interviewing responses and leads.

Gibbs, M. A. (1984). The therapist as imposter. In C. M. Brody (Ed.), *Women therapists working with women: New theory and process of feminist therapy.* New York: Springer. This chapter is a strong appeal to therapists to acknowledge their insecurities and inadequacies. Very well written, it provides insights into how experienced professionals can and do feel inadequate.

Hutchins, D. E., & Cole, C. G. (1986). *Helping relationships and strategies.* Monterey, CA: Brooks/Cole. This book has individual chapters that specifically discuss active listening, questions, clarification and reflection, silence, and confrontation.

Meador, B., & Rogers, C. R. (1984). Person-centered therapy. In R. J. Corsini (Ed.), *Current psychotherapies.* Itasca, IL: Peacock. This chapter contains an excerpt of Rogers' classic interview with the "silent young man."

6

DIRECTIVES: LISTENING AND ACTION RESPONSES

Directive Listening Responses
    Interpretive Reflection of Feeling
    Interpretation
    Feeling Validation
    Questions
    Confrontation

Directive Action Responses
    Explanation (Providing Information)
    Suggestion
    Giving Advice
    Agreement-Disagreement
    Urging
    Approval-Disapproval

Chapter Summary

Suggested Readings and Professional Recordings

In more than 700 operations, I rotated, reversed, added, subtracted, and scrambled the brain parts. I shuffled. I reshuffled. I sliced, lengthened, deviated, shortened, opposed, transposed, juxtaposed, and flipped. I sliced front to back with lengths of spinal cord, of medulla, with other pieces of brain turned inside out. But nothing short of dispatching the brain to the slop bucket—nothing expunged feeling.
           —P. PIETSCH, " 'Shuffle Brain' " (as quoted by
           R.D. Laing, 1982, The Voice of Experience)

Sometimes we go too far. In our efforts to "get at" something we become too directive, too analytic, too scientific. We end up dissecting our clients, their feelings, behavior, and thoughts, and the result is usually not what was intended. As the gentleman in the preceding excerpt discovered, no matter how much we treat our clients like objects, they refuse to become inhuman; they continue to feel.

This chapter outlines and discusses directive listening and action responses. These responses are referred to as directives because they place interviewers in the position of director, or choreographer, or expert. Directives may have a positive or a negative effect on clients, depending upon how and when they are used. To be used effectively, they require knowledge of psychopathology, clinical sensitivity, and diagnostic skill; in order to fix something, you must first be able to determine what is wrong.

In a sense, this chapter is out of sequence. The text's next section will focus on assessment interviewing, and throughout this text we emphasize how adequate assessment must precede psychotherapeutic intervention. Why then, do we include a description of responses such as interpretation, confrontation, and advice-giving before we discuss assessment techniques?

In order to conduct assessment interviews, interviewers must know the complete range of responses available to them. Assessment interviewing requires using some directive responses. Also, without knowing the range of responses available, beginning therapeutic interviewers may inadvertently use inappropriate advanced, directive technical responses. The purpose of this chapter is to provide you with *knowledge about* directive responses that can be used in therapeutic interviewing. The goal of the chapter is not to guide you toward mastery of directive psychotherapeutic techniques. Instead, it is designed to whet your appetite by letting you know more about what you will learn if you continue to pursue advanced therapeutic interviewing skills.

Directive Listening Responses

Directive listening responses focus on what clients have said, but also seek to move or direct clients toward a particular type of material (a particular topic or a specific emotional response). They may be primarily client-centered, or they may be primarily interviewer-centered, but they always are used to focus the interview on some aspects of issues in which both client and interviewer have interest. They can be viewed as involving a combination of what client and interviewer want to talk about or see accomplished.

Interpretive Reflection of Feeling
Interpretive feeling reflections are feeling-based statements made by interviewers that go beyond the client's obvious emotional expressions. The goal of interpretive feeling reflection is to uncover emotions within clients of which the clients themselves have only partial awareness. This type of listening response may produce a client insight (i.e., the client becomes aware of some-

thing, usually associated with strong emotion, that was previously unconscious or only partially conscious).

Interpretive feeling reflections have been referred to elsewhere as "advanced empathy" (Egan, 1986, p. 212). Egan states:

> Basic empathy [nondirective reflection of feeling] gets at relevant surface (not to be confused with superficial) feelings and meanings, while advanced accurate empathy [interpretive reflection of feeling] gets at feelings and meanings that are buried, hidden, or beyond the immediate reach of the client. (p. 213)

Consider, again, the example of the fifteen-year-old boy who was so angry with his teacher:

C: "That teacher pissed me off big time when she accused me of stealing her watch. . . . I wanted to punch her lights out."

I: "So you were pretty pissed off." (nondirective feeling reflection)

C: "Damn right."

I: "You know, I also sense you have some other feelings about what your teacher did. Maybe you were hurt because she didn't trust you." (interpretive feeling reflection)

The interviewer's second statement is in pursuit of deeper feelings, feelings that have not been directly articulated by this client. This type of feeling reflection can be very threatening to a client. However, it encourages further exploration of the meaning behind the client's expressed feelings, and when used appropriately, it may enhance client-interviewer rapport and interviewer credibility.

The reason an interpretive reflection of feeling is considered primarily a directive, interviewer-centered response may not be clear. You may also be wondering why such a response is labeled "interpretive" if it is based on the client's report of his personal experience. First, as Egan suggests, the interpretive feeling reflection is based on emotional material that is "buried" or "hidden" from the client (1986, p. 213). When an interviewer takes it upon herself to bring this buried or hidden material to a client's awareness, the interviewer is engaging in a directive or interviewer-centered activity. Second, an interpretive feeling reflection or Egan's "advanced empathy" assumes that unconscious or out-of-awareness processes are influencing the client's functioning. In making such an assumption, the interviewer is imposing a theoretical construct on the client. Third, the goal of an interpretation is to bring previously unconscious material into consciousness (Weiner, 1975). As George and Cristiani (1990) suggest, reflection of feeling can produce this effect: "The classic client-centered technique, reflection of feeling, can be viewed as an interpretation" (p. 162).

Interpretive feeling reflections are powerful techniques that may promote therapeutic breakthroughs or nontherapeutic defensiveness. As psychoanalytically oriented clinicians have emphasized, when it comes to effective interpretations, timing is extremely important (Freud, 1940/1949; Weiner, 1975). That is why in the example above the interviewer initially uses a nondirective feeling reflection and then, only after that reflection has been affirmed, moves to a more probing and interpretive response. Interpretive feeling reflections should be used only after an initial rapport and working alliance have been established, because these responses usually require a good relationship and previous knowledge of the client as a foundation for their effectiveness. In addition, as with nondirective feeling reflections, it is often best to word interpretive feeling reflections tentatively. (See chapter 7 for further discussion of nondirective and interpretive feeling reflections as they relate to empathy).

Interpretation

The goal of an interpretation is insight or increased client self-awareness. Fenichel (1945) states, "Interpretation means helping something unconscious to become conscious by naming it at the moment it is striving to break through." (p. 25). An interpretation is a statement made by an interviewer designed to help the client obtain greater self-understanding or a clearer or more accurate perception of reality (i.e., interpretations are supposed to help clients see themselves and their interpersonal relationships with more reality-based accuracy). When an interviewer provides an interpretation, the interviewer is in essence saying to the client, "This is how I see you and your situation."

Psychoanalytic or "Classical" Interpretations　According to the psychoanalytic tradition, an interpretation is based on the theoretical assumption that unconscious processes influence behavior. Further, it is believed that by pointing out unconscious patterns of feeling, thinking, and behaving, therapists help clients move toward greater self-awareness and higher levels of functioning. This is not to suggest that insight alone produces behavior change. Instead, insight is viewed as a phenomenon that begins moving clients toward more adaptive ways of feeling, thinking, and acting.

There are many forms of classical interpretation, but because it is an advanced skill, we will illustrate the technique only briefly here. Consider, one last time, our angry 15-year-old junior high school student.

> C: "That teacher pissed me off big time when she accused me of stealing her watch. . . . I wanted to punch her lights out."
>
> I: "So you were pretty pissed off." (nondirective feeling reflection)
>
> C: "Damn right."
>
> I: "You know, I also sense you have some other feelings about what your teacher did. Maybe you were hurt because she didn't trust you." (interpretive feeling reflection)

C: (Pauses.) "Yeah, well that's a dumb idea . . . it doesn't hurt anymore
    . . . after a while when no one trusts you, it ain't no big surprise to
    get accused again of something I didn't do."

I: "So when you respond to your teacher's distrust of you with anger,
    it's almost like you're reacting to your parents on those occasions
    they didn't trust you." (interpretation)

In this exchange the boy gives an indirect confirmation of the interpretive
feeling reflection's accuracy. He first demeans the interviewer's reflection and
then confirms it by noting "it doesn't hurt anymore." Notice that within this
phrase the boy gives the interviewer a signal to search for past traumatic
experiences (i.e., the word "anymore" is past-oriented; it is a comparative
reference to the past). This is not surprising. Accurate interpretations often
produce "genetic" material (i.e., material from the past). Thus, the interviewer perceives the client's "signal" and proceeds with a more basic interpretation.

Classical interpretations require knowledge of the client and the client's
past and present relationship experiences. In the example above, the interviewer knows from previous interviews that the boy was harassed and sometimes beaten by his parents despite the fact that he did not engage in the acts
his parents accused him of. The interviewer had the knowledge needed to
make the interpretation after the boy's first statement, but waited and made
the interpretation only after the boy responded positively to the first two
interventions. This illustrates the importance of timing when using interpretations. As Fenichel (1945) states, "The unprepared patient can in no way connect
the words he hears from the analyst with his emotional experiences. Such an
'interpretation' does not interpret at all" (p. 25).

As noted, classical interpretation is an advanced interviewing technique.
Much has been written about the technical aspects of interpretation—what
type of material to interpret, when to interpret it, and how to go about interpre-
ting it (Fenichel, 1945; Greenson, 1967; Weiner, 1975). We recommend that you
consult basic psychoanalytic texts before beginning to use classical interpretations. As with interpretive feeling reflections, poorly timed interpretations
usually produce resistance and defensiveness.

Reframing Other theoretical orientations do not view the effectiveness of
interpretation as based on unconscious processes. Instead, an interpretation
can be seen as an intervention that helps clients view their problems or complaints from another perspective. This approach has been labeled "reframing"
by psychotherapists from both family systems and cognitive orientations
(Borysenko, 1986; de Shazer, 1985; Greenberg & Safran, 1987; Watzlawick,
Weakland, & Fisch, 1974).

Reframing is used primarily when interviewers believe their clients are
viewing the world in an inaccurate or distorted manner. Distorted client perceptions are usually somewhat negative, and therefore interviewers provide an
alternative interpretation or reframing of the situation. Consider the following

exchange between two members of an outpatient group for delinquent youths and their counselor during a group session:

Peggy: "He's always bugging me. He insults me. And I think he's a jerk. I want to make a deal to quit picking on each other, but he won't do it."

Dan: "She's the problem. Always thinks she's right. Never willing to back down or admit there's another way of looking at things. No way am I gonna make a deal with her. She won't change."

C: "I notice you two are sitting next to each other again today."

Peggy: "So. I'd rather not be next to him."

C: "I think you two like each other. You almost always sit next to each other. You're always sparring back and forth. You must really get off on being with one another."

Others: "Wow. That's it. We always thought so."

In this actual case the two teenagers were constantly interacting with one another and labeling it mutual harassment. The interviewer suggested an alternative interpretation or reframing of mutual attraction. Although the two involved parties were unimpressed by the reframe, other group members agreed with it and began to use it in the group session (and beyond).

Effective reframing should be based on a reasonable alternative hypothesis. Reframes may be met initially with denial, but the process of having clients view their interactions or problems in a new way can reduce client anxiety and interpersonal tension by promoting flexibility in perceptions or actions.

Feeling Validation

Reflection of feeling is often confused with feeling validation. Beginning textbooks normally do not distinguish between these two very different responses (Ivey, 1988; Meier, 1989; Okun, 1987). Feeling validation occurs when an interviewer acknowledges and approves of a client's clearly stated feelings. Feeling validation can also be viewed as interpretive; clients are encouraged to look at their feelings from a more accepting and approving perspective.

The purpose of feeling validation is to help clients accept their feelings as a natural and normal part of human experience. Feeling validation can serve as an ego boost; clients feel supported and bolstered and more normal as a function of the interviewer's comments. Sometimes the process of telling clients to accept their feelings results in improved self-esteem. However, this is a controversial issue because directive and supportive techniques such as feeling validation may cause only temporary relief if the client becomes dependent on the interviewer for ego support; feeling validation contains approval and reassurance, both of which can foster dependent relationships.

There are many approaches to feeling validation, but all give clients basically the same message: Your feelings are acceptable and you have permission to feel them. In the following example, the interviewer openly states that it is acceptable for a client to feel a particular emotion:

C: "I've just been so sad since my mother died. I can't seem to stop myself from crying." (client begins to sob)

I: "It's OK for you to be sad. Go ahead and cry if you feel like it."

Notice that the interviewer goes beyond reflection of feeling to validation of feeling. A key point here is that the interviewer is no longer being person-centered or nondirective. By openly stating that feeling sad and crying is "OK" the interviewer has begun to judge the client's feelings and behavior. The interviewer has become an expert who has the power to judge whether or not a client's feelings and behavior are appropriate.

Two other variations to feeling validation are presented below:

C: "I get so anxious before tests you wouldn't believe it! All I can think about is how I'm going to freeze up and forget everything I've learned. Then, when I get in there and look at the test, my mind just goes blank."

I: "You know, I feel the same way about tests sometimes."

C: "I don't understand why I always doubt myself so much. I'm always comparing myself to everyone else . . . and I usually come up short. I wonder if I'll ever really feel a complete sense of confidence."

I: "You're awfully hard on yourself. Almost everyone has self-doubts sometimes. In fact I don't know anyone who feels a complete sense of confidence."

In these examples the interviewers are using authority or expertise to tell the clients that their feelings are normal. In the first example, the interviewer uses self-disclosure to demonstrate that he has felt similar anxiety. Although using self-disclosure to validate feelings can be very reassuring to clients, it is not without risk. In cases like the one above, clients may privately wonder whether counselors who sometimes feel anxiety can help them overcome their own anxiety; counselor credibility can be diminished.

In the second example, the interviewer is trying to convince the client that her feelings are normal by pointing out that everyone feels a sense of self-doubt sometimes. This approach is capitalizing on what Yalom (1985) has referred to as "universality":

Once I reviewed with a patient his 600-hour experience in . . . analysis. . . . When I inquired about his recollection of the most significant event in his therapy, he recalled an incident when he was profoundly distressed about his feelings toward his mother. Despite strong concurrent positive sentiments, he was beset with death wishes for her so that he might inherit a sizable estate. His analyst . . . commented simply, "That seems to be the way we're built." That artless statement offered considerable relief and furthermore enabled the patient to explore his ambivalence in great depth. (p. 8)

Feeling validation is a very common technique in interviewing and counseling. This is partly because people like to have their feelings validated, so feeling validation can greatly enhance rapport. In some cases clients come to therapy primarily because they want to know that it is OK or normal for them to feel a particular way. On the other hand, some therapeutic approaches hold that displays of open support, such as feeling validation, cheat clients from truly developing a positive attitude toward themselves. Below are some of the potential effects of feeling validation:

- Enhances rapport
- May increase or reduce client exploration of the problem or feeling
- Reduces client anxiety, at least temporarily
- Enhances client self-esteem or feelings of normality (again, perhaps only temporarily)
- Increases the likelihood of client-interviewer dependency

Questions

A question, sometimes called a "probe" (Cormier & Cormier, 1991, p. 112; Egan, 1986, p. 110), is a directive interviewer-centered response. Generally, questions are used to obtain information. Some clients like to be asked lots of questions because questions provide clear guidelines regarding what to say, while less directive techniques may produce anxiety because the client is unsure of how to proceed. A secondary function of questions is to provide the interviewer with control over the direction and course of the interview.

Many beginning and advanced interviewers rely heavily on questions to obtain information from clients (Spooner & Stone, 1977). Similarly, many clients rely heavily on the interviewer's questions for structure and guidance regarding what they should talk about. The obvious result is that clients end up talking about what interviewers want them to talk about, but perhaps not what they need or want to talk about. This is only one of many potentially negative side effects of using questions in a therapeutic interview. Egan (1986) describes another: "When clients are asked too many questions, it can interfere with the rapport between helper and client" (p. 112).

The use and abuse of questions by interviewers is covered in detail in chapter 9. For now, you need only be aware that questions are a very directive and interviewer-centered type of response with numerous potential benefits and liabilities. We suggest that beginning interviewers completely eliminate questions from their repertoire during initial practice interviews, partly because beginners tend to overuse questions (Sommers-Flanagan & Means, 1987; recall the activity on brief nondirective interviews in chapter 5).

It is important for interviewers to learn to function without questions and then learn questioning strategies later so that finally they are equipped to use questions when and if they want. Our reservations about questions parallel Benjamin's (1981):

> Yes, I have many reservations about the use of questions in the interview. I feel certain that we ask too many questions, often meaningless ones. We ask questions that confuse the interviewee, that interrupt him. We ask questions the interviewee cannot possibly answer. We even ask questions we don't want the answers to, and consequently, we do not hear the answers when forthcoming. (p. 71)

Confrontation

The goal of a confrontation is to help clients perceive and deal with reality more effectively. Clients often come to clinicians with distorted views of others, the world, and themselves. These distortions usually manifest themselves as incongruities or discrepancies. For example, clients often display discrepancies between what they say and how they appear to be feeling. Imagine a client with clenched fists and a harsh, angry voice saying, "I wish you wouldn't bring up my ex-wife, I've told you before that's over. I don't have any feelings toward her, it's water under the bridge." Obviously such a client still has strong feelings about his ex-wife. Perhaps the relationship is over and the client wishes he could put it behind him, but his nonverbal behavior clues the interviewer in to the existence of underlying emotions.

Confrontations are most effective when the interviewer has a solid relationship with the client and ample evidence to demonstrate the incongruity or discrepancy. In the preceding example we would not recommend using a confrontation unless the client had provided earlier concrete examples indicating unresolved feelings about his ex-wife. If such examples had been provided by the client, a confrontation such as the following might be tried:

> I: "You mentioned before that every time you think of her and how the relationship ended, you want to somehow get back at her. And now you say you don't have any feelings about her. But judging by your clenched fists, voice tone, and previous descriptions of how you felt she 'screwed you over,' it seems pretty clear that you still have very strong feelings about her. Perhaps you wish those feelings would go away, but it sure looks like they're still there!"

Notice how the interviewer cites evidence to support the confrontation. The interviewer has decided that the client would be better off admitting to and dealing with his unresolved feelings toward his ex-wife. In order to achieve that end, the confrontation must be supported by convincing evidence.

As with most techniques, there are a variety of ways to implement a confrontation. Confrontations can be gentle and almost imperceptible. Take for example the case of a young, newly married man who, after thirty-five minutes in his psychotherapy session, has not made a single reference to his wife, who left two days earlier for an extended stay on the other side of the continent. The young man is in the midst of working on his doctoral dissertation and mentioned to his therapist in their last session that his wife was to be leaving during the next week. A psychoanalytically oriented therapist's response might be gently confrontational: "I noticed you haven't mentioned your wife's leaving all hour."

In this case the therapist is actually using a reflection of content (or lack of content) to gently confront the young man's avoidance of discussing his wife. Certainly his wife's absence produces some feelings in the young man, and the therapist's goal is to get him to acknowledge these feelings and explore their effect on his life.

In some cases, particularly with individuals addicted to substances, confrontations must be not only convincing but also firm and repetitive—and sometimes even harsh. This is because addicted persons usually use denial, rationalization, and minimization to justify their use of substances. These defenses must be broken down in order to attain the goal of confrontation: getting the client to perceive reality more clearly and consequently deal with it more effectively. For example:

> C: "Doc, it's not a problem. I drink when I want to, but it doesn't have a big effect on the rest of my life. I like to party. . . . I like to put a few down on the weekends, doesn't everybody?"

> I: (looking straight into the eyes of the client) "You've had two DUIs [tickets for driving under the influence], three different jobs, and at least a half dozen fist fights over the past year. Sounds to me like you've got a major problem with alcohol. If you don't start admitting to it and doing something about it, you're going to continue to have legal trouble, job trouble, and relationship trouble. Now tell me again you think that's no problem!"

This is only a moderately firm confrontation. They can be stronger. Unfortunately, many people incorrectly believe that all confrontations must be harsh and aggressive. It is more therapeutic and more sensible to begin with gentle confrontations and become firmer and more aggressive as needed. As we often tell our assertiveness-training classes, there will be plenty of time to get obnoxious and aggressive later; begin by being gentle and assertive.

A final example of an incongruity worthy of confrontation involves a 42-year-old bisexual man who is describing how he has recently established a sexual relationship with a very attractive and much younger (23-year-old) schizophrenic man. The client's statement is followed by three potential interviewer responses, each progressively more confrontive:

C: "Yes, I recently got involved in a sexual relationship with a younger man. He's chronically mentally ill . . . schizophrenic. I'm expressing unconditional love. I don't think there's anything wrong with that. Do you?"

I-1:   "Simply the fact that you ask me if I think there's anything wrong with your relationship suggests that you're not completely resolved or comfortable with it."

I-2:   "Seems like you might be taking advantage of someone who is not totally capable of making reasonable and independent choices about his sexual behavior. I wonder what that says about your level of security in initiating sexual relationships?"

I-3:   "You call that unconditional love? That sounds like a situation where you're using someone much younger and much less mentally capable than you to fulfill your sexual needs. I suggest you re-evaluate this relationship and take a look at what it says about you. Why can't you initiate a relationship with someone nearer to you in terms of age and mental stability?"

A confrontation's effectiveness may be evaluated by examining your client's subsequent response (Ivey, 1988). For example, a client may blatantly deny the accuracy of your confrontation, partially accept it, or completely accept its accuracy and significance.

True confrontation does not contain an explicit prescription for change. Instead, the confrontation itself implies that change is needed; it implies that the client had best examine this incongruity and perhaps do something about it. Confrontation is the most extreme form of directive listening response; it implies that action is necessary, but does not prescribe it. In the next section we review technical responses that explicitly suggest or prescribe action.

Directive Action Responses

Directive action responses by therapeutic interviewers encourage clients to change the way they think, feel, or act. They are essentially persuasive techniques, pushing clients toward specific changes. Directives are usually used when interviewers believe, based on clinical judgment, that clients should change something about their life, attitudes, or behavior. Such responses are obviously interviewer-centered and involve the interviewer taking some responsibility in determining what type of changes might be desirable. This is somewhat true even in cases when interviewer and client are working together in a very collaborative manner, because even then the interviewer must decide when to offer an explanation or suggest, advise, or urge the client to take a particular action. Of course the client determines whether or not to listen and apply the interviewer's opinion, suggestion, or advice.

TABLE 6-1 Summary of Directive Listening Responses and Their Usual Effects

Directive Listening Response	Description	Primary Intent / Effect
Interpretive Reflection of Feeling	Statement indicating what feelings the interviewer believes are underlying the client's thoughts or actions	May enhance empathy and encourage emotional exploration and insight
Interpretation	Statement indicating what meaning the interviewer believes a client's emotions, thoughts, or actions represent. Often includes references to past experiences	Encourages reflection and self-observation of clients' emotions, thoughts and acitons. Promotes client insight
Question	Query. Words that directly elicit information from a client. There are many forms of questions.	Elicits information. Enhances interviewer control. May help clients talk or encourage them to reflect on something
Feeling Validation	Statement that supports, affirms, approves of, or validates feelings articulated by clients	Enhances rapport. Temporarily reduces anxiety. May cause the interviewer to be viewed as an expert
Confrontation	Statement that points out or identifies a client incongruity or discrepancy. Ranges from very gentle to very harsh	Encourages clients to examine themselves and their patterns of thinking, feeling, and behaving. May result in personal change and development

Directive action responses should be used primarily by advanced interviewers, because interviewers should be able to first evaluate *how* a client might make positive changes before employing a tactic designed to produce change. Many textbooks and graduate programs in counseling and psychology encourage the application of techniques or directives that foster client change (Cormier & Cormier, 1991; Egan, 1986; George & Cristiani, 1990; Hutchins & Cole, 1986; Ivey, 1988; Okun, 1987). While it is true that directive techniques are effective methods of producing client change, our position is similar to Seligman's (1990), interviewers should be well trained in evaluation and assessment techniques prior to applying technical interventions. Consequently, the following descriptions of directive action responses are provided primarily to help you differentiate between these types of responses and other less directive techniques.

The directive action responses described in this section are organized in order of intensity, from milder to stronger persuasive techniques. Milder persuasive techniques, such as some forms of explanation and suggestion, can be used effectively by both beginning and advanced interviewers. More powerful and potentially harmful persuasive techniques (e.g., disagreement, urging, and moralizing), can be inadvertently misused by less experienced interviewers.

Explanation (Providing Information)

An explanation is a descriptive statement that seeks to make something plain or understandable. With respect to interviewing, an explanation usually describes:

- The process of counseling
- The implications of a particular symptom
- The implementation of a specific piece of advice or therapeutic strategy

Often client questions are signals indicating that clients need an explanation because there is something they don't completely understand. Client questions often fall into the following three categories:

- How long will it take for me to feel better?
- Am I crazy?
- How do I change?

In our view, the most constructive use of explanation is in the service of role induction. Role induction consists of the interviewer explaining the process of interviewing or counseling to the client. Clients come to their initial sessions with little or no information about what a therapeutic interview entails. A significant body of research on role induction has indicated, not surprisingly, that role induction enhances the effectiveness of counseling and psychotherapy (Luborsky, 1984; Mayerson, 1984; Orlinsky & Howard, 1978).

Interviewing should not be a mysterious process, and almost all clinical practitioners periodically stop and explain a little bit about core concepts of the counseling process to their clients. Imagine that you, as an interviewer, have a client tell you at the beginning of the second session about her strong emotional reactions to the initial interview experience:

> C: "I'm not sure if I should tell you this, but after our session last Monday, I had these very strong negative feelings. Now this has nothing to do with you, but I just was thinking, 'Oh God, none of the things I talked with you about will ever change.' It isn't you ... don't take it personally, I like you."

This client statement provides an interviewer with several explanation issues to address. First, when clients begin their statements with "I don't know if I should talk about this" or "I'm not sure what I'm supposed to say" it is often a signal that some explanation is needed. If clients are confused or uncertain about the counseling process, it is the interviewer's job to provide information to reduce confusion.

Second, when clients are in doubt about whether to talk about a particular issue, they should be encouraged to discuss it so that the interviewer and client can decide together whether or not the material is of significance. Discussing issues together helps enhance the collaborative relationship.

Third, although the client is suggesting otherwise, her feelings may well have to do with the interviewer. It is important for clients to know they may occasionally have strong feelings toward therapy or toward the interviewer. These may be initial signs of transference and should not be ignored (neither should they be interpreted, but simply noted or explored).

Fourth, often clients initially feel worse before feeling better when coming for counseling. Consequently, explaining to clients that they may feel worse, hopeless, mixed up, or angry at having to confront their problems helps keep them in therapy when they might otherwise drop out due to negative feelings.

The following interviewer responses are appropriate explanations that might be used in response to clients who have reported strong negative feelings toward their interviewer:

- "If you're not sure whether you want to talk about something in here with me, it is a good idea to at least describe your feelings or describe the issue. Then we can decide together whether or not to spend time discussing it further."
- "Sometimes people develop strong feelings about their counselors or about counseling while they're going through it. Usually these feelings are important to talk about."
- "You know, it isn't all that unusual to have some negative feelings during the counseling process. Many people seem to feel worse before they feel better. I guess that's just part of what people experience when they begin facing their problems head on."

A second type of explanation is warranted when a client is experiencing a symptom but is puzzled about what the symptom means. Frequently when clients are experiencing symptoms, they lack a clear understanding of what their symptoms mean. Clients with anxiety disorders often report they believe they're "going crazy" or "losing their mind" or "dying" (Barlow & Cerny, 1988). They start to think and eventually believe that they have a psychotic disorder and that they will undoubtedly end up institutionalized. In reality, the prognosis for most anxiety disorders is fairly optimistic and this should be explained to the client.

"I know you're feeling like there must be something wrong with your mind, because the symptoms you have can be very frightening, but based on your personal history, family history, and the symptoms you've told me about, I think it's very safe to tell you that you're not going crazy, that the problems you're experiencing are not unusual, and that they respond very well to treatment."

Clients usually find such explanations very reassuring. For example, a young client whom author John Sommers-Flanagan once saw on an emergency basis had a fear that he'd "snap" and end up like a "zombie" sitting in a corner. Based on the information obtained from him in the interview, John judged the odds of such an event occurring to be extremely low. Therefore, although he did not downplay the very real and distressing nature of his symptoms, John simply reassured the client that his symptoms were not unusual and often responded well to counseling. The young man's sigh of relief was audible. Explanation can be particularly useful with clients who are highly distressed or experiencing an emotional crisis.

The third type of explanation involves giving a client information in order to facilitate the application of a particular therapeutic technique. Of course, this type of explanation should be used only after an assessment has been made to determine what type of therapeutic approach is most appropriate. An example of an explanation focusing on educating a client in the use of a specific cognitive-behavioral therapeutic technique is provided below:

C: "I don't know what causes my anxiety. . . . It just seems to come out of nowhere. Is there anything I can do to get in more control of these feelings?"

I: "The first step to controlling anxiety usually involves identifying the thoughts or situations that cause you to feel anxious. I'd like you to give the following experiment a try. Keep a log of your anxiety level. Maybe you could buy one of those pocket-sized notebooks to carry around and record times when you feel anxious. You should write down how anxious you feel on a scale of 0 to 100, 0 being not anxious at all and 100 being so anxious you think you're going to die. Then, right next to your anxiety rating, list the specific thoughts you're thinking and situation you're in. If you bring your anxiety log to the next session, maybe we can begin to figure out what's causing all this anxiety you're experiencing."

This is an example of the type of instruction or explanation a cognitive-behavioral therapist might give a client to initiate self-monitoring of anxiety. As you can see, giving information about the application of a specific therapeutic technique can become lengthy and involved. The interviewer becomes much more of an expert or dominant force within the session. In the preceding example it is likely that the client will ask questions about the self-monitoring technique in order to obtain additional information pertaining to its application.

The type of explanation an interviewer chooses to give is dictated, in part, by the interviewer's theoretical orientation. Specifically, behavioral therapists will explain to their clients the importance of behavior and self-monitoring; cognitive therapists will explain how thoughts influence or cause behavior and emotions; person-centered therapists will explain how sessions should consist of whatever they feel is important; and psychoanalytic therapists will explain to their clients the importance of "saying whatever comes to mind." Whether interviewers are describing free association or discussing benefits of guided imagery, they are still utilizing the same general interviewing response: explanation.

Suggestion

Suggestion is usually not discussed in introductory interviewing and counseling texts (Cormier & Cormier, 1991; Hutchins & Cole, 1986; Moursund, 1990). This may be because suggestion is traditionally associated with psychoanalytic or hypnotic approaches (Erickson, Rossi, & Rossi, 1976; Kihlstrom, 1985). It also may be because some authorities define suggestion as "a mild form of advice" and therefore discuss it in the context of advice giving (Benjamin, 1981, p. 134).

In our view, suggestion and advice are two distinct interviewer responses. Unfortunately, suggestion and advice are often considered interchangeable for at least two reasons. First, they are often used together. Second, the word suggest is often used when the speaker really means *advise*—for example, "I'm going to suggest that Bill ask Mary out on a date." What the speaker probably means is that she is going to *advise* Bill to ask Mary out on a date (although she could also use suggestion to try to accomplish the same goal). Keep in mind that to suggest is to "insinuate, imply, or hint indirectly" while to advise is "to give recommendation or counsel" (Webster's Ninth New Collegiate Dictionary, 1985).

A suggestion is an interviewer statement directly or indirectly suggesting or predicting a particular phenomenon will occur in a client's life. The purpose of using suggestion is to move clients consciously or unconsciously toward engaging in a particular behavior, changing their thinking patterns, or experiencing a specific emotion.

Although suggestions are often given when clients are in a hypnotic trance, they may also be given when clients are fully alert and awake. Take, for example, the following interviewer-client interaction:

> C: "I have never been able to stand up to my mother. It's like I'm afraid of her. She's always had her act together. . . . She's stronger than I am."

> I: "If you look closely at your interactions with her this next week, I think you'll discover ways in which you're stronger than her."

Perhaps a more classic example of suggestion is when the interviewer suggests that client will have a dream about a particular issue. This example is classic in the sense that psychoanalytically oriented interviewers have often directed suggestions toward what they believe to be unconscious processes:

C: "This decision is really getting to me. I have these two job offers but I don't know which one to take. I feel frozen. I've analyzed the pros and cons for days and I just swing back and forth. One minute I think I want one job and the next minute I'm thinking of all the reasons that job is totally wrong for me."

I: "If you relax and think about the conflict as clearly as possible in your mind before you drop off to sleep tonight, perhaps you'll have a dream that might help clarify your feelings about this decision."

In this example, suggestion is mixed with advice. The interviewer is advising the client to relax and clearly think about the conflict before falling asleep and suggesting that a dream will subsequently occur.

One last word of caution when using suggestion: Suggestion can be viewed as sneaky or manipulative. From a psychoanalytic perspective, it is based on the belief that unconscious processes influence us in our waking lives (Haley, 1973; Watkins, 1989). Thus, one potential response that it can evoke in clients is opposition. All of the suggestions used in examples from this section could backfire, producing the following results:

- Bill will oppose his friend's suggestion by refusing to ask Mary out on a date.
- The woman will continue not to see ways in which she is stronger than her mother and may continue to insist that her mother is stronger.
- The client will not recall his dreams or will not be able to make any connections between his dreams and his decision-making process. (This result might be viewed as resistance by psychoanalytically oriented therapists.)

Giving Advice

Giving advice involves telling clients what they should do. Advice essentially consists of a statement designed to communicate the message, "Here's what I think you should do." Giving advice is very much interviewer-centered; it clearly casts interviewers in the role of expert.

It is important to avoid giving advice in early stages of interviewing. Giving advice is easy, and as the old saying goes, advice is cheap. If simple advice is all a client needs, it should be surprising that the client did not already receive it before coming for counseling. Usually friends and relatives freely give advice to one another, sometimes effectively, other times less so. You may wonder, if advice is so available to people outside of therapy, why would it ever be used by an interviewer?

The answer to this question is fairly simple: sometimes advice works, and that's why some interviewers choose to use it as a change technique (Haley, 1973). Nonetheless, advice remains a controversial issue in therapeutic interviewing; many interviewers use it, but many others avoid it with a passion (Benjamin, 1981; Rogers, 1957).

As you might guess, our advice is for you to become aware of when and why you feel the need to give advice to a client. Although we are not strong advocates of giving advice, we are less concerned with whether interviewers give advice than we are with when and why they give it and how they go about doing so.

In many cases clients try to pull ideas or advice from their interviewers during their first session. However, premature problem solving or advice giving in a therapeutic interview is usually ineffective (Egan, 1986; Meier, 1989). Interviewers should seek to thoroughly explore a specific issue with a client before trying to solve the problem or render advice. A good basic rule is to find out everything the client has tried in an effort to resolve the problem before jumping in with prescriptive advice.

Sometimes restraining yourself from giving advice can be difficult. Imagine yourself with a client who tells you, "I'm pregnant and I don't know what to do. I just found out two days ago. No one else knows. Well . . . I guess now you know too." You may have some good advice for this young woman. In fact, you may have gone through a similar experience or known someone close to you who struggled with what to do about an unplanned pregnancy. The woman in this scenario may also desperately need information from you and she may even need some constructive advice. However, all this is speculation, because based on what she has said, we don't know whether or not she needs information or advice. All we know is that she's stated she "doesn't know what to do." We can be assured that if she discovered she was pregnant two days ago that she's probably spent nearly forty-eight hours thinking about the options available to her. At this point to tell her what we think she should do would be ineffective and inappropriate.

Giving premature advice tends to shut down further problem exploration and exploration of potential alternative solutions. We recommend starting off nondirectively: "So this is pretty new news for you, and you haven't told anyone yet, except me. And if I understand you correctly, you're feeling maybe you should be taking some particular action, but you're not sure what."

As we noted above, clients may also push you for advice: "What do you think I should do?" In many cases, an explanation and an open-ended question should be used when you are feeling pressure from the client to provide advice. For example: "Before we talk about possible options or actions, it's best for us to explore what you've been thinking and feeling about your situation. What kinds of things have you thought about and felt since discovering you're pregnant?" Or, in this case, simply an open-ended question might be appropriate: "What kinds of alternatives have you thought of on your own?"

Clients are typically more complex, thoughtful, and full of constructive ideas than we give them credit for, or than they give themselves credit for. Therefore it is an injustice to them to provide specific advice before you have explored all the ways in which they've tried to solve their own problems. In addition, providing advice that others have previously provided, or that the client has already tried, can damage your credibility. We've made a practice of routinely asking clients about advice they've already received from friends, family, and past counselors.

Agreement-Disagreement

Perhaps one of the most common directive action responses used by beginning interviewers is agreement. Agreement occurs when an interviewer makes a statement indicating he is in harmony with the client's opinion. Agreement is usually rewarding to both interviewer and client, partly because, as studies from social and clinical psychology have shown, people like to be in the presence of others similar to themselves (Hatfield & Walster, 1981; Kurdek & Smith, 1987; Yalom, 1985).

As with advice giving, if you find yourself wanting to agree with your clients, explore your motives for doing so. Why do you want clients to know that you agree with them? Is the expression of agreement a therapeutic response, or are you agreeing simply because it feels good to let someone else know your opinions are similar? If you are agreeing with your clients in an effort to affirm their viewpoint, are there any other ways you can help affirm their viewpoint?

Using agreement has several potential effects. First, agreement tends to enhance rapport. Second, if your clients view you as a credible authority, agreement can serve to affirm the correctness of their opinion (i.e., "if my therapist agrees with me, then I must be right"). Third, agreement will put you in the role of expert, and your opinion, agreement or disagreement, will be sought in the future. Fourth, agreement tends to reduce client exploration (i.e., "why explore my feelings or belief any longer; after all, my therapist agrees with me").

Wherever there is agreement, there is also the possibility of disagreement. If you are viewed as someone who can agree with your client, you will also be viewed as someone who can potentially disagree. It is simple, rewarding, and somewhat natural to openly express yourself when you are in agreement with someone else. On the other hand, disagreement is often seen as socially unacceptable or at least socially undesirable. People sometimes muffle their disagreement, because to disagree is to promote conflict and tension between two individuals. Many people avoid disagreeing with others in social situations because they are unassertive; they fear the other person will have a stronger argument or they fear rejection. In a therapeutic interview, however, interviewers are in a position of power and authority. Consequently, interviewers sometimes lose their inhibition and disagree openly with clients. Depending upon the issue, the result can be devastating to clients and may approach abuse of the interviewer role.

Disagreement may also be subtle. Sometimes clients may interpret silence, lack of head nods, or lack of open agreement as a sign of disagreement. Although some clients may mistakenly interpret their interviewer's lack of agreement as a sign of disagreement, others may accurately interpret subtle interviewer behaviors as indicative of disagreement. It is important for interviewers to examine themselves to determine if they are communicating disagreement (or disapproval) in a subtle way.

The purpose of disagreement is to change client opinion. The problem with disagreement is that countering one opinion with another opinion usually deteriorates into a personal argument, resulting in increased defensiveness on the parts of both interviewer and client. Therefore, interviewers should not use disagreement. The cost is too high, and the potential benefit can be achieved through other means. Two basic guidelines apply when you feel impelled to use disagreement:

- If you have a different opinion than a client regarding a philosophical issue (e.g., abortion, mixed-race marriage, sexual practices, etc.), remember that it is not your job to change the client's opinion; disagreement is inappropriate.
- If your professional judgment indicates that the client's belief or opinion is maladaptive (e.g., is causing stress, is ineffective, etc.), then you may want to provide the client with better information. In such a case, you would employ the technique of explanation or providing information rather than disagreement.

A good example of when an interviewer should employ explanation instead of disagreement is in the area of child rearing. Clients often report using ineffective child-rearing techniques, but support such techniques by citing their opinion or experience. Interviewers should avoid bluntly rushing in and telling clients they are "wrong," that is, using disagreement. Rather, interviewers should help clients examine the effectiveness of their technique by asking, for example, whether the client is accomplishing what she wants by her particular method of discipline or whether that method produces some significantly deleterious side effects:

C: "I know some people say that spanking children isn't alright. Well, I was spanked when I was young and I turned out just fine."

I: "Even though you weren't adversely effected by being spanked, there are some children who are. Sometimes spanking is simply not the most effective method of accomplishing what you want. Let's talk about what you're trying to accomplish by spanking your daughter. Maybe there are more efficient methods through which you can accomplish your goal."

In this case there is empirical evidence indicating that the behavior discussed (spanking or physical punishment) may produce a number of undesirable consequences (Dodson, 1987). Both the American Psychological Association and the American Medical Association oppose physical punishment of children (Strong & Devault, 1989). Therefore, it is the interviewer's professional responsibility to inform clients of physical punishment's undesirable consequences as well as other discipline alternatives.

Urging

Urging is a step beyond advice giving. It involves pressuring or pleading with a client to take a specific action. When an interviewer chooses to urge a client to take a specific action, the interviewer has completely taken on the role of expert or director.

Urging is not a particularly common interviewing technique, but there are situations when its use is appropriate. These situations primarily involve some type of crisis: when the client is in danger or dangerous. For example, in cases involving battered women, often the woman needs to be urged to take her children and move to a battered women's shelter for safety. Similarly, in cases of child abuse, if you are interviewing the abuser, you may urge him to report himself to the local agency responsible for protecting children.

Author John can recall only one noncrisis situation when he used urging as a therapeutic technique. A 20 year-old male client was suffering from obsessive-compulsive disorder. His family situation was clearly affecting his condition in a negative way, and he came to therapy one day outlining a plan to move away from his parents:

> C: "My plan is to move into the college dorms next fall [in six months]."
> I: "Why wait?"

The interviewer's response was brief and simple. "Why wait?" was designed to urge him to consider *why* he was putting off the move when, in reality, there were no good reasons to not move earlier. In essence, the interviewer was urging him to reconsider his decision. The choice of this particular change-oriented intervention was also based on empirical data that indicates encouraging (and helping) obsessive-compulsive clients confront their anxieties is a productive approach (McCarthy & Foa, 1990).

Approval-Disapproval

Approval refers to an interviewer's sanction of clients' thoughts, feelings, or behavior. To give one's approval is to render a favorable judgment. To use approval and disapproval as interviewing responses, interviewers must have the knowledge, expertise, and sensitivity to render judgments on their clients' ideas and behavior. Approval and disapproval are sometimes avoided (or utilized) because of the vast power they place in the interviewer's hands. Obviously, such power can be abused by interviewers. Most interviewers would rather that clients judge, accept, and approve of their own thoughts, feelings, and behavior rather than rely on someone else's evaluation of themselves.

As you may have noticed, the concept of approval-disapproval is similar to agreement-disagreement. An interviewer's inclination to agree or disagree with a client, however, generally comes from the desire to be in social harmony; approving or disapproving is a step further in that the interviewer is taking on a greater degree of authority. That is, approval may involve the interviewer communicating that she not only agrees with a client's belief, attitude, feelings, or behavior, but also approves of the client as a person.

Many clients come to therapeutic interviewers in order to seek approval. In this regard clients are vulnerable; they need or want a professional interviewer's stamp of approval. As interviewers we must ask ourselves

TABLE 6-2 Summary of Directive Action Responses and Their Usual Effects

Directive Action Response	Description	Primary Intent / Effect
Explanation	Statement providing factual information usually about the interview process, client problem, or implementation of a treatment strategy	Clarifies client misconceptions. Helps clients attain maximal benefit from counseling
Suggestion	Interviewer statement that directly or indirectly suggests or predicts that a particular phenomenon will occur	May help clients consciously or unconsciously move toward engaging in a particular behavior, thinking a specific thought, or experiencing a particular emotion
Advice	Recommendation given to the client by the interviewer. A prescription to act, think, or feel in a specific manner	Provides the client with ideas regarding new ways to act, think, or feel. If given prematurely, can be ineffective and can damage interviewer credibility
Agreement-Disagreement	Statement indicating harmony or disharmony of opinion	Agreement may affirm or reassure a client, enhance rapport, or shut down exploration of thoughts and feelings. Disagreement can produce conflict and stimulate arguments or defensiveness
Urging	Technique of pressuring or pleading with a client to engage in specific actions or to consider specific issues	May produce the desired change or may backfire and stimulate resistance. May be considered offensive by some clients
Approval-Disapproval	Favorable or unfavorable judgment of the thoughts feelings, or behavior of a client	Approval may enhance rapport and foster client dependency. Disapproval may reduce rapport and produce client feelings of rejection

BOX 6-1 ━━

Interviewer Response Analysis

Now that you are familiar with the majority of technical responses available to therapeutic interviewers, it is useful to review the initial interviewing video- or audio-tape that we suggested you produce at the end of chapter 4. As you review the ten- or fifteen-minute interview, stop the tape after each of your verbal responses and try to categorize it as one of the technical responses discussed in chapters 5 and 6. In this manner you can accomplish two important objectives. First, you will become more familiar with your own basic response tendencies. For example, you may discover you have a tendency to agree with clients, question clients, or primarily rely upon feeling reflections. Second, by analyzing your own taped interviews (or interviews conducted by others), you become more familiar and knowledgeable of responses utilized by various interviewers. In fact, we recommend that you take time to listen to other professionally taped recordings of interviews. Your instructor or campus media service may have professional recordings available for you to review.

━━━

whether we should accept the responsibility, power, and control that needy and vulnerable clients try to give us. In some ways choosing to bestow approval or disapproval on clients is similar to playing God. Who are we to decide which feelings, thoughts, or behaviors are good or bad?

Clients who seek their interviewer's approval may be feeling temporarily insecure or suffering from longstanding needs for approval. Such needs for approval may stem from feelings of being unaccepted and not approved of as a child. As a consequence, giving or awarding approval can be a powerful therapeutic technique. Interviewer approval can enhance rapport and increase client self-esteem. It also tends to foster dependent relationships. When a client's search for approval is rewarded, the client is likely to resume the search for approval when or if the insecure feelings begin again.

In some cases it is difficult for interviewers to avoid feeling disapproval toward some clients. Not only is it difficult to maintain a sense of professional neutrality when your client is talking about child abuse, wife battering, rape, murderous thoughts and impulses, deviant sexual practices, and so on, but it is also difficult to restrain your personal and moral abhorrence for such behavior. Keep in mind the following facts:

- Clients who engage in deviant or abusive behavior have been disapproved of before, usually by people who mean very much to them and sometimes by an entire society. Nonetheless, they have not stopped engaging in deviant or abusive behavior. This suggests that disapproval is ineffective.
- Your disapproval will only alienate you from someone who desperately needs to change.
- By maintaining a sense of objectivity and neutrality, you are not implicitly approving of your client's behavior. There are other responses besides disapproval (e.g., explanation and confrontation) that will show the client you believe change is needed.

- If you cannot accept the client's behavior well enough to allow you to continue with your professional duties, you should refer the client to another qualified professional.
- Obviously, disapproval is associated with reduced rapport, client feelings of rejection, and premature termination of counseling.

Approval and disapproval can be communicated subtly to your clients. For example, responding with the words "OK" or "right" can be interpreted by clients as approval when you may simply be using these words as a means of verbal tracking. When engaging in specific interviewing assignments, pay close attention to your verbal and nonverbal behavior so you can determine whether or not subtle messages of approval or disapproval are being communicated.

There are other categories of interviewer responses that are not discussed here. Some, such as scolding and rejection, are even more interviewer-centered than approval and disapproval (see Benjamin, 1981). Others, such as humor and self-disclosure, are difficult to place along a continuum of interviewer responses or are discussed elsewhere in this text.

Chapter Summary

Directive interviewer responses are defined as responses that not only focus on what clients have said, but also bring into the session the therapeutic interviewer's perspective. Interviewers can be too directive, leaving clients feeling like they've been analyzed or dissected. They also can be too nondirective, leaving clients feeling lost and sensing that the interviewer is evasive or manipulative. Generally, directive interview responses are advanced techniques that encourage clients to change their thinking, feeling, or behavior patterns. Therefore, most directives should be used only after adequate clinical assessment has occurred.

Interpretive feeling reflections are designed to encourage clients to uncover and explore their feelings—personal feelings that clients may have been only partially aware of before. As with less directive feeling reflections, interpretive feeling reflections can be threatening or too personal for clients to tolerate. Therefore, such reflections are utilized most effectively after an initial rapport and collaborative relationship have been established.

Interpretation is an advanced therapeutic intervention designed to bring unconscious conflicts to awareness. When used appropriately, interpretation is a powerful technique that often results in the client experiencing an emotional insight. When used inappropriately, interpretation usually results in increased client defensiveness. Timing is a very important factor associated with effective interpretations.

Beginning interviewers often rely heavily on questions to obtain information from their clients. Although questions can be effective in eliciting information, they are less useful in establishing rapport and have other potentially negative side effects. Questions are discussed in greater detail in chapter 9.

Feeling validation is a supportive interviewer response that can help clients feel accepted and understood. Unfortunately, feeling validations also tend to foster dependency and may reduce client exploration of personal issues or problems. Interviewers should be able to discriminate between feeling reflection and feeling validation so that they can use feeling validations intentionally rather than inadvertently.

Confrontations range from gentle to firm or harsh and are used when interviewers want their clients to take a hard look at a personal discrepancy or inconsistency. Confrontations imply that clients should examine their discrepancies, but they do not prescribe specific changes. The effect or impact of confrontations can be determined by observing whether or not clients respond to them by examining the meaning of their personal inconsistencies. If clients deny the existence of the inconsistency pointed out by an interviewer, then the confrontation has been ineffective.

Directive action responses are designed to make it more likely for a client to think, feel, or behave in a particular manner. Directive action responses are used only when interviewers believe it would be therapeutic for a particular client to think, feel, or behave in a particular manner. Consequently, this type of interviewer response should be used primarily by experienced counselors after adequate client assessment has been conducted. Sometimes action responses are used as a part of client evaluation.

Interviewers use explanation to provide information to their clients, usually about one of three topics. First, interviewers should explain interviewing and counseling processes. This type of explanation has been referred to as role induction, and research indicates it enhances the interview process and outcome. Second, sometimes clients do not completely understand their symptoms and need a knowledgeable professional to provide an explanation. This type of explanation can be very reassuring (or threatening) to clients. Third, helping interviewers sometimes advocate specific change strategies that must be explained to clients. Explanations are useful tools, but care should be taken in their application because they take away from client talk time.

Suggestion is a therapeutic technique generally associated with psychoanalytic and hypnotic approaches to psychotherapy. Nonetheless, interviewers can subtly or directly suggest to clients that they will engage in a specific behavior or have a particular experience. Suggestions are sometimes viewed as sneaky or manipulative by clients and consequently resisted. Suggestions should be distinguished from advice, as they are less directive *and* less direct.

Some interviewers strictly avoid the giving of advice because they believe it is inappropriate or ineffective. Other interviewers are more liberal in their advice giving. For your advice to be maximally effective, it is important that you first have rapport and a collaborative relationship with your client. It is also important to explore all of the advice clients have already received from friends and family, before giving your own advice.

Interviewers are often tempted to agree or disagree with clients. Agreement and disagreement occur in natural social contexts, and many interviewers naturally extend this social custom to interviewing. Agreement and disagreement may have positive or negative effects. Because these responses are opinion-based, they can either help people feel justified in their beliefs and actions or they can stimulate arguments. It is important to remember that if you express agreement with your clients, you may later have to decide whether to express disagreement.

Urging is a strong form of advice giving. Interviewers use urging when they want to push their clients toward a particular thought, feeling, or action. Urging is most commonly used in crisis situations, such as when the client is threatening suicide or being physically mistreated. However, urging may also be used to help clients deal more effectively with clinical issues. This type of response is obviously very directive.

Approval and disapproval generally should be avoided by interviewers. They can be very powerful influencing strategies when applied to vulnerable and needy clients. Although approval may strengthen client self-esteem, it also fosters dependency and is suggestive of moral judgment. Disapproval can be especially damaging to clients. The other technical responses available to interviewers are preferred to approval and disapproval.

After you read chapters 4, 5, and 6, we recommend that you examine your own technical response tendencies by listening or watching recordings of yourselves. It can also be helpful to listen to or watch recordings of professionals conducting therapeutic interviews.

Suggested Readings and Professional Recordings

Cormier, W. H., & Cormier, L. S. (1991). *Interviewing strategies for helpers: Fundamental skills and cognitive behavioral interventions* (3rd ed.). Monterey, CA: Brooks/Cole. Chapters 11 through 20 provide extensive information on cognitive and behavioral intervention strategies.

Greenson, R. R. (1967). *The technique and practice of psychoanalysis* (Vol. I). New York: International Universities Press. This classic work provides good ground rules for the use of interpretation.

Rogers, C. R. (1951). *Client-centered therapy*. Boston: Houghton Mifflin. This text includes Rogers' original discussion of feeling reflection (chapter 4).

Weiner, I. B. (1975). *Principles of psychotherapy*. New York: John Wiley & Sons. This is a good general text on psychoanalytically oriented psychotherapy. It provides clear examples and descriptions of interpretations, free association, and other concepts.

Yalom, I. D. (1985). *The theory and practice of group psychotherapy* (3rd ed.). New York: Basic Books. Chapters 1 and 2 discuss therapeutic factors in group psychotherapy. These factors are extremely relevant to individual psychotherapy and help illustrate the importance of specific responses, such as feeling validation.

Several famous psychotherapists have produced professional recordings of therapeutic interviews, among them Aaron Beck, Donald Meichanbaum, Fritz Perls, Carl Rogers, and Hans Strupp. Videotapes have also been produced as components of interpersonal skills training programs; Robert Carkhuff, Gerard Egan, George Gazda, and Allen Ivey have developed such programs. You can obtain information on ordering these tapes from media centers on most college campuses.

_7_

RELATIONSHIP VARIABLES AND THERAPEUTIC INTERVIEWING

Rapport
  Common Client Fears
  Putting the Client at Ease

Carl Rogers's Core Conditions
  Congruence
  Unconditional Positive Regard
  Accurate Empathy
  The Relationship Among Rogers's Core Conditions

Psychoanalytic and Interpersonal Relationship Variables
  Transference
  Countertransference
  Identification and Internalization
  Resistance
  Working Alliance

Relationship Variables and Behavioral and Social Psychology
  Expertness (Credibility)
  Attractiveness
  Trustworthiness

Feminist Relationship Variables
  Mutuality
  Empowerment

Integrating Relationship Variables

Chapter Summary

Suggested Readings

One brief way of describing the change which has taken place in me is to say that in my early professional years I was asking the question, How can I treat, or cure, or change this person? Now I would phrase the question in this way: How can I provide a relationship which this person may use for . . . personal growth?
                                                    —*CARL ROGERS, On Becoming a Person*

In his counseling work, Carl Rogers grew disillusioned with traditional psychoanalytic and behavioral methods of personality and behavior change. Instead, he began to focus on a "certain type of relationship" (1961, p. 33) that seemed to facilitate personal development. Rogers came to view this relationship as all-important to the success of counseling, psychotherapy, teaching, and even international peacekeeping. He boldly claimed that the psychotherapeutic relationship he envisioned provided *all* that was necessary *and* sufficient for positive personal development.

Most clinicians today would heartily agree with only part of Rogers's bold claim. A good psychotherapeutic relationship is considered a necessary, but perhaps not always *sufficient* ingredient for positive client personal development. The purpose of this chapter is to discuss a variety of relationship variables and how they influence the clinical interviewing process and therapy outcomes.

In the years following Rogers's early publications on the importance of relationship in counseling (*Counseling and psychotherapy*, 1942 and *Client-centered therapy, 1951)*, an immense amount of research has addressed this issue. We begin this chapter by exploring the concept of rapport in therapeutic interviewing. We then move to the core relationship conditions that Rogers considered so crucial to therapeutic success. Lastly, we examine therapeutic relationship variables commonly associated with psychoanalytic, feminist, and social-behavioral approaches to therapeutic interviewing.

Rapport

Rapport is a generic relationship variable; interviewers of all orientations generally acknowledge the importance of having good rapport with their clients. However, the concept of rapport has probably been popularized more by behavioral, humanistic, and feminist clinicians than by psychoanalytically oriented psychotherapists. Rapport is defined broadly as "relation" and "good"

rapport is more specifically considered a "relation marked by harmony, confor-
mity, accord, or affinity" (*Webster's*, 1985, p. 976).

Effective interviewers take specific steps to establish good rapport with
their clients. Many technical responses discussed in chapters 5 and 6 are associated with developing good rapport (e.g., paraphrase, reflection of feeling,
and feeling validation). Othmer and Othmer (1989) outline six strategies for
developing good rapport.

1. Put the patient and yourself at ease.
2. Find the suffering; show compassion.
3. Assess insight; become an ally.
4. Show expertise.
5. Establish authority.
6. Balance the roles (Othmer & Othmer, 1989, p. 15).

Portions of Othmer and Othmer's six strategies will be referred to and
discussed throughout this chapter.

Common Client Fears

Most people are not comfortable coming to a therapist for personal assistance.
Recognizing and effectively dealing with client discomfort constitutes the first
step of establishing rapport.

Clients have many fears and doubts when first consulting a professional
interviewer or counselor. It is impossible to address all of these fears and
doubts in an initial session; establishing the type of rapport necessary to make
clients comfortable working with you is a lengthy and involved process (Weinberg, 1984). On the other hand, therapeutic interviewers can begin initiating
rapport by acknowledging and sensitively addressing at least some of their
clients' fears. Common client fears and doubts are listed below (adapted from
Othmer & Othmer, 1989; Pipes & Davenport, 1990; Wolberg, 1988):

1. Is this interviewer competent?
2. More importantly, can she help me?
3. Will she understand me and my problems?
4. Am I going crazy?
5. Will she be honest with me (can I trust her)?
6. With whom will she discuss my situation?
7. I feel embarrassed about my problems, is she someone with whom I can
   talk openly or will she ridicule me?
8. Will this interviewer share my values (or religious views)?
9. Will I be pressured to say things I don't want to say?
10. Will she think I am a bad person?
11. What if my friends or family find out I'm here?
12. Will I like my interviewer (too much or not enough)?

Sometimes new clients are intimidated by interviewers, whom they view
as authority figures. Remember that as a therapeutic interviewer, you *are* an
authority figure, whether you like it or not. Some forms of therapy take advan-

tage of the authority associated with being a professional interviewer (e.g., rational emotive therapy; see Corey, 1991), while others, such as feminist therapy and person-centered therapies (Brody, 1984; Rogers, 1961) seek to establish a more egalitarian working relationship. The fact remains that in most therapy situations, at least initially, the therapist is seen as an authority. When clients come to see you, they may believe they should act as they do when around other authority figures, such as physicians or teachers, or they may perceive you as they perceived previous authority figures in their lives, such as harsh, cold, or rejecting. In order to address the fact that many clients come into counseling with conscious or unconscious assumptions about the interviewer as an authority figure, therapeutic interviewers strive to help clients view their interviewers as partners in the therapeutic process.

Putting the Client at Ease

An important part of putting clients at ease involves convincing them you are a "different kind" of authority figure. You must encourage new clients to be interactive, to ask questions, and to be open; these are behaviors that they may have avoided with previous authority figures. Once we have sat down with clients and explained confidentiality, we often use a statement similar to the following:

> "You know, this is kind of an unusual situation. We're strangers—I don't know you, and you don't know me. So really, this first session is mostly a chance for us to get to know one another better. My goal is to listen as well as I can to you as you describe yourself and the concerns that have brought you here. I may ask some questions during this process in order to get more information about particular aspects of your life. This first session is also a chance for you to get a sense for how I work with people in counseling and determine if that feels comfortable to you. If you have any questions as we proceed today, feel free to ask them. I like to keep things as clear as possible, so if something isn't clear, let me know."

This introduction may seem long and rambling, but it usually serves to put clients at ease. It acknowledges the fact that interviewers and clients are initially strangers and gives the client permission to evaluate the interviewer and ask questions about therapeutic processes.

Othmer and Othmer (1989) consider introduction, conversation, and initial informal chatting as methods to help put clients at ease. These efforts may involve some of the following.

- "You must be Steven Green." (initial greeting)
- "Do you like to be called Steven, Steve, or Mr. Green?" (clarifying how the client would like to be addressed, or how to correctly pronounce his name)
- "Were you able to find the office (or a place to park) easily?" (small talk and empathic concern)

- "Where are you originally from?" (geographical origin is usually a safe place to start an interview; this question can be answered successfully and may allow for interviewer comment regarding what it was like to have been from a particular place)
- (with children or adolescents) "I see you've got a Los Angeles Lakers hat on . . . you must be a Lakers fan." (small talk; an attempt to connect with the client's world)

Of course, chatting is usually held to a minimum with adult clients, unless they are uncooperative and resistant, in which case it may constitute your primary interviewing technique. On the other hand, initial casual conversation can easily make or break an interview with a child or adolescent. For example, author John Sommers-Flanagan is convinced that one interview with a ten-year-old client succeeded primarily because at the beginning of the first session John took time to discuss with the boy his views on Ninja Turtles (i.e., "So who's your favorite Ninja Turtle?"). Similarly, in interviews with adolescents or preadolescents, John usually discusses what slang words are "in" and how to use them appropriately (e.g., "Now I want to make sure I'm using the right words here. Is it cool, radical, fresh, or sweet? What's the right word to use now?").

Interviewers who are good at putting their clients at ease are usually sensitive and flexible. They sense their clients' discomfort by reading signals. For example, they may notice a client chooses a distant chair in the interviewing room, or, conversely, that a client sits too close and seems to intrude on the interviewer's personal space. Flexible interviewers respect their clients' interpersonal styles; they do not insist a client sit in a particular chair or at a certain distance. They try to speak the client's nonverbal language.

Carl Rogers's Core Conditions

The core therapeutic conditions identified by Rogers (1942) extend the importance of relationship issues beyond that of rapport. Rogers believed that establishing a therapeutic relationship constituted all of what is therapeutic about counseling. Rogers's three core conditions are:

- Congruence
- Unconditional positive regard
- Accurate empathy

In Rogers's own words,

Thus the relationship which I have found helpful is characterized by a sort of transparency on my part, in which my real feelings are evident; by an acceptance of this other person as a separate person with value in his own right; and by a deep empathic understanding which enables me to see his private world through his eyes. When these conditions are achieved, I become a companion to my client, accompanying him in the frightening search for himself, which he now feels free to undertake. (Rogers, 1961, p. 34)

Congruence

Congruence means that one's thoughts, feelings, and behavior match. There are no discrepancies; congruent interviewers think, feel, and behave in a consistent manner. Terms used interchangeably with congruence include genuineness, authenticity, and being real. The congruent interviewer is genuine, authentic, and real in interactions with clients.

Congruence implies spontaneity and honesty. Rogers was clear in his writing that congruence requires expression of "various feelings and attitudes which exist in me" (1961, p. 33). He also emphasized that congruent expression was important even if it consists of attitudes, thoughts, or feelings that do not, on the surface, appear conducive to a good relationship. On the surface it might appear that Rogers is an advocate of self-disclosure in the service of congruence.

Implications of Congruence   When discussing congruence in our courses on therapeutic interviewing, we have been barraged by student questions regarding the implication of this concept for interviewer behavior. Typical questions about congruence include:

- Does congruence mean I can say what I *really* think about the client right to her face?
- If I feel sexually attracted to a client, should I be "congruent" and tell her?
- If I feel like touching a client, should I go ahead and do so? Am I being ingenuine if I restrain myself?
- What if I don't like a client or something a client does? Am I being incongruent if I don't tell him?

These are important questions, and some of them are controversial within the fields of interviewing, counseling, and psychotherapy. Although they do not have simple answers, our typical response to each of these questions is *no*. To be excessively transparent or congruent with clients can be damaging; sometimes the cost of complete congruence outweighs the benefit. For example, Luborsky (1984) states:

> In trying to gain a good measure of trust and rapport, therapists typically experience a natural temptation to impart to the patient information about themselves. . . . This temptation generally should be resisted since, on balance, it provides fewer benefits than it does potential long-term problems. (p. 68)

Before you assume we are advocates of incongruence or phoniness, let us explain our position.

To evaluate and utilize the concept of congruence, it is useful to view this idea from Carl Rogers's perspective. When counseling, Rogers became deeply absorbed with his clients. He strove for the goal of completely understanding his clients, from *their* points of view, which is precisely why he named his approach "client-centered" or "person-centered" centered therapy. Consequently, Rogers's role or stance when interviewing greatly reduced his need to judge or express negative feelings toward his clients. Moreover, Rogers (1958) was clear that the aim of client-centered therapy was not for interviewers to talk about their own feelings:

> Certainly the aim is not for the therapist to express or talk about his own feelings, but primarily that he should not be deceiving the client as to himself. At times he may need to talk about some of his own feelings (either to the client, or to a colleague or superior) if they are standing in the way . . . (pp. 133-134)

This statement suggests Rogers believed good judgment should be used before self-disclosing with clients. Sometimes discussing your feelings about a client with peers or supervisors is more appropriate than discussing those feelings directly with your client.

Rogers believed that when congruence and empathy or unconditional positive regard conflicted, congruence should be maintained. He believed congruence or genuineness was the most important of the core conditions. Yet for Rogers, even more important than maintaining the core relationship conditions was his emphasis on being truly present and committed to listening to and helping clients. Rogers was a remarkable individual who rarely needed to deal with a conflict between congruence and unconditional positive regard because he was almost always genuinely interested in listening to what his clients were saying; he was committed to his clients' personal growth and development. After decades of counseling, he reported only rarely feeling anger or irritation toward his clients (1972).

Tempering Your Congruence   When it comes to evaluating whether or not you should be spontaneously expressive in a session, Gazda, Asbury, Balzer, Childers, and Walters (1984) provide excellent advice. Although Gazda et al. are referring to the use of touch in counseling, their advice is sound with respect to most potentially spontaneous interviewer behaviors: "Whom is it for—me, the other person, or to impress those who observe" (p. 111).

In other words, explore motives underlying your potentially spontaneous behaviors. When it comes to touch, we take a stance that might be considered even more conservative than that of Gazda and his associates. As we usually tell our students, if you are going to touch a client, you had better be absolutely sure you are doing so purely for the client's benefit and not for your own gratification. In addition, you need to be absolutely sure your touch will not feel invasive or overbearing and that it will not be misinterpreted. If you have any doubts, *do not touch your client.*

In his book *The Road Less Travelled*, M. Scott Peck (1978) outlines his controversial view on sexual relations with clients; a view in which expressive action is tempered by clinical judgment and a personal and professional commitment to client growth:

> Were I ever to have a case in which I concluded after careful and judicious consideration that my patient's spiritual growth would be substantially furthered by our having sexual relations, I would proceed to have them. In fifteen years of practice, however, I have not yet had such a case, and I find it difficult to imagine that such a case could really exist. (p. 176)

We have never come across a case in which an interviewer or psychotherapist had sexual relations with a client based upon completely unselfish motives. The fact is that sexual relations between therapist and client are *always* inappropriate and unacceptable; the result of therapist-client sex is victimization and trauma (Folman, 1991; Sonne & Pope, 1991). We agree with Pope's (1990) terminology for sexual relations between therapists and clients: sexual abuse of clients. When such terminology is used, it becomes obvious that sexual abuse of clients can *never* be a therapeutic endeavor.

Although congruence suggests spontaneous expression, we recommend consideration of the following guidelines before expressing yourself spontaneously. In other words, temper your spontaneity with good clinical judgment.

1. Examine your motives. Are you expressing yourself solely for your client's benefit?
2. Consider if what you want to say or do will be therapeutic. Are there any possibilities that your client will respond in a negative or unpredictable manner to your expression?
3. Congruence does not mean that you say whatever comes to mind. It means that whenever you do choose to speak, you do so with honesty and integrity.

Currently, feminist therapists probably are the strongest advocates of congruence, or authenticity, in interviewer-client relations. Brody (1984) describes the range of responses that an authentic interviewer might use:

> To be involved, to use myself as a variable in the process, entails using, from time to time, mimicry, provocation, joking, annoyance, analogies, or brief lectures. It also means utilizing my own and others' physical behavior, sensations, emotional states, and reactions to me and others, and sharing a variety of intuitive responses. This is being authentic. (p. 17)

Brody advocates the use of a wide range of sophisticated, advanced, and sometimes directive therapeutic strategies. It is important to note that she describes herself as using such approaches more often as she becomes more experienced. As we noted above, such an authentic or congruent approach to interviewing is best if combined with good clinical judgment, which is obtained, in part, through clinical experience.

A final example from Peck (1978) illustrates the struggle between psychoanalytic and person-centered or feminist perspectives when it comes to congruence:

> After a year of this [therapy], she (the client) asked me the middle of a session, "Do you think I'm a bit of a shit?"
>
> "You seem to be asking me to tell you what I think of you," I replied, brilliantly stalling for time.
>
> That was exactly what she wanted, she said. But what did I do now? What magical words or techniques or postures could help me? I could say, "Why do you ask that?" or "What are your fantasies about what I think of you?" or "What's important, Marcia, is not what I think of you but what you think of yourself." Yet I had an overpowering feeling that these gambits were cop-outs, and that after a whole year of seeing me three times a week the least Marcia was entitled to was an honest answer from me as to what I thought of her. (p. 170–171)

At some point as a therapeutic interviewer you will be faced with similar questions. With certain questions, like the one Peck is facing above, you will need to decide within yourself how you should respond. Do you deny your client a human and congruent response for the sake of preserving neutrality, professionalism, and technical correctness? Or do you forsake professional and technical neutrality and respond to your client as another real human being? Interviewers with psychoanalytic orientations tend to stay with professional neutrality, while person-centered, existential, and feminist interviewers choose a more open and humanistic approach.

Unconditional Positive Regard

Unconditional positive regard is also referred to as "acceptance" or "respect" (Rogers, 1961, p. 34). Rogers defines this construct: "By acceptance I mean a warm regard for him as a person of unconditional self-worth—of value no matter what his condition, his behavior, or his feelings" (p. 34). Unconditional positive regard suggests warmth, caring, respect, and a nonjudgmental attitude. No one knows clients better than they know themselves. Therefore, as interviewers, we are not in a good position to judge our clients. Usually, all we know is a thin slice or sample of their lives and behavior. Consequently, our judgments would be necessarily based on incomplete or inadequate information. We have not lived with our clients, we usually have not observed them at great length, and we cannot directly know their internal motives, thoughts, or feelings. Even if it were possible to have complete information on clients and we did obtain that information, rendering judgment on good or bad qualities of clients' thoughts, feelings, or behavior would be inappropriate.

The term unconditional positive regard also suggests more than a neutral acceptance of clients. Rogers (1961) stated that "the safety of being liked and prized as a person seems a highly important element in a helping relationship" (p. 34). Rogers is referring to positive or affectionate feelings interviewers need to have in order for their clients to feel safe enough to explore their self-doubts, insecurities, and weaknesses. Research shows that clients improve more when their therapists have positive feelings toward them (Moras & Strupp, 1982; Strupp & Hadley, 1979).

An important question for interviewers to consider is, How can I express or demonstrate unconditional positive regard toward my clients? It is tempting to try to express positive feelings directly by either touching clients or making statements such as "I like (or love) you," "I care about you," "I will accept you unconditionally," or "I won't judge you."

To express unconditional positive regard directly can be ineffective or even dangerous for several reasons. First, direct expressions may be interpreted by clients as phony or inappropriate. Second, direct expressions of affection may imply that you want to establish a friendship or loving relationship with your client outside of counseling. In other words, such expressions may be viewed as unprofessional in the sense that they imply that you have, or want to have, more than a professional relationship with your client. Third, even professional interviewers sometimes have negative evaluative feelings toward their clients. If you claim you will maintain "unconditional acceptance," you are promising something that is impossible. You can't like all of the people all of the time, so you should avoid making any claims of that nature.

The question remains, "How do you express liking, acceptance, and respect to your clients indirectly?" First, simply by keeping appointments, by asking how your clients like to be addressed and then remembering to address them that way, and by listening sensitively and compassionately, you establish a relationship characterized by affection and respect. Second, by allowing clients freedom to discuss themselves in their natural manner, you communicate respect and acceptance. This involves using a significant amount of nondirective technical responses (see chapters 4 and 5). Third, by demonstrating that you have heard and that you remember specific parts of a client's story, you communicate respect. This usually involves the use of paraphrase, summary, and sometimes interpretation. Fourth, by responding with compassion or empathy to clients' emotional pain and intellectual conflicts, you express liking and acceptance. This is what Othmer and Othmer (1989, p. 26) mean when they refer to "find the suffering" and "show compassion" as strategies for building rapport. Fifth, clinical experience and research both point to the fact that clients are often sensitive to an interviewer's intentions. Thus, simply by clearly making an effort and *intending* to accept or respect your clients, you are communicating a message that may be more powerful than any technique you might utilize (Hill, Helms, Tichenor, Spiegel, et al., 1988). In the following example, the interviewer uses a feeling oriented summary along with a gentle interpretive comment.

> "Earlier in the hour you mentioned how you felt hurt and rejected
> when a woman whom you cared about turned away from you. Now
> you're talking about your mother and how you felt she abandoned you
> in your youth to take care of your father and his alcoholism. It seems
> like there's a connection or pattern here."

Although this type of response is designed to facilitate insight into patterns of interpersonal relationships (Luborsky, 1984), it also can serve to let your client know how closely you're listening. As a result of such a response, your client may feel honored and respected and the relationship may take on a sense of intimacy; remembering what your client says requires an intimate attentiveness (Hanson, 1991).

Accurate Empathy

Empathy is a popular concept in therapeutic interviewing, counseling, and psychotherapy. When Othmer and Othmer (1989) discuss their rapport-building strategy of finding "the suffering" and showing "compassion, (p.26)" they are referring to empathic responding. Empathy is crucial to initial rapport and, according to some schools of thought, eventual psychotherapeutic change (Kohut, 1984; Rogers, 1951). Unfortunately, empathy is as complex as it is popular. Take, for example, the definition of "empathy" in *Webster's Ninth New Collegiate Dictionary*:

> . . . the action of understanding, being aware of, being sensitive to, and vicariously experiencing the feelings, thoughts, and experience of another of either the past or present without having the feelings, thoughts, and experience fully communicated in an objectively explicit manner. (1985, p. 407)

According to this definition, empathy requires inference. Because we cannot know "in an objectively explicit manner" the feelings, thoughts, and experience of another, we must use our intellect to infer what this other person might be feeling, thinking, and experiencing. Consequently, empathy is *both* an intellectual and affective process.

While the Webster's definition may seem complex, even more in-depth efforts have been made to define the empathic process. For example, Buie (1981) suggests four components of empathy:

1. Cognitive or intellectual understanding of the client.
2. Low intensity feelings, memories, and associations experienced by the interviewer in response to client communications.
3. Imaginative imitation empathy (similar to Carkhuff's empathy question; see below).
4. Affective contagion or a resonating with clients emotional expressions (Watkins, 1978).

Empathy is a complex affective-cognitive-experiential concept that continues to stimulate analysis and research (Margulies, 1984).

Carkhuff (1987) refers to the intellectual part of empathy as "asking the empathy question" (p. 100). Specifically, he states, "By answering the empathy question we try to understand the feelings expressed by our helpee. We summarize the clues to the helpee's feelings and then answer the question, How would I feel if I were Tom and saying these things?" (p. 101).

Asking the empathy question, as defined by Carkhuff, is a very useful strategy for enhancing empathic sensitivity. However, it also tends to oversimplify the empathic process in at least two ways. First, it assumes that the interviewer (or helper) has an accurately calibrated affective barometer within, allowing for objective readings of client emotional states. The fact is, clients and therapists may have had such different personal experiences that the empathy question produces completely inaccurate results; that you "would" feel a particular way if you were having a client's experience, doesn't necessarily mean that the client feels the same way. As Pietrofesa and associates state, "Some skeptics suggest that an empathic response is a projection" (1984, p. 238). If interviewers rely solely on Carkhuff's empathy question, they run the risk of projecting their own feelings onto their clients. For example, consider what might happen if an interviewer tends to view events somewhat pessimistically, while her client usually uses rationalization, denial, or repression to put on a happy face. The following exchange might occur:

> C: "I don't know why my dad wants us to come into therapy now . . . . After all, we've never been able to communicate effectively. It doesn't even bother me anymore."
>
> I: "It must feel sad for you to have never felt you and your Dad communicated effectively."
>
> C: "Not at all. I'm letting go of my relationships with my parents. Really, I don't let it bother me."

In this case, thinking about how it would feel to never communicate effectively with her own father may indeed make the interviewer feel sad. But her comment is a projection because it is based on her feelings and not on the client's feelings. Accurate empathic responding stays close to client word content and nonverbal messages. If this client had previously expressed sadness or was currently *looking* sad (e.g., by staring downward, tearing, and talking in low voice tones), then the interviewer would have been more justified in her choice of empathic response. However, her comment is an inaccurate reflection of feeling, and as such, it is rejected by the client. The interviewer could have stayed more closely with what her client had expressed both verbally and nonverbally by focusing on the key words never and anymore.

> "Coming into therapy now doesn't make much sense to you. Maybe you used to have some feelings about your lack of communication with your dad, but it sounds like you feel pretty numb about the whole situation now."

This second response is more accurately empathic. It touches on how the client used to feel and how he presently thinks, as well as the numbed affective response. There may be some unresolved feelings of sadness, anger, or disappointment, but for the interviewer to connect with these buried feelings requires an interviewer interpretation, which would need to be supported with strong evidence before it could be convincing enough to the client to be empathic. Recall from chapter 5 that interpretations and interpretive feeling reflections must be supported by adequate evidence to be maximally effective.

Instead of focusing solely on what you would feel if you were in your client's shoes, it is more effective to reflect intellectually on how other clients (or other people you know) might feel and think in response to this particular experience. Rogers (1961) emphasized that feeling reflections should be stated in a tentative manner so that the client feels able to freely accept or dismiss them. Also keep in mind the defensive style of your clients. If they are using a defense mechanism such as rationalization or denial, you need to first acknowledge, in an empathic manner, their use of defensive thinking. For example:

C: "I don't know why my dad wants us to come into therapy now . . . . After all, we've never been able to communicate effectively. It doesn't even bother me anymore."

I: "Coming into therapy now doesn't make much sense to you. Maybe you used to have some feelings about your lack of communication with your dad, but it sounds like you feel pretty numb about the whole situation now."

C: "Yeah, I guess so. I think I'm letting go of my relationships with my parents. Really, I don't let it bother me."

I: "Maybe one of the ways you're protecting yourself from how you felt about your lack of communication with your dad is to distance yourself from your parents. Otherwise, it could still bother you I suppose?"

C: "I, yeah. I suppose if I let myself get close to my parents again, my dad's lame communication style would bug me again."

Obviously, this client still has deep feelings about his father's poor communication skills. However, only through gentle empathic responding can the interviewer begin to help him admit such feelings.

A second way in which Carkhuff's empathy question is simplistic is that it treats empathy as if it had only to do with accurately reflecting client *feelings*. Certainly, accurate feeling reflection is an important part of the empathic process, but, as Rogers (1961), Webster's (1985) and others (Buie, 1981; Margulies, 1984) indicate, empathy involves not only *feeling* with clients, but also *thinking* and *experiencing* with clients. This is why empathic acknowledgment of clients' defensive styles is important to empathic responding. Clients seek to protect themselves from emotional pain through defense mechanisms (i.e., largely unconscious patterns of distorting reality that are ego-protective; A. Freud, 1946). Consequently, to be maximally empathic, interviewers need to address not only the clients' feelings, but also the way in which clients try to shield themselves from such feelings. As Sigmund Freud (1921/1955) suggested, "[empathy] plays the largest part in our understanding of what is inherently foreign to our ego" (p. 108).

Accurate and effective empathic responding is usually based on a combination of at least the following four strategies:

1. Acknowledging and reflecting surface or buried feelings as clients express them through word content and nonverbal messages. This strategy may include matching of representational systems, mirroring, paraphrase, reflection of feeling, interpretation, and other responses (see chapters 4 and 5).

2. Noting how clients are thinking about, coping with, and defending against their emotional pain.

3. Coming up with an answer to Carkhuff's empathy question, How would I feel if I were in the client's shoes?

4. Demonstrating to clients that you are interested in discussing issues important to them and trying actively to comprehend, through a variety of listening and attending techniques, how clients experience these issues from their own perspectives.

The Effects of Empathy   Obviously, empathy enhances rapport. Empathy has a number of other positive effects. First, empathy helps clients explore personal issues more freely. When clients feel understood, they also tend to feel more open and willing to talk about their concerns in greater detail; empathy elicits information (Egan, 1986).

Second, as Rogers (1961) emphasized, empathy, combined with unconditional positive regard, allows clients to explore themselves more completely than they would otherwise: "It is only as I see them (your feelings and thoughts) as you see them, and accept them and you, that you feel really free to explore all the hidden nooks and frightening crannies of your inner and often buried experience" (p. 34). Rogers is suggesting that accurate empathy helps clients become aware of previously unconscious material. Thus, he also is suggesting that the effect of an accurately empathic response is similar to an accurate interpretation in that it results in increased client self-awareness.

Third, empathy enhances the working alliance (Greenson, 1967). Empathic responding helps clients feel that the interviewer is on their side, a perception that also can considerably increase levels of client trust and motivation (Krumboltz & Thoresen, 1976).

Misguided Empathic Attempts   In order to identify how interviewers can behave empathically, it is important to examine empathic strategies that are usually in part ineffective (Sommers-Flanagan & Sommers-Flanagan, 1989). Reading and hearing about empathy is much different than experiencing empathy, and experiencing empathy for someone provides no guarantee that effective empathic communication will occur. Usually, early interviews are filled with self-disclosures and other attempts to let clients know they're understood. Classic empathic statements that beginning interviewers often use, but should avoid, include the following:

1. "I know how you feel" or "I understand." In response to such a statement, clients may wonder, "How could she know how I feel; she's only known me for fifteen minutes," or they may reason, "If she really knew how I felt, or had been through what I've been through, there's no way she would have been able to get where she is."

BOX 7-1

Empathy and Other Theoretical Orientations

Writers and clinicians of various professional perspectives and theoretical orientations have emphasized the importance of empathy in interviewing, counseling, and psychotherapy. Below is a brief sampling from some prominent writers and clinicians.

Psychoanalytic Psychotherapy
"Empathy is the operation that defines the field of psychoanalysis. No psychology of complex mental states is conceivable without the employment of empathy" (Kohut, 1984, pp. 174–175).

Psychiatric Interviewing
"When the patient reveals his suffering, tell him that you understand, show your empathy, and express your compassion" (Othmer & Othmer, 1989, p. 27).

Feminist Theory
"We have a long tradition of trying to dispense with, or at least to control or neutralize, emotionality, rather than valuing, embracing, and cultivating its contributing strengths . . . . However attained, these qualities bespeak a basic ability that is very valuable. It can hardly be denied that emotions are essential aspects of human life" (Miller, 1986, pp. 38–39).

Behavior Therapy
"Any behavior therapist who maintains that principles of learning and social influence are all one needs to know in order to bring about behavior change is out of contact with clinical reality . . . . The truly skillful behavior therapist is one who can both conceptualize problems behaviorally and make the necessary translations so that he interacts in a warm and empathic manner with his client" (Goldfried & Davison, 1976, pp. 55–56).

Marriage Counseling
"A major design of the treatment is to enable each spouse to receive empathic understanding when he or she communicates with the therapist, and for the task of the spouse who is listening to be defined as an attempt to put aside his or her complaints and empathically enter the world of the other" (Lansky, 1986, p. 562).

---

2. "I've been through the same type of thing." Clients may respond with skepticism or ask you to elaborate on your experience. Suddenly the roles are reversed—the interviewer is being interviewed.

3. "Oh God, that must have been terrible." Clients who have been through traumatic events are sometimes unsure about how objectively traumatic such events really were, and therefore to hear a professional exclaim that what they've lived through and coped with was "terrible" can have a deleterious effect. The important point here is whether you are leading or are tracking the client's emotional experience. If the client is giving you a clear indication that she senses the "terribleness" of her experiences, then reflecting that the experiences "must have been terrible" is acceptably empathic. However, such a statement is not nondirective empathy but a judgment of the terribleness the client felt. A nondirective empathic response would remove the judgment of

"must have" and might be, "Sounds like you felt pretty terrible about what happened."

4. "Gee, you poor thing" or "That's awful. You must be a strong person to have made it through that." Again, these statements contain judgments and offer inappropriate sympathy. The client may feel complimented temporarily but may subsequently feel unable to disclose other emotions or weaknesses, for fear of further judgments by the expert. The interviewer must encourage open communication rather than shape the client into presenting things in certain ways. Once someone is rewarded for looking strong, they may choose to try to present all their material in the same light.

Clients often have ambivalent feelings about their experiences. Take for example, the following interviewer-client interaction:

I: "Can you think of any times in your past when you felt you were unfairly treated? Perhaps punished when you didn't deserve it?"

C: "No not really. (fifteen-second pause) Well I guess there was this one time. I was supposed to clean the house for my mother while she was gone. And it wasn't done when she got back, and she broke a broom over my back."

I: "She broke a broom over your back?" (stated with just a slight inflection, indicating interviewer disapproval or surprise)

C: "Yeah. I probably deserved it though . . . the house wasn't cleaned like she had asked."

In this situation the client is experiencing incompatible feelings toward her mother. On the one hand, the mother is someone who treats her unfairly, while on the other hand, the client feels herself to be guilty because she is a bad girl who did not follow her mother's wishes. The interviewer is trying to convey empathy through voice tone and inflection. This technique is appropriately chosen because focusing strongly on either the client's guilt or indignation and anger would prematurely shut down exploration and appreciation of the client's ambivalent feelings. By not openly saying "How could she do such a thing to an eleven-year-old girl?" the interviewer is able to retain the ability to explore the client's victim guilt. Despite the interviewer's tentative and minimal expression of empathy, the client's response is to defend her mother's punitive actions. This suggests the client had already accepted (by age 11, and still accepted in this session, at age 42) her mother's negative evaluation of her. A stronger supportive statement such as "That's ridiculous, mothers should never break brooms over their daughter's backs" would probably have closed off any exploration of the client's opposing feelings of guilt over the incident. Gustafson (1986) discusses the importance of "double appreciation": "There is something quite extraordinary about someone's realizing that one has tried so hard to be what the family has needed, yet, in spite of one's best efforts, one has had other feelings, which would appear to be incompatible. Yet they are there" (p. 14).

Minimally empathic, nondirective responses that communicate empathy through voice tone, facial expression, and feeling reflection are usually recommended as initially more advantageous than open support and sympathy. There is always time for open support later, after the client has had an opportunity to explore both sides of the issue (in this case guilt and indignation or anger).

The Relationship Among Rogers's Core Conditions

Rogers believed that the need to judge clients or respond to them out of his own needs was greatly diminished with an empathic stance. He found that believing in the interrelatedness of empathy, unconditional positive regard, and congruence helped modify the spontaneity associated with congruence. Accurate empathy also serves to diminish the tendency to judge clients, and thus enhances unconditional positive regard. Empathy, unconditional positive regard, and congruence are not competing individual constructs (in statistical terms, they are not orthogonal). Instead, they form a single triarchic construct; they complement one another.

Psychoanalytic and Interpersonal Relationship Variables

The following interviewing relationship variables are derived from psychoanalytic, object relations, and interpersonal theoretical perspectives.

Transference

Sigmund Freud defined transference as a process that occurs when "the patient sees in his analyst the return—the reincarnation—of some important figure out of his childhood or past, and consequently transfers on to him feelings and reactions that undoubtedly applied to this model" (1940/1949, p. 66). Subsequently, Harry Stack Sullivan (1970) defined a similar process that he referred to as parataxic distortion: "The real characteristics of the other fellow at that time may be of negligible importance to the interpersonal situation. This we call parataxic distortion" (p. 25).

One way to explain transference is to compare it to the process of applying an old map to a new road. The client transfers onto the interviewer characteristics of others with whom the client has been in significant relationships and responds to the interviewer in ways he used to respond to them. Transference is characterized by inappropriateness; that is, the client responds to the interviewer by acting, thinking, or feeling in an inappropriate manner. Freud (1912/1958) stated that transference "exceeds anything that could be justified on sensible or rational grounds" (p. 100). Sometimes, but not always, intense and obvious transference issues can come right to the surface, early in an interview or early in the therapeutic process. For example, author Rita Sommers-Flanagan once had an angry, confused young man become verbally violent during an initial screening interview. During his tirade, he said over and over, "Women. You *&%$# women are all the same." Since it is unlikely that Rita behaved in a manner that warranted such a strong reaction, it is likely this client was displacing "feelings, attitudes, or impulses" from previous relationships he had experienced with females (Weiner, 1975, p. 203).

More commonly, like most relationship variables, transference will be abstract, vague, and elusive. To notice it, you usually have to pay specific attention to idiosyncratic transactions clients initiate with you. One clue is when clients seem to respond emotionally to you in ways that are out of proportion with respect to the situation or material at hand. Another clue is when clients begin to make assumptions about you that have little or no basis in reality and about which they have no information. Another sign has to do with clients expressing expectations regarding you or therapy that are unfounded and unrealistic—that have no basis in reality.

A fairly common "old map on new terrain" is the client's unspoken belief that you too will evaluate him, find him lacking, and reject him. A client we once knew expressed evaluation anxiety regarding her performance on a psychological test and cognitive-behavioral homework assignment: "You know, some of those things the test says about me don't seem accurate. I must have done something wrong when I took the test." This comment is especially revealing because when most clients are provided with psychological test feedback that seems inaccurate, they begin to question the test's validity, rather than their own performance. Similarly, she stated, "I did the assignment you gave me, but I'm not sure if I really had the right idea." Again, she makes this statement when, in fact, she is turning in one of the most thorough homework assignment we had ever had a client complete. She did exactly what was instructed, but her self-doubt was activated because she was exposed to an authority figure who might evaluate her negatively. Her expectation of criticism suggests she had been harshly, and perhaps inappropriately, criticized before. In this sense her reaction is similar to the child who flinches when approached by an adult whose arm is extended. The reason the child probably flinches is because of previous physical abuse. The flinch may be an automatic and unconscious response. Similarly, clients who have been exposed to excessive criticism have an automatic and unconscious tendency to prepare themselves (or flinch) when exposed to evaluative situations. This is an enactment of transference.

Transference reactions may become self-fulfilling prophecies. The client who expects rejection, negative evaluation, or lack of empathy is usually scanning for this particular interpersonal pattern. Therefore, every subtle rejection, every frown, and every missed opportunity at empathic responding is interpreted by the client, who is an expert at detecting these transgressions, as fulfilling her unconscious assumptions of how people treat her. The client may then begin to respond negatively to these small but magnified errors on the part of the interviewer by harshly rejecting the accuracy of the interviewer's paraphrases or feeling reflections. Soon the interviewer will be thinking, "I don't know what it is about her, but she is getting under my skin." If the interviewer fails to pick up on this pattern, this misplaced map, the client stands a good chance of making the map fit, and may eventually succeed in eliciting a negative evaluation of herself.

As Freud (1940/1949) stated, "Transference is ambivalent" (p. 66). Transference may manifest itself in positive (e.g., affectionate, liking, or loving) or negative (hostile, rejecting, or cold) attitudes, feelings, or behaviors. Each can be a productive area to work through with the client as therapy progresses. However, during initial stages, the wisest course for interviewers is to be astute observers, noting responses and behaviors that seem to come from old terrain and past relationships in the client's life. It is tempting to attribute overly positive, warm, complimentary attitudes as being legitimate responses by the client to the interviewer's good work, while attributing hostile, rejecting, cold attitudes to a defect in the client's character. Neither attribution should be made early, and probably neither should be made at all. Instead, interviewers need to use their knowledge about transference responses to sharpen their observational skills and to remain accepting and neutral whether transference responses are positive or negative.

We recommend against interpretation of transference early in the therapeutic relationship. Development of adequate rapport and a working relationship should always precede interpretation (Meissner, 1991). Further, interpretation of transference at any point in therapy requires advanced skills and firm theoretical grounding that should be obtained from specialized texts and professional supervision (Weiner, 1975). A generally accepted rule is to notice but ignore mildly positive transference reactions and to deal first with negative transference reactions. Of course, interpretation of both positive and negative transference should be delayed until evidence for the inappropriateness of these reactions becomes clear and more easily interpreted.

Simply being aware that a client is exhibiting transference reactions provides interviewers with potentially important information. A statement of hostility or warmth or some other feeling on the part of the client toward the interviewer can provide an opportunity to explore the client's problem areas more deeply. One can simply respond by saying, "When are some times you have felt similar feelings in the past?" This neatly deflects the comment back to the client rather than necessitating a direct or defensive response by the interviewer such as, "Well, you make me nervous too" or "Sounds like that's an old problem from your past!" After all, if the client is really manifesting a transference reaction, it pertains more to the client and her history than it does to her real relationship with you. The client's reaction can provide an opportunity to explore significant past relationships.

Examining a client's transference reaction gives the interviewer a special opportunity to glimpse the nature of a client's past relationships, and possibly contemporary relationships within the interview hour. Psychoanalytic, interpersonal, and even behavioral clinicians have commented on this distinct advantage of transference reactions (Goldfried & Davison, 1976; Sullivan, 1970). Fenichel (1945) states, "The transference offers the analyst a unique opportunity to observe directly the past of his patient and thereby to understand the development of his conflicts" (p. 30).

One final bit of bottom-line advice about transference. When clients respond to you with strong positive or emotions, *try not to take it personally*. Instead, explore your clients thoughts and feelings about you while maintaining your professional stance. Psychoanalytically oriented interviewers usually refrain from self-disclosure because to talk about one's own real feelings tends to muddy the transference. If clients press psychoanalytic interviewers for a congruent or genuine response, such interviewers usually avoid direct responses by taking shelter behind the professional relationship. For example:

> C: "I like being with you so much that I wish we could get together outside of therapy. I wish we could go out to lunch and do the kinds of things together that friends do."

> I: "I want you to know how important it is for us to maintain our professional relationship. Even if I did have the feelings and impulses you speak of, I wouldn't act on them, because to do so would adversely affect our professional work together."

The psychoanalytic response is much cooler and distant than the person-centered or feminist response in similar situations. Although person-centered and feminist interviewers also would be likely to maintain professional client-therapist boundaries, they would probably be more warm and disclosing in the process:

> C: "I like being with you so much that I wish we could get together outside of therapy. I wish we could go out to lunch and do the kinds of things together that friends do."

> I: "I enjoy our time together here too, and sometimes wish we could extend our time together as well. However, I think to do so would be, in a sense, cheating you out of the opportunity of establishing the kind of relationship we have here outside of therapy. After all, our purpose here is to help you fulfill your relationship potentials outside of therapy, to apply what we've attained here to your current personal life."

As noted above, whether positive or negative, it is important to take your clients' reactions to you with a grain of salt. If you take your clients' emotional reactions to you too personally, you will probably experience strong emotional reactions. In other words, personal reactions to clients often constitute counter-transference.

Countertransference

Countertransference is the inverse of transference; it happens to interviewers rather than clients. Countertransference, like transference, stems from unconsciously held conflicts, attitudes, and motives and is generally outside an interviewer's conscious awareness. Countertransference also consists of emotional, attitudinal, and behavioral responses that are inappropriate in terms of their intensity, frequency, and duration. It is a challenge for professional interviewers to become aware of their own patterns of countertransference (Beitman, 1983; Robbins & Jolkovski, 1987).

While countertransference has some of the same qualities as transference, there are some important differences. Originally, Freud identified the phenomenon as one in which psychotherapists respond to client transference issues. This is certainly the case sometimes. On occasion, clients will treat their interviewer with such open hostility or admiration that the interviewer finds himself caught up in the transference and behaves in ways that are very unusual for him. For example, when author John was a psychology intern, a hospitalized patient once unleashed an unforgettable accusation against him: "You are the coldest, most computerlike person I've ever met. You're like a robot! I talk and you just sit there . . . nodding your head like some machine. I'll bet if I cut open your arms, I'd find wires, not veins!" In most cases, this type of accusation might be considered pure transference. Perhaps the client was responding to John in this manner because historically she had experienced males as emotionally unavailable. On the other hand, as the saying goes, "it takes two to tango." As interviewers, it is important to examine our personal contributions to how our clients react to us.

As John analyzed his reactions to this particular client, he took a hard look at how he was behaving with her and also consulted with colleagues and a supervisor to obtain some objective input. His colleagues reassured John that he was not emotionally cold and aloof, and the supervisor suggested there was something happening in the relationship between John and the patient that was affecting John's behavior during sessions. John was also given an article on countertransference reactions to borderline patients by one colleague, who shared that intellectualizing about his reactions to clients sometimes helped him (Bornstein, 1985).

After thoroughly exploring the issue, John came to several conclusions. First, he was indeed behaving cooler and less emotionally with the client than he generally did with clients. Second, he was frightened of her constant demands for emotional intimacy. He felt inadequate in the face of such demands. Because he believed he could not adequately comfort her, his response was to protect himself by becoming more inhibited and "robotic." Third, countertransference reactions to severely disturbed patients are not unusual. John took solace in the fact that he was not alone in manifesting a countertransference reaction; therapists far more experienced and skilled than he had succumbed to similar reactions.

The manner in which interviewers respond to transference reactions will be unique manifestations of their own unconscious conflicts. Their reactions in turn will elicit unique responses from each client. So the specific relationship distortions produced by transference and countertransference are imbedded in the unique transactions between each interviewer and each client. In the preceding example, some men had truly been emotionally unavailable to the client. Her outraged response usually drew emotional (and sometimes physical) counterattacks from men with whom she had relationships. Her therapist's withdrawal into emotional neutrality was unique for her. In fact, his response to her was the most unemotional she had ever encountered and certainly the most emotionally neutral the therapist had ever provided.

Many theorists go beyond Freud's definition of countertransference to define it more broadly as "any unconscious attitude or behavior on the part of the therapist which is prompted by the needs of the therapist rather than by the needs of the client" (Pipes & Davenport, 1990, p. 161). In other words, countertransference may primarily pertain to an interviewer's unconscious agenda. For example, let's say an interviewer lost his mother to cancer when he was an adolescent and his father's grief was very severe. As a consequence, little emotional support was available to this interviewer for several years when he was a child. The situation eventually improved, his father recovered, and the interviewer's conscious memory consists of a general sense that losing his mother was very difficult. Now, years later, he is a graduate student, conducting his first interviews. Things are fine until a very depressed middle-aged man comes in because he recently lost his wife. What reactions might you expect from the interviewer? What reactions might catch him by surprise?

Freud originally considered transference an impediment to psychotherapy, but later modified his position, suggesting that the analysis of transference, conducted properly, is a crucial therapeutic tool. In contrast, Freud always considered countertransference to be an impediment to psychotherapy. That is, Freud viewed good psychotherapists as having dealt with their own inner conflicts through analysis, so their high levels of self-awareness reduced the likelihood of them experiencing countertransference reactions: "Recognize this counter-transference . . . and overcome it" because "no psycho-analyst goes further than his own complexes and internal resistances permit" (Freud, 1910, p. 145). In fact, research has shown that therapists reputed as excellent are also rated as having better self-awareness and less countertransference potential than therapists considered "average" (Van Wagoner, Gelso, Hayes, & Diemer, 1991, p. 411).

Many contemporary psychoanalysts and object relation theorists have broken with Freud's wholeheartedly negative view of countertransference and believe much is to be gained through the analysis of an interviewer's countertransference reactions (Beitman, 1983; Weiner, 1975): "Any exaggerated, inappropriate feelings, behaviors, thoughts, and fantasies about patients may indicate countertransference distortions which probably deserve self-scrutiny" (Beitman, 1983, p. 83). For example, if a client provokes within you strong and somewhat unusual feelings of fear, disappointment, or sexual attraction, then it may be worthwhile to scrutinize yourself to determine if your emotional response is derived from your own personal history or issues. Only after examining yourself can you assume that your client's behavior is an indicator of the client's usual effect on other people outside of the interview. Countertransference reactions can also teach us much about ourselves, and our underlying conflicts and issues. We believe that countertransference is best viewed as a source of information about ourselves and our clients. Although it may be a hindrance to the interviewing and psychotherapy process and may make it difficult to distinguish our own personal issues from those of our clients, countertransference also has the potential of facilitating the therapeutic process.

Clinicians from various theoretical orientations acknowledge the reality of countertransference. Goldfried and Davison (1976), the authors of *Clinical Behavior Therapy*, offer the following advice: "The therapist should continually observe his own behavior and emotional reactions, and question what the client may have done to bring about such reactions" (p. 58).

Similarly, Beitman (1983) suggests that technique-oriented counselors may fall prey to countertransference and believes that "any technique may be used in the service of avoidance of countertransference awareness" (p. 83). In other words, a clinician may respond to her largely unconscious personal discomfort by repetitively applying a particular therapeutic technique to her clients (e.g., progressive muscle relaxation, mental imagery or thought stopping) without realizing the extent to which she is applying the techniques to deal with her own discomfort (see Box 7-2).

Identification and Internalization

The terms identification and internalization come primarily from psychoanalytic and object-relations theory. However, concepts that share very similar meanings can certainly be found in other schools of thought, a fact that underscores the importance of identification and internalization and their central role in therapeutic relationship development and treatment outcome. For example, behaviorists emphasize the importance of modeling in behavior therapy (Bandura, 1969). And according to social learning theory, we adopt many

---

BOX 7-2 ▄▄▄

Coping with Countertransference

The following guidelines are provided to assist you in coping with countertransference reactions.

1. Recognize that countertransference reactions are normal and inevitable. If you experience strong emotional reactions, persistent thoughts, and behavioral impulses toward a client, it does not mean you are a "sick" person or a "bad" interviewer.
2. If you have strong reactions to a client, consult a colleague or supervisor.
3. Do some additional reading about countertransference. It is especially useful to obtain reading materials pertaining to the particular type of client you're working with (e.g., eating disorder clients, depressed clients, or antisocial clients).
4. If your feelings, thoughts, and behavioral impulses remain despite efforts to deal with them, two options may be appropriate: refer your client to another therapist, or obtain personal psychotherapy to work through the issues that have been aroused within you.

specific behavior patterns because we have watched others perform such behavior previously (i.e., we have seen the behavior modeled). Furthermore, as Myers (1989) states, "we more often imitate those we respect and admire, those we perceive as similar to ourselves, and those we perceive as successful" (p.251). Obviously, parents can be important models to children, but interviewers and psychotherapists may also teach their clients specific behavior patterns through explicit, as well as subtle, modeling procedures.

Psychoanalytic and object-relations theorists use the concepts of identification and internalization to describe what learning theorists consider to be the process associated with modeling (Eagle, 1984; Greenberg & Mitchell, 1983). Specifically, individuals identify with others whom they love, respect, or view as similar to themselves. Through this identification process, individuals come to incorporate or internalize unique and specific ways in which that loved or respected person thinks, behaves, or feels. In a sense, the process of identification and internalization results in the formation of identity; we become like those we have been near, but also those whom we love, respect, or view as similar to ourselves.

The process of identification is enhanced when a client feels his interviewer or therapist has the capacity to understand him at those points where his values run deepest or his distress is most poignant. If this identification is achieved, then superficial dissimilarities will not detract from the therapy relationship. In other words, empathy enhances identification and reduces the importance of surface differences. The client can say internally, "I can identify with this person. Even though we are different in some ways, she understands where I am coming from." More importantly, the client also can then say to himself, "Since she understands and has heard the worst of my fears, *and* she hasn't said it is hopeless, then maybe she will be able to help me figure out my problems." If differences between you and a given client are large and central, identification may be difficult or impossible.

For instance, one client wanted to work on deeply troubling issues she had because she had chosen not to marry, which is unacceptable in her family. She carefully selected a middle-aged female therapist, thinking she would find the basic understanding there that she needed to work on her feelings. Unfortunately, after a few sessions, the therapist interpreted the woman's no-marriage decision as held-over adolescent rebellion. Clearly, there were some basic differences between the therapist's world view and our friend's, which made rapport, empathy, and eventual identification very unlikely.

Identification is the precursor to internalization. Object-relations theorists hypothesize that as we develop as human beings, we internalize components of our various caretakers and others in our early environment. These internalizations then serve as the basis for how we feel about ourselves and how we interact with others (Fairbairn, 1952; Kernberg, 1976; Kohut, 1972, 1977). If we internalize "bad objects" (i.e. abusive parents, neglectful caretakers, vengeful siblings), we then may experience distressing self-perceptions and interpersonal relationships. Psychotherapy is seen as involving a relationship that has the potential to replace maladaptive or bad internalizations with more adaptive or good internalizations, derived primarily from a relatively healthy psychotherapist. Strupp (1983) states:

> [I have] stressed the importance of the patient's identification with the therapist, which occurs in all forms of psychotherapy. Since the internalization of "bad objects" has made the patient "ill," therapy succeeds to the extent that the therapist becomes internalized as a "good object." (p. 481).

Despite the fact that identification and internalization are concepts that emerge primarily in ongoing psychotherapy relationships, these concepts do have some practical relevance for beginning interviewers. We recommend that you explore what types of relationships and interpersonal behaviors you believe are important to the process of identification and internalization. Think about yourself and who you have chosen to emulate. Why have you chosen those particular people? Then, think about yourself and the traits and behaviors you have that clients might consciously or unconsciously adopt.

As Strupp (1983) has pointed out, "since the patient tends to remain loyal to the early objects of his childhood, defending these internalizations against modification, therapy inevitably becomes a struggle" (p. 481). Therefore, the process of identification and internalization is most relevant in long-term psychotherapy cases in which interviewer-client contact is fairly consistent and extensive. For clients to give up their loyalties to early childhood objects and develop loyalties to new, more adaptive objects, long term therapy is required.

Resistance

At times we are at odds with our clients. We want them to talk about their life history, and they want to talk about their last trip to the mall, the Olympic games, or some other matter that seems distant from the therapeutic task. If clients are indeed avoiding the treatment task, yet at the same time wanting its benefits, it is likely that resistance is occurring.

Perhaps the best examples of resistance come from medical science. We avoid going to the dentist even though our tooth aches because we do not want to face the pain involved in drilling or extracting a tooth. We have physical aches and pains, lumps, bumps, or other symptoms, but we do not go to the physician. Perhaps we fear discovery of a disease or disorder, perhaps we fear the potential treatment (e.g., medicine, traction, or surgery), and perhaps we simply do not recognize the severity of our symptoms. Whatever the case, we are engaging in resistance. Children provide excellent examples of resistance (see Box 7-3). They resist shots and bad-tasting medicine, even though some part of them would like to recover from their illness.

Changing one's ways of viewing the world, solving problems, or relating to other people is never easy. People need to proceed at their own pace and to feel safe as they take each step. Resistance often develops when change feels too hard or too fast. Clients slow down, shut down, retreat, engage in meaningless chatter, cry incessantly, don't cry at all, or just drop out of therapy. Since

BOX 7-3

Resistance and the Terrible Twos

Our two-year-old is a master at resistance. It is as natural as breathing for her, and at times, we even have to outsmart her and use her strong resistance to get things done. For instance, we may say "Rylee, you cannot drink any milk with your supper, because only big girls can drink milk." This increases the likelihood that she will drink the milk. While you may not agree with our parenting style, this anecdote may begin to give you a sense of the meaning of resistance. With some clients who are particularly oppositional (such as most two-year-olds or most adolescents), techniques based on reverse psychology or paradoxical intention are often effective (Frankl, 1960).

Resistance occurs in many forms and for many reasons. According to some critics of Freud, resistance was the explanation Freud resorted to when therapy wasn't going well. Whenever client and interviewer are at odds, the problem can casually be attributed to client resistance; this releases the interviewer from responsibility for providing effective treatment.

To return to our two-year-old: We feel her resistance comes from her need to assert her independence. Adolescents often exhibit a similar need; they define themselves not by virtue of who they are but by virtue of who they oppose. Our daughter needs to test her will against something or someone. Being a "big girl" is a powerful motivator, especially since her neighbor friend (someone with whom she has enough rapport, empathy, and similarity to foster identification) is a year older. Rational conversation about why she should drink milk is ineffective. Forcing her to sit until she drinks her milk is aversive, exhausting, and time-prohibitive for everyone involved. So, at times we use her natural need to resist parental commands to turn things around, and we *engage* her resistance to achieve our goals (e.g., "I bet you can't go pee in the big toilet."). On other occasions we utilize her identification with the neighbor to similarly enhance her motivation and achieve our goals (e.g., "The girl next door goes pee-pee on the big toilet.") Of course there are times in the test of wills that our will needs to assert itself directly, but this is not always true when it comes to raising two-year-olds; neither is it always true when interviewing an oppositional client.

resistance, like defense mechanisms, is a method of coping learned early in life and applied when feelings of fear or anxiety are present, it is not easily overcome. One must first recognize that resistance is occurring and then begin looking for the reasons. Unless resistance is noticed and discussed and underlying feelings and fears are addressed, opposing resistance will be futile or counterproductive.

Recognizing Resistance Recognizing behaviors that represent resistance is both simple and complex. It is simple because almost any behavior can represent resistance. Resistance may entail talking too little or too much. It can be manifested in focusing only on the present or by dwelling too much on the past. Recognizing resistance is complex for the same reason: almost any specific behavior pattern, if engaged in excessively, can constitute resistance.

Weiner (1975) identifies five common forms of resistant behavior: "(a) reducing the amount of time spent in the treatment; (b) restricting the amount or range of conversation; (c) isolating the therapy from real life; (d) acting out; and (e) flight into health" (p. 178).

Managing Resistance   With clients who seem resistant right away, sometimes subtly or blatantly paradoxical techniques are useful. For example, an interviewer can indicate that it is quite common for people to feel frightened or reluctant about discussing especially personal or painful topics and therefore it certainly isn't necessary for them to take such a risk right away. This approach encourages resistant clients to prove you wrong, and they may begin working on deeper material. At the same time, clients may come to believe that you know how hard it is for them, and they may begin to feel that their reluctant feelings are normal. This feeling, in turn, may serve to allay client anxiety and thereby remove resistance. More blatant paradoxical techniques are risky, and you should study their use extensively before you attempt them. Even then, we recommend close, experienced supervision.

Another method for dealing with resistance is to talk about the resistance itself, rather than probing more deeply into underlying conflicts or anxieties. Classic psychoanalytic psychotherapists refer to this as interpretation of defense. For our purposes it is sufficient to describe this process as "noticing" the resistance. For example, if resistance is manifest through discussion of irrelevant or inane topics, you may choose to say, "I notice that when we begin talking about your spouse's role in your depressive feelings, you usually begin talking about television shows, how this office is decorated, international issues, and other things that seem unrelated to your relationship with your spouse." Sometimes simply noticing the pattern of resistance functions somewhat like a confrontation and encourages clients to examine their behavior and begin to make constructive changes.

A third method for dealing with resistance involves discussion of what makes the resistance needed. This approach is sometimes easier for clients to tolerate because you are stepping back from the difficult issue itself. To use this technique, ask your clients to talk about what they're experiencing that makes talking openly so difficult. You could say, "Obviously you don't want to talk about your father's death. Rather than talk about it directly, maybe we could talk about what makes talking about it so hard" or "What might happen if you did start talking about your father's death?" Clients may respond to such strategies by continuing to discount the importance of the topic (e.g., "My father died two years ago; it isn't a big deal now.") Or they may be able to acknowledge that "talking about my dad's death makes me feel sad, and I don't want to feel that right now."

Sometimes the most prudent approach is to avoid dealing with resistance during initial interviews. Especially if you are going to have further contact with a particular client, it may be best to simply recognize areas in which the client seems reluctant or resistant and make note of them for later work.

One final point on resistance: It is *not* "bad behavior" on the part of the client. We believe resistance emanates from the very center of a person and is part of the force that gives people stability and predictability in their interactions with others. Without resistance, we would change with each passing whim, ever at the mercy of those around us. Resistance exists because change is often frightening and more difficult than retaining our old ways of being, even when they are maladaptive.

Working Alliance

In addition to involving a real human relationship and sometimes a transference relationship, all professional interviewing involves a working alliance. The term working alliance refers to the explicit or implicit professional contract between client and interviewer. The client consults an interviewer in an effort to reduce symptoms of distress or to achieve a personal goal. Ordinarily, the professional relationship is not established because of social, friendship, or pleasure needs. There is work to be done, and the word alliance suggests collaboration toward reaching a mutually agreed upon goal. Therapeutic interviewing may be experienced as social, friendly, and pleasurable as well as cold, unfriendly, and threatening, but in order to achieve a client's goal, a partnership or alliance must be present. Clients and interviewers need to work together to achieve common goal.

Strupp (1983), among others, has pointed out that the ability of a client to enter into a therapeutic or working alliance is to some extent predictive of the client's amenability to psychotherapy and of the extent of her potential to eventually grow and change, as a function of psychotherapy. In other words, if the client cannot or will not engage in a working alliance of some sort with an interviewer, there is little hope for productive change. Conversely, the more completely the client can enter into such a relationship, the greater her chance for significant change. Many researchers and theorists agree that ironically, people's abilities to enter into productive relationships are determined in large part by the quality of their early interpersonal relations (Mallinckrodt, 1991). Therefore, those most in need of a curative relationship are those least able to enter into one (Strupp, 1983).

Ainsworth and Bowlby's work on attachment has shed light on components of the therapy process (Ainsworth, 1984, 1989; Bowlby, 1969, 1988). As infants begin to explore and learn from their environment, they venture away from their caretakers for short periods, then return to reassure themselves that they are safe and secure and that their caretakers are to be trusted. This venturing and returning is the mark of a secure, healthy attachment. Similar to a caretaker, a therapist provides a safe base from which clients can explore and to which they can return. In optimal situations, all of the relationship factors discussed in this chapter come into play to help interviewers serve as a "safe base" to which clients can return for comfort, support, and a sense of security.

Relationship Variables and Behavioral and Social Psychology

Social and behavioral psychology have contributed to our understanding of interviewer-client relationships. Components of each approach will be discussed in this section, but further reading is necessary to gain a full understanding of the components we mention and the broader concepts underlying them.

Stanley Strong (1968) identified three counselor or interviewer characteristics that make it more likely that clients will accept suggestions and recommendations put forth by their interviewers. Goldstein (1980) has referred to the same characteristics as relationship enhancers because they enhance the therapeutic relationship. These characteristics are expertness, attractiveness, and trustworthiness.

Expertness (Credibility)

As Othmer and Othmer (1989) suggest, empathy and compassion are important, but effective interviewers must also "show expertise" and "establish authority" (p. 34). In other words, no matter how understanding and respectful you are of your client, at some point you must demonstrate you are competent at your craft; you must be perceived by your client as a competent professional who can act, if necessary, with authority. Behaviorists generally refer to this concept as establishing credibility. Goldfried and Davison (1976) state, "The principle underlying this utilization technique is that it reinforces the client's perception of the . . . [therapist's] credibility" (p. 62). Interviewers who are highly credible are usually viewed as being highly expert.

There are many methods for establishing expertness or credibility. Cues to indicating expertness are signs of an interviewer's competence that clients can readily observe (Cormier & Cormier, 1985). These include:

- Your credentials (e.g., certificates, licenses, diplomas, etc.) displayed on office walls
- Shelves of professional books and journals in the office
- An office arrangement that appears conducive to open dialogue
- Professional grooming and attire

Specific interviewer behaviors also communicate expertise, credibility, and authority. Interviewers who use questions liberally tend to be viewed as more controlling and authoritative than those who do not. Interviewers must ask themselves if they want to be viewed as controlling and authoritative; too much expertise and authoritativeness tends to diminish empathy and rapport. Interviewers who use interpretation, confrontation, and other directive techniques are usually viewed as experts, although such techniques can backfire (e.g., clients may discount or discredit such an interviewer if the clients view the techniques as offensive or if the clients find themselves in frequent disagreement with the interviewer).

Othmer and Othmer (1989) identify three strategies for showing expertise. First, they suggest interviewers help clients realize they are not alone with their problems by putting the problems in perspective. For example, you may want to reassure your clients that their problems, although unique, are similar to problems other clients have had and that have been successfully treated. Second, they recommend that interviewers "show knowledge" by communicating to clients an awareness of or familiarity with their particular disorder (p. 35). This strategy often involves naming the client's disorder (e.g., panic disorder, obsessive compulsive disorder, or dysthymia) and helping the client identify symptoms frequently associated with such a disorder. Othmer and Othmer state, "Your knowledge is reassuring for the intellectual, obsessive, or educated patient who bases his trust in you more on how much you know than how much you care . . ." (Othmer & Othmer, 1989, p. 36). Third, they note that interviewers need to deal effectively with their client distrust. For example, when clients express distrust by questioning your credentials, you should be able to manage such challenges effectively (see chapter nine).

Finally, when it comes to expertness, Cormier and Cormier (1985) express an appropriate warning: "Expertness is not in any way the same as being dogmatic, authoritarian, or 'one up.' Expert helpers are those perceived as confident, attentive, and, because of background and behavior, capable of helping the client resolve problems and work toward goals" (p. 50).

Attractiveness

With interviewing, as it is with love, beauty is in the eye of the beholder. However, again as it is with love, there are some standard features that most people view as attractive. Rather than discussing specific behaviors or characteristics of attractive helpers, we thought it would be more useful for you to explore what behaviors and characteristics you would find attractive if you went to a professional interviewer. Note that when we speak of what is attractive, we are referring not only to physical appearance but also to behaviors, attitudes, or personality traits that may or may not be considered attractive. Reflect on the following questions:

1. How you would like your interviewer to look? Would your ideal interviewer be male or female? How would he or she dress? What type of facial expressions would you like to see? Lots of smiles? Do you want an expressive interviewer? One with open body posture? A more serious demeanor? Imagine all sorts of details (e.g., use of make-up, type of shoes, length of hair, etc.).

2. What types of technical interviewing responses would your "attractive interviewer" make? Would she use plenty of feeling reflections, or would she be more directive (e.g., using plenty of confrontations or explanations)?

3. How would an attractive interviewer respond to your feelings? For example, if you started crying in a session, how would you like him to act and what would you like him to say?

4. In your opinion, would an attractive interviewer touch you, self-disclose, call you by your first name, or stay more distant and focus on analyzing your thoughts and feelings within the session?

It is important to be sensitive to issues of interpersonal attractiveness in interviewing. After you think about how you would answer these questions, you may want to ask them of a fellow student or a friend or family member. Although you may find initially that you and your friends or family don't seem to have specific criteria for what constitutes interviewer attractiveness, after discussion people usually discover they have stronger opinions than they originally thought.

Trustworthiness

Trust is defined as an "assured reliance on the character, ability, strength, or truth of someone or something" (Webster's, 1985, p. 1268). Establishing trust is crucial to effective interviewing. Strong (1968) emphasized the importance of interviewers being perceived as trustworthy by their clients, finding that when interviewers are perceived as trustworthy, clients are more likely to believe what they say and to follow their recommendations or advice.

It is not appropriate to express trustworthiness directly in an interview. That is, it is not convincing to tell your clients, "You can trust me." A person saying "trust me" is interpreted by many people as a signal that perhaps the person is not to be trusted. As are empathy and unconditional positive regard, trustworthiness is an interviewer characteristic that is best implied; clients interpret it from interviewer behavior.

Perceptions of interviewer trustworthiness begin with initial client-interviewer contacts. These contacts may be over the telephone or during an initial greeting in the waiting room. We have found the following interviewer behaviors to be associated with trust:

1. Initial introductions that are courteous, gentle, and respectful.
2. Clear and direct explanations of confidentiality and its limits.
3. Acknowledgment of the difficulty associated with coming to a professional interviewer (e.g., Othmer and Othmer's "putting the patient at ease").
4. Manifestations of congruence, unconditional positive regard, and empathy (as discussed previously).

Throughout interviewing and counseling relationships, clients periodically test their interviewers (Fong & Cox, 1983; Horowitz, Marmar, Krupnick, Wilner, Kaltreider, and Wallerstein, 1984). In a sense, clients "set up" their interviewers to determine whether they are trustworthy. For example, children who have been sexually abused often immediately behave seductively when they meet an interviewer. They may sit in your lap, rub up against you, or tell you they love you. Some, once left alone with an interviewer for the first time, even request the interviewer to undress. These behaviors can be viewed as blatant tests of interviewer trustworthiness (i.e., the behaviors serve to ask, Are you going to abuse me too?).

Feminist Relationship Variables

Feminist theory and psychotherapy emphasizes the importance of establishing an "egalitarian relationship" between client and interviewer (Brown & Brodsky, 1992, p. 52). The type of egalitarian relationship preferred by feminist interviewers is one characterized by mutuality and empowerment.

Mutuality

Mutuality refers to a sharing process; that is, power, decision making, goal selection, and learning, are shared. Although various psychotherapy orientations (especially person-centered) consider treatment a mutual process wherein clients and therapists are open and human with one another, nowhere are egalitarian values and the concept of mutuality emphasized more than in feminist theory and therapy (Nutt, Hampton, Folks, & Johnson, 1990).

The following example illustrates this concept: Betty comes in for an initial interview. The interviewer has been trained in traditional psychoanalytic techniques and is supervised by a psychoanalytically oriented supervisor. The interviewer says, "Tell me about what brings you in at this time."

Betty begins crying almost immediately and says roughly the following: "My mother is dying of cancer. She lives two hundred miles away but wants me there all the time. I am finishing my Ph.D. in Chemistry and my dissertation chair is going on sabbatical in three months. I have two undergraduate courses to teach, and my husband has decided he isn't sure he wants this relationship. I don't know what to do. I don't know how to prioritize. I feel like I am disappearing. There is hardly anything left of me. I am afraid . . . . I feel like a failure being in therapy, but . . . " Betty cries a while longer.

The interviewer feels the overwhelming sadness and fear and confusion of these situations. She is tempted to cry herself. Instead, she says something like, "All of these things leave you feeling diminished, afraid, perhaps like you're losing a sense of who you are. Being in therapy adds to the sense of defeat."

Betty says, "Yes, my mother always said therapists were for weak folks. Her term was 'addle-brained'. My husband refuses to see anyone. He feels if I would stay home and drop this education thing, we could be happy together again. Sometimes I feel that even my dissertation chair would be happier if I just gave it up."

The interviewer has a host of choices regarding an interpretation, but she chooses, "The important people in your life somehow want you to do things differently than you are doing."

The preceding interactions are not necessarily bad. However, if both Betty and the interviewer stayed with this modality, Betty would finish up the interview perhaps seeing a bit more about herself and her patterns in life, but she would know very little about her therapist and she would feel, generally, that the therapist was the provider of insight, while she, Betty, was the provider of material (i.e., problems).

In a more mutuality-oriented interaction, when the interviewer felt overwhelming sadness, fear and confusion, she might say something like, "You know, those are some very difficult situations. Just hearing about all that makes me feel a little bit of what you must be feeling."

Betty might then say, "Really? Geez, that makes me feel better. See, my mom says people who come to therapy are 'addle-brained', and my husband thinks the whole thing is just because I am too busy outside the home . . . and I even get the same sort of thing from my dissertation chair."

The interviewer might then say, "It is hard to decide to work out some of your problems in therapy, or to even keep going when you feel those close to you disapprove somehow."

The differences in responses may not seem huge, but the underlying framework of the interviewer-client relationship being built in mutuality-oriented therapies contrasts sharply with traditional frameworks. The client is not excluded from the emotional reactions of the interviewer. She is not given the message that she is the bearer of problems while the interviewer is somehow the bearer of insight. Instead, the groundwork is being laid for a relationship that includes honest self-disclosure on the part of the interviewer and that may, later in therapy, even include times when the client observes and comments on patterns in the interviewer's behavior. In a mutuality-oriented relationship, interviewers and therapists are ready to respond to such offers from clients in a genuine manner that neither merely reflects back client statements nor interprets them as coming from client pathological needs.

When interviewers engage in mutuality, they usually do so for the ultimate purpose of empowering clients. Their clients will see therapy as a working relationship in which they are equal members rather than subordinates. While mutuality does not entirely alter the fact that a certain amount of authority must rest with the therapist, it actively works to teach clients how to respond to that authority with a sense of personal worth, and, in fact, with their own personal authority. These types of interactions often result in a growing sense of personal power within clients.

Empowerment

Most therapies have as underlying goals the eventual well-being, health, and growth of clients. However, therapies vary in the routes they take to reach these goals, and therefore different approaches will inevitably leave clients with different beliefs as to how they "got better." The interviewer who begins therapy with an emphasis on authenticity and mutuality usually has, as an ultimate goal, the hope that clients will attribute their gains, growth, and life improvements to their own efforts and to the strength and potential that reside within them. Rather than set up an atmosphere that separates client from therapist along the lines of dependency or neediness versus authority or expertise, the interviewer who is interested in empowerment actively works to affirm that both participants in the therapy process are human and therefore more similar than different.

While interviewers certainly have skills and knowledge that clients may not have, in feminist therapy these skills are viewed as useful tools clients can avail themselves of to help themselves grow. Clients understand that there are no magical formulas and no authority figure to instruct them, to be obeyed, or to offer mysterious insights previously unavailable to them. Instead, interviewers interact with clients in ways that serve to validate clients' life experiences and attempts at solving their own problems. Interviewers recognize that often people who come to therapy do so in part because of the pressures, discrimination, and mistreatment we all experience in varying degrees as we interact with society at large. These experiences of disenfranchisement are acknowledged for what they are rather than interpreted as something intrapsychically askew in the client.

Initially, incorporating mutuality, authenticity, and empowerment into the interviewing relationship may be threatening to the interviewer. In some ways it is a very advanced skill, requiring knowing how to be authentic without burdening the client; being able to welcome and enhance a sense of mutuality while maintaining enough control so that the hope for change via the vehicle of therapy is not lost; and finally, having the patience and wisdom to allow clients to find their own way, thus empowering them, rather than issuing edicts on how to become empowered.

Integrating Relationship Variables

The therapeutic interviewing relationship variables discussed in this chapter should not be considered an exhaustive list. And, since the variables discussed are advocated by different schools of thought, it should not be surprising that some of the variables oppose one another. For example, although mutuality and expertness are not exact opposites, a high level of interviewer expertness is usually associated with a low level of interviewer-client mutuality. The purpose of this chapter is to enhance your awareness of important relationship variables in interviewing, rather than convince you that a single type of therapeutic relationship is preferred. We believe that person-centered, feminist, and behavioral-oriented interviewers should all be sensitive to potential transference, countertransference, and other reactions within sessions. Similarly, psychoanalytic interviewers enhance their effectiveness if they are at least attentive to issues involving congruence, empathy, and empowerment.

Chapter Summary

The early work of Carl Rogers (1942, 1951, 1961) articulated the importance of relationship variables in psychotherapy. Similarly, therapeutic interviewing is characterized, to some degree, by the formation of a special type of relationship between interviewer and client. This chapter explores many different aspects of the therapeutic relationship that are sometimes important in therapeutic interviewing.

All theoretical orientations emphasize the need for establishing rapport with clients. There are many different tactics or strategies interviewers utilize to establish rapport. Some of these strategies address client fears about therapy through education, reassurance, courteous introductions, conversation, and flexibility.

Rogers identified three core conditions that he believed were necessary and sufficient for personal growth and development to occur: congruence, unconditional positive regard, and accurate empathy. Each of these concepts is complex and difficult to put into operation. In this chapter specific examples and guidelines are provided to help interviewing students understand how to implement these important behaviors with clients. For the most part, it is inappropriate to be completely congruent or authentic with clients all of the time. It is also inappropriate to try to communicate unconditional positive regard and accurate empathy directly to clients.

Several relationship variables derived from interpersonal and psychoanalytic theories are potentially greatly influential in therapeutic interviews. These include, but are not limited to, transference, countertransference, identification, internalization, resistance, and working alliance. Each of these variables is defined, and examples are provided to help interviewers detect and manage them. Further reading and supervised clinical experience is needed before interviewers should be expected to deal effectively with these particular relationship variables. Consequently, this chapter aims primarily to help interviewers recognize when these variables are affecting the therapeutic process.

Behavioral and social psychologists also have examined interviewing processes and identified several variables associated with effective interviewing and counseling. Specifically, it is very important for interviewers to be perceived as credible experts who are personally and professionally attractive and trustworthy. This chapter explores methods that interviewers can use to present themselves as having high levels of expertness, attractiveness, and trustworthiness.

Finally, feminist theorists and psychotherapists emphasize the importance of establishing relationships between interviewers and clients that incorporate the concepts of mutuality and empowerment. They believe open, mutual relationships facilitate therapeutic processes and help empower clients to be their own advocates and to attribute their growth to the power that resides within themselves.

It is impossible for interviewers to have high amounts of all of these relationship variables in any single interview. Therefore, it is suggested that interviewers examine the variables described in this chapter and develop an awareness of their presence (or absence) in the clinical setting.

Suggested Readings

Fitzgerald, L. F., & Nutt, R. (1986). The Division 17 principles concerning the counseling/psychotherapy of women: Rationale and implementation. *Counseling Psychologist, 14,* 180–216. APA's Division of Counseling Psychology addresses issues of women who receive counseling or psychotherapy.

Fong, M. L., & Cox, B. G. (1983). Trust as an underlying dynamic in the counseling process: How clients test trust. *Personnel and Guidance Journal, 62,* 163–166. This article lists and describes six common ways in which clients test their counselors' trust.

Greenson, R. R. (1965). The working alliance and the transference neurosis. *Psychoanalytic Quarterly, 34,* 155–181. This article presents Greenson's now classic discussion of the working alliance.

Othmer, E., & Othmer, S. C. (1989). *The clinical interview using DSM-III-R.* Washington DC: American Psychiatric Press. Chapter 2 of this very practical text discusses strategies for developing rapport.

Rogers, C. R. (1961). *On becoming a person.* Boston: Houghton-Mifflin. This text contains much of Rogers's thinking regarding congruence, unconditional positive regard, and empathy.

8

AN OVERVIEW OF THE INTERVIEW PROCESS

Structural Models

The Introduction
    Telephone Contact
    Initial Face-to-Face Meeting
    Conversation and Small Talk
    Educating Clients and Evaluating Their Expectations

The Opening
    The Interviewer's Opening Statement
    The Client's Opening Response
    Evaluating Client Verbal Behavior During the Opening

The Body
    Sources of Clinical Judgment: Making Inferences
    Defining Psychological and Emotional Disorders

The Closing
    Reassuring and Supporting Your Client
    Summarizing Crucial Themes and Issues
    Instilling Hope
    Guiding and Empowering Your Client
    Tying Up Loose Ends

Termination
    Watching the Clock
    Guiding or Controlling Termination
    Facing Termination

Chapter Summary

Suggested Readings

It is good to have an end to journey towards; but it is the journey that matters, in the end.—URSULA K. LE GUIN, The Left Hand of Darkness

The therapeutic interview cannot be and should not be an interaction that runs along a prescribed path from point A to point B. True, we can dissect each component of the interview, and in fact, we do so in this book; but in the end, an interview should be a smooth and continuous process. As we have suggested before, conducting an interview is in many ways like learning other new skills, such as dancing or driving an automobile. This is particularly true when it comes to analyzing structural components of an interview. Most beginning interviewers rigidly conform to taking the proper step at the proper time. Alexander (1990) refers to this conformance as a "lock-step approach." For example, as an interviewer you may find yourself thinking, I need to establish rapport here. . . . Now it is time to elicit information. . . . Time to prepare for closing. In actual interviewing, therapists do not clearly shift from rapport building to information gathering; experienced interviewers gather information, maintain rapport, and begin to deal with closure at the same time, but they did not begin their careers with such an ability (Tracey, Hays, Malone, & Herman, 1988).

Human interaction is guided by spoken and unspoken rules that vary depending on variables such as setting, purpose, individual differences, and cultural differences. Most of the time we are unaware of the sequences involved in negotiating our way through the day. We don't sit down and think about it, we just know the correct steps to take when we get to work or go to the laundromat or attend a surprise party. When meeting someone, we know when to say what and when to stand or sit or offer a hand for a handshake. On those occasions when we are not so sure of what is expected, we are ill at ease; we may even actively avoid such situations. The way we handle each step of these interactions reveals things about us, and while we are revealing parts of ourselves, we are also monitoring other people's choices and making judgments about them. This chapter helps clarify some of the unspoken rules associated with therapeutic interviewing. If you know the rules, you will expend less energy wondering what you should be doing next and more energy on understanding, evaluating, and helping your clients.

Structural Models

Just as many of our social interactions have a normal, implicit sequence, ritual, or set of phases, so does the therapeutic interview. Shea (1988) has identified these phases as:

1. The introduction
2. The opening
3. The body
4. The closing
5. The termination

We find Shea's five-part distinction helpful partly because it enlarges on the more common "beginning, middle, and end" schema sometimes referred to in training texts (Benjamin, 1981; Moursund, 1990). Shea's model also remains fairly generic and atheoretical; it may be applied to virtually all interviewing situations, regardless of the interviewer's orientation. Therefore, we will use Shea's five phases as a basis for this chapter. We will outline and discuss the interviewer tasks and potential pitfalls associated with each interview phase.

In adopting Shea's format, we are not implying that his is the most important, inclusive, or descriptive of those available in the literature. Several other models are worth scrutiny. For example, Foley and Sharf (1981) describe sessions as involving five sequential interviewer duties that act as criteria for effective interviewing:

1. Putting the patient at ease
2. Eliciting information
3. Maintaining control
4. Maintaining rapport
5. Bringing closure

Like all models in the literature, Foley and Sharf's (1981) model is similar to the model developed by Shea.

One of the more descriptive stage approaches to interview structure has been put forth by Ivey (1988), who identifies five stages or components within a typical therapeutic interview:

1. Establishing rapport and structuring
2. Gathering information, defining the problem, and identifying assets
3. Determining outcomes (setting goals)
4. Exploring alternatives and confronting client incongruities
5. Encouraging generalization of ideas and skills to situations outside therapy

As you compare the three models presented above, you probably notice similarity but not uniformity among them. The variety is fortunate because interviewers and clients vary in their approaches and responses to therapeutic interviews; each has an individual sense of timing and propriety.

The astute interviewer allows her clients to set the pace as much as possible because observing this process yields valuable information to the interviewer. Setting the pace themselves also provides clients with a sense of control and safety; they do not feel rushed from stage to stage. Ideally, interviewers guide clients gently forward through each step of the interview while allowing them to rush through or linger on a given point as much as they need. The interviewer is responsible for managing the essential elements of a good interview, seeing that it does not run overtime, and ensuring that it covers what is necessary given the setting and the expectations. However, the less overtly and rigidly this responsibility is exercised, the better. In other words, be organized and attentive to interview structure while remaining flexible.

The Introduction

Shea (1988) defines the introduction phase of an interview as follows: "The introduction begins when the clinician and the patient first see one another. It ends when the clinician feels comfortable enough to begin an inquiry into the reasons the patient has sought help" (p. 56). The introduction phase of an interview mainly involves "putting the patient at ease" (see Foley & Sharf, 1981; Othmer & Othmer, 1989; and chapter 7 of this text), or, as Shea (1988) words it, "decreasing the patient's anxiety" (p. 56).

Telephone Contact

In some situations the introduction phase actually begins before you see the client. You may set up your initial contact with the client by telephone. Whether you do this yourself or it is done by a receptionist, you must be aware that the therapeutic relationship all begins with the initial contact. The phone call, the paperwork, and the clarity and warmth with which clients are greeted can serve to put them at ease or to confuse and intimidate.

Interviewers vary greatly in how they inform their clients of financial arrangements, session lengths, and intake procedures. Some leave these duties to the receptionist. Some provide the information in written form; some go over it verbally with the client themselves before the first session; others consider providing these facts as part of the interview or therapy process and deal with it during the interview. One therapist we knew put great emphasis on the manner in which his clients inquired about fees. The important point is that the very first contact, whether via mail, phone, or questionnaire or in person, is a process that may crucially affect your relationship with potential clients.

The following brief transcript illustrates a typical initial telephone contact:

I: Hello, I'm trying to reach Barry Johnson.

C: That's me.

I: Barry, this is Chelsea Elander, I'm a therapist at the university counseling center. I understand you might be interested in counseling, and I'm calling to see if you'd like to set up an appointment.

C: Yes, I filled out a questionnaire, I guess you got my number from that.

I: That's right. If you're still interested in coming for counseling we should set up a time to meet. Do you have any particular days and times that are best for you?

C: I guess Tuesday or Thursday afternoons look best . . . after 2 p.m., but before 6 p.m.

I: How about this Thursday, the 24th, at 4 p.m.?

C: Sounds fine to me.

I: I guess since you were in the counseling center to fill out a questionnaire, you know how to find the center.

C: Yep, I just go to the same building.

I: Yes. Just be sure to check in with the receptionist when you arrive. In fact, you might want to come a few minutes early. There are a few forms to fill out. Is that OK?

I: Sure.

C: OK, then, I guess we're all set. I'll look forward to meeting you on Thursday the 24th at 4 p.m.

C: OK, see you then.

Note several points in the dialogue. First, scheduling the initial appointment is the first collaborative activity that occurs between interviewer and client. This activity begins the process of establishing a working alliance. You will find it is very difficult to schedule an appointment with some prospective clients, perhaps because of the common difficulty of finding a meeting time for two busy people, or perhaps because of client issues such as rigidity, resistance, or ambivalence about coming for counseling. The preceding dialogue illustrates a simple, straightforward scheduling procedure. Such will not always be the case.

Second, the interviewer clearly identifies herself, her status (i.e., therapist), and her place of employment. Depending upon the situation, you may want to be even more clear about these facts. For example, when students in our upper-level interviewing courses must contact the volunteers they are to interview, we have the students say "I'm a student in Psych 455, and I received your name and number from Dr. Sommers-Flanagan."

Third, the interviewer checks to make sure the client knows how to get to the interview location. If you are calling a new client and there is a possibility the client will not know how to reach the interviewing office, you should prepare clear directions before getting on the telephone.

Fourth, the interviewer asks the potential client what days and times would be best for him. If your schedule is particularly busy, you may want to first identify days and times when you have openings. Whatever the case, it is not necessary to disclose specific information regarding why you cannot meet at a particular time. For example, you should *not* say, "Oh, I can't meet then because I have to pick up my daughter from school" or "I'm in class then." Such disclosures are not necessary and are not facilitative during an initial telephone contact. They set a more social than professional tone. Especially at first, it is better to say as little as possible about yourself personally.

Fifth, the interviewer closes by repeating the appointment time and noting that she's looking forward to meeting the client. She also clarifies exactly what the client should do when arriving at the center (i.e., check in with the receptionist). Avoid saying things like, "Check in with the receptionist and I'll be right out to meet you," because you don't know when the client will arrive. If he arrives twenty-five minutes early, you're stuck—either you meet him twenty-five minutes early or you end up not following through with what you said over the telephone.

Overall, be organized and prepared when making initial telephone contact with potential clients. You may want to practice telephone conversations in class or with a supportive friend or family member. If you are prepared and have practiced, you can attend to how clients present themselves and to the task of working together to schedule an appointment.

Initial Face-to-Face Meeting

Privacy is one of the first issues to consider when you first meet a client face to face. Most clinics and agencies have public waiting rooms with seating for more than one person at a time. It is more difficult to keep one's identity anonymous in these settings than in the surroundings maintained by single clinicians in private practice. It is incumbent upon interviewers who work in relatively public settings to give consideration to how they can best respect their clients' needs for privacy. The preference of author Rita Sommers-Flanagan is to have the receptionist point out or describe a new client so she can walk up and say the client's name in a quiet, friendly voice not easily overheard by others in the room. Rita then smiles and says "I'm Rita," or "I'm Dr. Sommers-Flanagan." She assesses quickly if the client might welcome a handshake, and if so, offers her hand. Otherwise, she simply says "Come back this way," and leads the client to the office.

An array of issues are associated with first impressions. You need to be aware of how much hinges on the first impressions and how much information you can gain by being especially observant of your client's behavior during the first few moments of your meeting. It is likely that your client will be nervous, although some may be excited, some may be angry, and some might like you to believe they couldn't care less about seeing a therapist. The reaction depends partly on whose idea it was for the client to be there. Let's assume a new client of yours is nervous. You have the opportunity to observe how she expresses nervousness. Is she quiet? Loud? Is she smoking or clinging to a coffee cup? Is she chewing her nails? Is she formal, informal, talkative, withdrawn, pale, or flushed? These are among behaviors that you can use to begin to form your composite impression of the client. The initial meeting may begin to give you a sense of how your client deals with anxiety and stress.

As you are observing your client's behavior, the client is sizing up you and the situation. In order to increase the consistency of how various clients perceive them, some professionals always follow an introductory ritual that includes

- Shaking hands
- Offering coffee
- Chatting about the weather or some other trivial subject as they go to the interview room

A ritual can be comforting, and because you can follow it without thinking, it frees you to be more observant. A ritual also involves standardization. Standardization (described in more detail in Box 8-1) strengthens your ability to make inferences from your observations. You can design your ritual to reflect a warm, welcoming, professional image. Not every interviewer uses a standardized ritual, however. Author Rita has never established an exact ritual; she likes to size up clients individually and offer what seems to be called for. Sometimes, this is a firm handshake. On other occasions, less contact seems wiser.

This issue leads to the issue of how to address your clients. The first rule is to go with the "base rates"—the known norm for the group of which the client is a part. For example, when you are meeting with a middle-age or older man, it is a safe bet that he will be comfortable being addressed as "Mr." Later when you sit down in the room with your client, if you're not sure whether you've addressed him in a proper manner, it may be appropriate to ask how he likes to be addressed. If he answers with a sexually suggestive nickname, you should be aware this is a very unusual phenomenon, and one about which you should notify a supervisor right away.

Other groups have less clear base rates. For example, women over forty may strongly prefer being referred to as "Ms." or "Mrs." so it is difficult to know in advance which to try. You may choose to go with the woman's entire name: "You're Susan Smith." "Ms." may offend less women over forty than "Mrs." Finally, if you sense you've used the wrong strategy, you should ascertain once you are in the interviewing room whether you've offended your client (e.g., "I noticed you corrected me when I referred to you as Ms. Smith; you'd rather be called Mrs. Smith?"). The effort to address clients as they would like to be addressed communicates respect and acceptance.

The second rule of addressing clients is when in doubt about what introductory approach the client might prefer, choose the least offensive alternative.

BOX 8-1 ——

Standardized Introductions

In some ways, it is best to have a standardized introductory procedure to use with all clients, because the more consistent you are, the more certain you can be that individual differences in how clients present themselves reflect actual differences in their personality styles. If you vary your introduction ritual based on your mood or other factors, then clients may have different reactions to you based on differences in *your* approach to them. In other words, their reactions to you may represent something about you rather than something about them. Standardization is a part of good psychological science. If you have a standard approach, you increase the reliability of your observations.

On the other hand, as an interviewer, you do not want to be sterile, mechanistic, and ingenuine in your approach to clients. A strictly standardized approach probably comes across to clients as ingenuine or distant. Similarly, it is important to respond not only to each client's unique individual characteristics, but also to typical differences found within social or cultural groups. For example, the exact same introductory approach would usually not be equally effective with male adolescents and female senior citizens. Individuals in these two groups usually have significantly different styles of relating to others. To assume you can treat them identically during the introduction phase of an interview is a mistake. Keep in mind the fact that the introductory phase is crucial to establishing rapport with clients. Excessive standardization will adversely affect rapport. As noted previously, when dealing with different types of individuals in the introductory phase of an interview, you should follow two general guidelines:

- Go with the base rates.
- Choose the least offensive alternative.

Some beginning interviewers are eventually put off by the fact that standardization and routine creep into the interviewing process. After all, we are dealing with unique individuals and shouldn't we give each of them a unique and human response? Our answer to that question is "no" and "yes." No, it is not necessary to give each client a completely different response just for the sake of avoiding ritual or consistency. And yes, we should give each client a human response.

For example, author John almost always begins first sessions with a description of the limits of confidentiality and a discussion of how an initial interview is sometimes uncomfortable because it involves two strangers getting to know one another (see chapter 7 for a sample of this introductory statement). Although this is part of his standardized introduction, he sincerely means what he is saying each time; he genuinely wants each client to understand the concept of confidentiality and its limits. Simply because John says virtually the same statement to hundreds of clients does not mean he is being ingenuine in saying it.

We advocate a balance between standardization and flexibility. Be consistent and yet be genuine, which means you must feel free to deviate from your standard routine when it seems clinically appropriate.

——

Addressing a woman over forty by first and last name is an example of a least offensive alternative. Another example, this time with regard to shaking hands, is to wait until the client either reaches out for your hand or simply stands up and begins moving toward your office. Author John Sommers-Flanagan's usual approach is to wait for the client to reach forward. This strategy has helped him avoid trying to shake hands with people who prefer not to. When his clients are children, however, John almost always reaches out and shakes hands or asks for a high five. This choice is based on a combination of the base rate and least offensive principles.

Conversation and Small Talk

There are a number of topics of small talk that we feel are relatively safe and nonjudgmental and that serve to put the client at ease. Some of these are the weather, recent news events, sporting event outcomes, changes in office decor or location, and parking availability. However, *no* comment is without "baggage" in terms of meaning. Some topics that people commonly address in social situations should not be discussed in the interview situation as icebreakers. Comments on clients' clothing can seem innocuous to you, but in fact may be interpreted as judgmental, parental, or overly personal. After you are well acquainted with a client, a change in clothing style may be useful therapy material. Initially, it is wise to stay away from comments on clothing, hair style, perfume, or jewelry.

Also, comments regarding similarities between you and your client usually are not warranted, as such comments may be based on your own social needs and not on the client's therapeutic needs. In social situations, it is common to share and compare ages of offspring, marital status, likes and dislikes of food, exercise, political figures, and so on. You may feel an urge, upon seeing the wife of your client holding a toddler, to say something like, "We have a little one at home too," or "Our little girl likes that same Sesame Street book." If your client is carrying a bike helmet, you may feel tempted to say, "I commute on my bike too." Again, interviewing does not constitute a normal social situation. While you must try to put your client at ease and present a warm, reassuring image, you must do so through a rather narrow selection of appropriate comments and actions. We do not mean to say that interviewers should never comment on similarities between themselves and their clients. We simply mean that interviewers should exercise restraint in terms of their own social urges or impulses, because following through on every social urge or impulse does not constitute the most therapeutically effective approach. For example, Weiner (1975) states:

> Just as a patient will have difficulty identifying the real person in a therapist who hides behind a professional facade and never deviates from an impersonal stance, so too he will see as unreal a therapist who ushers him into the office for a first visit saying, "Hi, my name is Fred, and

I'm feeling a little anxious because you remind me of a fellow I knew in college who always made me feel I wasn't good enough to compete with him." (p. 28)

Educating Clients and Evaluating Their Expectations
The final tasks of the introduction phase involve client education and evaluation of client expectations. Several rules apply. First, as we have noted previously, clients should be informed of the limits of confidentiality. This process should be simple, straightforward, and interactive. You should be clear about the concept of confidentiality prior to beginning an interview so that you can explain it clearly (see chapter 3, Box 3.4). You should check with clients to determine if they understand the nature of confidentiality and its limits. A conversation similar to the following is recommended:

I: "Have you heard the term confidentiality before?"

C: "Uh, I think so."

I: "Well, let me briefly describe what counselors mean by confidentiality. Basically it means that what you say in here stays in here. It means that what you talk about with me is private; I won't be discussing the information with other people. However, there are some limits to confidentiality that counselors and psychotherapists adhere to. For example, if a client tells me information that leads me to believe she is a danger to herself or someone else, then I am obligated to break confidentiality and inform the proper authorities of the situation. Similarly, if I am given information pertaining to child abuse or neglect, I am also required to report such information. Also, if you and I agree that it would be useful or necessary for me to provide information about you to another person, usually a professional, such as an attorney or physician, then I can go ahead and provide information if you give me your written permission. So although there are some specific limits, basically what you say in here is private. Do you have any questions about what I've said about confidentiality?

In some cases after such an explanation, clients make a joke (e.g., "Well, I'm not a child abuser.") to lighten up the situation. Other times they will respond with specific questions (e.g., "Will you be keeping records about what I say to you?" or "Who else has access to your files?"). When clients ask questions about confidentiality, it may mean they are especially conscious of trust issues. It may also mean they have had some suicidal or homicidal thoughts and are wanting to further clarify the limits of what they can say to you. Whatever the case, as a professional interviewer you should respond to their questions directly and clearly (e.g., "Yes, I will be keeping records about our meetings, but only myself and the receptionist have access to these files. And the receptionist has agreed to abide by the same ethical principles regarding confidentiality as I have."). Finally, if you are being supervised and your supervisor has access to your case notes and tape recordings, you should make that clear in your initial statement to your client. For example:

> "Because I'm employed in a training clinic, I have a supervisor who checks over my work, and sometimes there are group discussions of particular cases. However, in each of these situations the purpose is to enable me to provide you with the best services possible. No information about you will leave this clinic."

The second rule with regard to client education and evaluation of client expectations is that clients should be informed of the purpose of the interview. Perhaps the classic line to avoid in this respect was offered by Benjamin (1981): "We both know why you are here" (p. 14). As Benjamin (1981) suggests, this type of introductory line can destroy any hope of initial rapport. Instead of a cryptic statement about the purpose of the interview, strive to be clear, straightforward, and honest.

Obviously, the type of explanation you provide regarding the purpose of an interview varies depending upon the type of interview you are conducting. A general statement regarding the purpose of the interview helps put clients at ease by clarifying their expectations of what might be a new experience. Author John once conducted an assessment interview to help determine whether or not a particular couple would make suitable adoptive parents. Although the clients already knew the purpose of the interview, John made the following statement:

> "The purpose of this interview is for me help the adoption agency you're working with evaluate qualities that might affect your performance as adoptive parents. I like to start this type of interview in an open-ended manner by having you describe why you're interested in adoption and having each of you talk about what kind of person you are, but eventually I'll get more specific by inquiring about your own childhoods. Finally, toward the end of the interview, I will ask you specific questions about your parenting attitudes and abilities. Do you have any questions for me before we begin?"

The third rule is checking to see if client expectations for the interview are consistent with your expectations or purpose. Usually a simple direct question, such as the one at the end of the previous example, serves this purpose. You may also ask, "Do you see the purpose of the interview as similar to what I've stated?" In essence, you want to be sure not only that your clients understand the purpose of the interview but that they feel free to ask any questions about the process you've outlined.

TABLE 8-1 Checklist For Introduction Phase

Interviewer Task	Relationship Variables
___ 1. Schedule a mutually agreed upon meeting time.	Working alliance, positive regard, mutuality
___ 2. Introduce yourself.	Congruence, attractiveness, positive regard
___ 3. Identify how the client likes to be addressed.	Positive regard, empowerment
___ 4. Engage in conversation or small talk.	Empathy, rapport
___ 5. Direct client to an appropriate seat (perhaps let the client choose).	Expertness, empathy, rapport
___ 6. Present your credentials or status (as appropriate).	Expertness
___ 7. Explain confidentiality.	Trustworthiness, working alliance
___ 8. Explain the purpose of the interview.	Working alliance, expertness
___ 9. Check client expectations of interview for similarity to or compatibility with your purpose.	Working alliance, mutuality, empowerment

The Opening

Shea (1988) writes that the opening begins with an interviewer's first questions about the client's current concerns and ends when the interviewer begins determining the focus of the interview by asking specific questions about specific topics.

In Shea's model, the opening is a nondirective phase of the interview lasting about five to eight minutes. During this phase the interviewer utilizes mainly basic attending skills and nondirective listening responses to encourage client disclosure. The main task of the interviewer is to stay out of the way so that clients can tell their story in their own words.

You arrive in the office. You allow the client to choose a seat. As discussed previously (see chapter 3) even this choice can provide information. (Once author Rita Sommers-Flanagan had a client choose to sit down at her desk.) There are no universal interpretations of behaviors clients engage in during any of the interview phases, especially the introduction; that is, no single behavior holds the same meaning for all clients. All interpretations (or in more scientific terms, inferences) require substantial data or evidence from several sources or behaviors. The purpose of closely observing client behavior is to begin making hypotheses. It is through forming hypotheses regarding the meaning of your clients' behavior that you eventually come closer in your understanding of what clients are communicating to you about themselves.

The Interviewer's Opening Statement

The opening statement is a signal to the client that small talk, introductions, and information giving about confidentiality and purpose of the interview are over and it is time to begin the interview. An opening statement consists of the interviewer's first direct inquiry into what has brought the client to seek professional assistance. The statement can usually be delivered in a calm, easy manner, and in such a way that it does not feel like an interruption in the flow of your contact. However, occasionally, you will need to be assertive in stopping the chatter and focusing the interview.

One of our mentors had a phrase he invariably used as his favorite opening statement. It was "Tell me all of what brought you here at this time." The elements of import include:

1. *Tell Me:* The interviewer is expressing personal interest in hearing what the client has to say. In addition, the interviewer is making it clear that the client is the one responsible for doing the telling.

2. *All of What:* The interviewer is being inclusive, that is, signalling that it is alright to include the details. The client is not directed to tell about only one issue.

3. *Brought You Here:* This phrase acknowledges that coming to the clinic or to see you is an action that is out of the ordinary. It suggests the client tell you about a precipitating event that stimulated the client to seek help.

4. *At This Time:* This helps the client direct her comments to the pertinent factors leading up to the decision to come in. The interviewer is aware that the decision to seek help has been made based not only on causes but on timing. Sometimes a problem will have existed for years, but the time was never quite right to seek help until now.

While you may not be comfortable with these exact words, it is important to think about what you can say to begin that will convey some or all of these elements to your clients.

There are a variety of approaches to formulating the opening statement. Essentially, the opening statement should be composed of either an open question (i.e., a question beginning with "what" or "how") or a gentle prompt. The opening statement described above is an example of a gentle prompt, which is a request that usually begins with the words "tell me."

Other popular opening statements include the following:

1. What brings you here?
2. How can I be of help?
3. I would like it if you began by telling me some things about yourself, or your situation, that you believe are important.
4. So, how's it going? (Ivey, 1988).
5. What are some of the stresses you have been coping with recently? (Shea, 1988).

As you examine these potential openings, think about how you would respond to each one. You may also want to try them out in practice interviews or role-plays. The important point to realize is that your opening statement will influence how your clients begin talking about themselves or their problems; therefore, you should consciously choose what statement you will use for your opening. For example, if you want to hear about stressors and coping responses, use the sample opening provided by Shea (1988). The opening recommended by Ivey (1988) is much more social in nature and communicates more of an informal, perhaps even chatty, style. "How can I be of help?" communicates an assumption that the client needs help and that you'll be functioning as a helper. No opening is completely nondirective. Generally speaking, the purpose of the opening statement is to help your clients begin talking freely about the personal concerns that have caused them to seek professional assistance.

The Client's Opening Response

After you have made your opening statement, the spotlight is on the client. How will she respond? Will she take your opening statement and run with it or will she hesitate, struggle for the right words, and perhaps ask for more direction or structure? As we have noted, some clients come to a professional interviewer expecting authoritative guidance. Therefore, they may be taken by surprise by the general and nondirective nature of your opening statement. Usually their first response will give you some clues to how they respond to unstructured situations. Some clinicians consider this initial behavior to be of great significance in understanding the client's personality.

Rehearsed Client Responses. Sometimes clients will begin in a manner that suggests they have rehearsed for their part in the interview. For example, we have heard clients begin with:

1. "Well, let me begin with my childhood."
2. "Currently, my symptoms include . . . "
3. "There are three things going on in my life right now that I'm having difficulty with."
4. "I'm depressed about . . . "

There are both advantages and disadvantages to working with clients who begin in such a straightforward and organized manner. The primary advantage is that these clients are trying to get to the point as quickly as possible. If they are relatively insightful and have a good grasp of the reasons they are seeking professional assistance, then you are at a distinct advantage and the interview should proceed smoothly. On the other hand, sometimes client openings characterized by too much directness and organization may indicate the beginning of what Shea (1988) refers to as a "rehearsed interview" (p. 76). In such cases the client may be defensive and constricted in terms of what he is willing to talk about. He may give factual and informative but emotionally distant accounts of his problems. Emotional distance may in fact be a major part of the problem (e.g., the client may have trouble being emotionally connected to his daily life experiences). A very organized and direct opening response may also reflect general discomfort with situations that lack structure; the client may be reacting to your opening statement by utilizing excessive structure and organization to cope with your vagueness. Your noting this initial behavior may lead you to wonder how the client responds to situations for which he has been unable to adequately prepare.

Helping Clients Who Struggle to Express Themselves   Other clients respond to opening statements by struggling because you have not provided clear directions and they are uncertain about how to proceed. For example, your client may fall silent, look at you with a pained expression, and ask, "So what am I supposed to talk about?" or "I don't know what you want me to say." If you are faced with clients who appear initially uncomfortable with an unstructured opening, we recommend you try the following:

1. Let them struggle for a few moments (while you evaluate their coping methods).
2. Provide emotional support regarding the difficulty of the task.
3. Provide additional structure.

Letting clients struggle with an unstructured opening provides a unique opportunity to assess general expressive abilities. If a client responds to your opening by asking, "What should I talk about?", respond with "Whatever you would like." This places the responsibility for identifying an appropriate "place to start" back on the client and provides an excellent test of the client's inner expressive resources. In essence, you are learning how much help the client needs to express herself.

Another reason it is important to let clients struggle with an unstructured opening is that it allows them an opportunity to overcome their faltering start and recover by adequately identifying a place to begin their communications with you. If you assist them too soon by providing support or structure, you do not allow them to demonstrate their ability to recover and express themselves adequately. Perhaps the client is simply a slow starter; you should not deprive her of the opportunity to demonstrate her actual abilities.

If your client falters a second time or begins to become visibly irritated with your unstructured opening, then you may want to provide some mild support:

C: "Come on, really, I don't know where to start."

I: "Sometimes its difficult to know what you should say in here, but once you get started, it gets easier."

This interviewer statement is designed to acknowledge the difficulty of beginning an interview and to provide hope that the interview process will become smoother or easier.

Finally, if your client simply cannot seem to productively begin a description of herself and her problem independently, then you should help by providing additional structure:

C: "I still can't think of what to say."

I: "Sometimes it helps to begin with how things have been going at home [or work or school]."

By defining and narrowing the client's opening task, this interviewer statement provides structure and simplifies the demand placed on the client. In some cases the interviewer may need to become exceptionally structured in order to help a client succeed in expressing himself (e.g., "Maybe you could begin by telling me exactly what you were doing today before coming to the interview").

Other Client Responses to the Interviewer's Opening Statement Still other clients will begin in an odd manner that gives you reason to wonder about the "normality" of their current functioning. For example, we have had clients begin sessions by stating:

- "I am the Lord Jesus Christ; believe in me or burn."
- "You're the doc, you tell me what's wrong with me."
- "It's by the grace of Allah that I'm sitting before you right now."
- "I have this deep ache inside of me. It comes over me sometimes like a wave. It's not like I have been a well-spring of virtue and propriety, but then really . . . I ask myself constantly, do I deserve this?"

Judging the normality or level of disturbance of your clients is a difficult and demanding task that requires good clinical judgment (see Box 8-2).

Some of the best client responses to your opening statement usually reflect thoughtfulness and the initiation of a working alliance. For example:

"I'm not really sure of all the reasons I'm here, or why I chose to come right now. I guess I'll start with a few things that have been bothering me, and maybe you can let me know if I'm talking about the kind of things that will help you know what you need to know about me."

Evaluating Client Verbal Behavior During the Opening

As clients proceed during the opening phase of the interview, you should evaluate their approach and begin to modify your responses accordingly. For instance, with clients who are very verbal and tend to ramble, you need to be ready to "leap into" the interview whenever you get the chance. With such individuals, toward the end of the opening you may be thinking about how to exercise additional control over the client's verbal behavior. Specifically, you may consider using more closed questions in an effort to direct an overly rambling client.

Similarly, it will become apparent that some clients are using an internal frame of reference to describe their problems. For example:

"I don't know what's wrong with me. I feel anxious all the time . . . like someone's watching me and evaluating me, but I know that's not the case. And I feel so depressed. Nothing I do turns out quite right. I'm underemployed. I can't seem to get involved in a good relationship. I pick the wrong type of women, and I can't figure out why anyone who has anything going for them would want to go out with me anyway . . ."

Such clients tend to be self-critical and self-blaming. They may begin criticizing themselves and not stop until the end of the session. They are sometimes referred to as internalizers because they describe their problems as having an internal cause. Internalizing clients seem to be saying, "What's wrong with me?" or "There's something wrong with me."

On the other hand, some clients are better described as externalizers. They communicate the message "What's wrong with them?" or "There's something wrong with them." For example: "My problem is that I have a ridiculous boss. He's rude, stupid, and arrogant. In fact, men in general are insensitive, and my life would be fine if I never had to deal with another man again." Externalizing clients tend to believe that the cause of their troubles stem from others. While certainly there may be truth to their complaints, it usually becomes difficult to get them to focus on their own feelings, thoughts, and behavior in a constructive manner.

Realistically, client's problems usually stem from a combination of personal (internal) and situational (external) factors. It is useful, especially during the opening phase, to listen for whether your clients tend to take too much or too little responsibility for their problems.

As we mentioned previously, interviewers must observe their clients consistently speak or behave in a particular way before tentatively concluding what a particular client opening response means about a particular client. However, client opening responses provide you with an initial glimpse of how clients perceive themselves and their problems. It is helpful to examine your clients' openings with respect to the following questions.

1. Does the client express himself in a direct and coherent manner?
2. Is the opening response overly structured, organized, and perhaps rehearsed?
3. Does the client struggle excessively with lack of structure?
4. If the client does struggle with lack of structure, what is the nature of the struggle (e.g., does he ask you directly for more structure, does he become angry or scared in the face of low structure, does he digress into a disordered communication style)?
5. Is the client's speech characterized by oddities?
6. Does the client's response focus on external factors (other people or situations that are causing distress) or does it consider internal factors (ways in which the client may have contributed to his own distress)?

The Body

The body of an interview is characterized primarily by information gathering. The quality and quantity of information to be gathered depends almost en-

TABLE 8-2 Checklist for Opening Phase

Interviewer Task	*Technical Approaches*
___ 1. Continue working on rapport.	Nondirective listening
___ 2. Focus on client's view of her life and problems	Open-ended questioning. gentle prompting
___ 3. Provide structure and support if necessary	Feeling reflections, clarify purpose of opening phase, narrow focus
___ 4. Help clients adopt an internal, rather than external frame of reference, if necessary.	Nondirective listening, mild confrontation
___ 5. Evaluate how the interview is proceeding and think about what approaches might be most effective in the body of the interview.	Paraphrasing, summarization, role induction

tirely upon the interview's purpose. Shea (1988) states, "Like the Chinese artist, the goals of the clinician vary during the body of the interview depending upon the various therapeutic landscapes with which the clinician is presented" (p. 93). Sometimes the interview's purpose dictates the therapeutic landscape, while at other times, as suggested by Shea, the therapeutic landscape shapes clinical goals.

If a particular interview is designated with the purpose of you ascertaining whether the client will make a good candidate for psychoanalytic psychotherapy, then during the body of the interview you will direct the client toward disclosures designed to help you judge, among other things, whether the client is psychologically minded, motivated, and capable, both financially and psychologically, to seek such treatment. On the other hand, if the purpose of the interview is to determine the nature and extent of a client's distress in order to formulate an appropriate treatment plan, the data gathered during the interview's body will focus much more on diagnostic clues and criteria. As information is gathered, however, the purpose or focus of the interview body may change. For example, you may discover that your client has been contemplating suicide. Consequently, your general goal and clinical approach will likely shift to assessing the likelihood of your client acting on suicidal thoughts and plans (see chapter 11).

The body is the heart of the interview. As an interviewer you will want to obtain certain information so you will be able to formulate the case and make recommendations. Your ears are tuned to pick up information, while you use the range of nondirective and directive responses discussed in earlier chapters to encourage your client to elaborate on some areas and avoid others. At times you will need to ask direct questions, but you should do so only when necessary and with the knowledge that it inhibits the client's freedom of expression. Sometimes the only way to obtain specific diagnostic information is to use direct and precise questioning. In such cases you should tell the client that you will be asking specific questions in order to obtain necessary information. Informing the client of a change in approach will help decrease the potential negative effect that direct questioning may have on rapport.

Sources of Clinical Judgment: Making Inferences

A major objective of the body of a therapeutic interview is to generate information from which you can make inferences about client behavior. Depending upon the interview's purpose, the inferences you want to be able to make at the conclusion of an interview may result in some of the following:

1. Statements about client personality style and functioning
2. Recommendations on whether psychotherapy is needed
3. Recommendations regarding the most appropriate psychotherapeutic approach
4. Statements about the client's level of psychopathology or psychological dysfunction
5. Estimates of client intellectual or cognitive functioning
6. Statements pertaining to parenting ability, attitudes, and adequacy
7. Diagnostic impressions

The task of making statements, recommendations, estimates, or predictions based on a clinical interview is risky. Describing, explaining, and especially predicting human behavior is a challenging task that is often fraught with sources of error. Nonetheless, after having conducted an assessment-oriented interview, interviewers usually are asked to make some type of statement or decision about their clients. The purpose of this section is *not* to describe the specific activities interviewers engage in during the body of an interview; chapter 9 is devoted to discussing such activities. Instead, in this section we will examine how interviewers become capable of making statements or decisions about their clients' functioning. These decisions are referred to as clinical inferences.

Perhaps the most general question interviewers must answer after an interview is, "How is normal and healthy emotional or psychological functioning distinguished from disturbed or disordered functioning?"

There are several sources of judgment upon which interviewers base their clinical inferences, including:

- Personal experiences and opinions
- Experiences and opinions of friends or family
- Books, movies, television, radio, and other media
- Supervisors
- Research data
- Colleagues
- Previous therapeutic interviewing experiences
- Intuition

In order for therapeutic interviewers to make reasonable judgments about their clients, they need to have knowledge of norms. In other words, interviewers need to have a normative standard to which they can compare their client's interview behavior.

In many cases interviewers rely upon their own accumulated clinical experience to evaluate clients' behavior. Although relying upon one's own clinical judgment can be very helpful, it may also be problematic because all interviewers have idiosyncratic personal biases that adversely affect their judgment (Murphy & Davidshofer, 1988); interviewers also have imperfect memories that can further bias or distort what clients have said. Most beginning interviewers do not have any previous clinical experience or internalized standards to help them in evaluating their clients. They must rely on other information to support or bolster their own judgment.

It is tempting and natural for beginning interviewers to base their inferences on their own personal experiences. However, inferences are more accurate when interviewers utilize research reports, colleagues, and supervisors to enhance their clinical judgment. We recommend that beginning as well as advanced interviewers become aware of the norms they use as sources of clinical judgment. Awareness of normal functioning helps interviewers come to more valid conclusions about whether dysfunctional or abnormal behavior is present.

Defining Psychological and Emotional Disorders

All interviewers must be able to distinguish normal and healthy emotional or psychological functioning from disturbed or disordered functioning. The *Diagnostic and Statistical Manual of Mental Disorders*, third edition, revised (DSM-III-R), published in 1987, is the standard reference in the United States for diagnoses of mental disorders. The *International Classification of Disorders*, ninth edition, (ICD-9) is the world standard for classification of mental disorders. Before you use these manuals to identify specific clinical diagnoses, however, you must be able to judge whether a client's behavior indicates a psychological disorder (disordered way of thinking, feeling, and behaving) at all. What follows are some facts about psychological disorders in general that can help you judge whether a client is experiencing a disorder. These criteria are *not* to be used to establish diagnoses. Instead, they are general guidelines you can use to aid your clinical judgment.

A Disorder Is Abnormal or Statistically Infrequent   Any behavior that your client experiences or engages in is subject to objective evaluation. Engaging in or experiencing a behavior that is statistically infrequent or atypical is one way of defining disordered behavior (also referred to as psychopathology). For example, your client may report to you how many hours he sleeps each night, or how many beers he drinks each week. In each of these cases, as a therapeutic interviewer you can compare his reports with what is considered statistically normal. If your client reports sleeping twelve hours nightly and drinking three cases of beer weekly, you can begin to establish that your client is behaving in an unusual or abnormal manner.

Obviously, it is inappropriate to view all statistically infrequent behavior as disordered. Such reasoning is too simplistic and can result in classifying exceptional, creative, or culturally divergent people as disordered (e.g., it would result in classifying most professional basketball players as having a height disorder and most published poets as having a thinking disorder). Behavior should never be considered disordered simply on the basis of its statistical infrequency. Statistically infrequent behavior should be further examined for the following conditions.

A Disorder Is Disturbing to Self or Others   An individual might choose to sleep twelve hours nightly and drink large quantities of beer and feel just fine about that behavior. Other individuals may feel extreme personal distress because they slept more than nine hours two nights in a row or because they drank excessively on a single occasion. It is difficult for evaluators to predict what behaviors might produce personal distress within particular individuals. Therefore, when it comes to judging whether or not clients are personally disturbed by something they do or experience, interviewers should ask clients directly whether they are bothered by their own behaviors.

Disordered behavior may also be characterized by the fact that it disturbs or bothers others. It is difficult to imagine how a family member would not be at least a little concerned, if not severely distressed, to observe a loved one sleeping and drinking alcohol excessively. In the case of personality disorders, (one of the diagnostic categories identified in DSM-III-R), it is often the people around the disordered person who experience distress and eventually insist the person obtain some sort of treatment. Therefore, when evaluating clients for disordered behavior, be sure and ask whether anyone in your clients' immediate environment is disturbed or bothered by their behavior.

A Disorder Is Maladaptive   Engaging repeatedly in behavior, holding particular beliefs, or having repeated emotional experiences that are self-defeating or damaging to others are behavior patterns commonly viewed as disordered. Usually such patterns of thinking, feeling, or acting serve some function in the life of the person experiencing them, but for the most part the effect of the patterns is negative or dysfunctional. For instance, a parent may sincerely want to teach a teenager to keep her room clean, but constantly screaming and arguing about it may end up damaging the parent-child relationship and not achieve the goal of a clean room. In fact, our experience is that screaming, yelling, and striking children, especially teenagers, are maladaptive behaviors in that they are ineffective means of attaining the goals that are usually desired. Similarly, a man may sincerely want to be in an intimate relationship, but his overly enthusiastic behavior alarms potential partners and keeps them from becoming close to him. The man's intent is positive, but his approach is maladaptive; it results in his scaring potential partners away and, consequently, his increased loneliness. By definition, a behavior pattern is maladaptive when it interferes with effective occupational, social, physical, or recreational functioning.

A Disorder Is Rationally Unjustifiable If a client's behavior, thought, or feeling is unusual or maladaptive, you should also ascertain whether there is any reasonable excuse or justification for it. Author John Sommers-Flanagan once had a client who claimed that his wife was unable to determine when she was hungry or sleepy; therefore, he saw it as his responsibility to force her to eat or sleep when he judged it necessary to do so. Think about this scenario. Are there any rational justifications that a man might have for forcing his spouse to eat or sleep? In such a case it is appropriate to focus on whether or not the spouse is capable of caring for herself. John asked his client several questions: How old is she? Is she able to work or perform other functions effectively? Does she have Alzheimer's or another brain disease or deficiency? Then John asked him to what he attributed his wife's inabilities. The answers were revealing. His wife was capable of working outside the home. She was in her mid-forties. She did not have any identifiable brain disease or damage. He attributed her inability to monitor her own needs for sleep and food to the fact that she had a brother who was "mentally retarded"; therefore, he concluded, she probably had similar genetic deficits (although she was a fully functioning person in virtually every sense of the word).

In this case it was obvious, after conducting a thorough interview, that the client was behaving in a disturbed or disordered manner. His behavior was rationally unjustifiable, statistically infrequent (not many people believe they need to regulate their spouse's eating and sleeping patterns), disturbing (to his wife), and maladaptive (it had precipitated a marital crisis).

These standards may be applied to almost any type of clinical observation that takes place in an interview. For example, if a client exhibits symptoms of depression or sadness during an interview, you might ask yourself the following questions:

1. Is this person's sadness unusual or extraordinary as compared to the emotional states of most people?
2. Is the sadness disturbing or upsetting to the client? Is it particularly disturbing to other people in the client's environment?
3. Is the sadness adversely affecting the client's ability to function at work, to carry on in interpersonal relationships, or to enjoy usually pleasurable recreational activities?
4. Is there a rational explanation for the client's sadness? That is, did an event occur that is logically associated with your client's sadness (e.g., the death of a loved one).

In summary, it might be useful for you to conceptualize potentially disordered behavior in the following manner. During or perhaps after an interview, ask yourself; Is the client's behavior statistically infrequent? Is it disturbing to the client or others? Is it maladaptive in terms of the client's social, occupa-

BOX 8-2 _____

What is Your Favorite Interviewing Phase?

When author John Sommers-Flanagan first began teaching therapeutic interviewing skills, he was convinced that the most important phase of a therapeutic interview was the opening. He believed sensitive clinicians could glean incredible insights simply by listening to the first two or three sentences a client uttered. Consequently, when teaching interviewing skills, he emphasized the opening phase by requiring students to play the beginning of tapes they had made of analogue interviewing sessions. Every week in class students would play their tapes and after the client had said the first few statements, he would stop the tape and ask the class, "OK, now what can you tell me about this person?" After about three or four weeks of this activity, students began asking, "How about if we listen to the middle of a tape? Or maybe the end?" Somewhat grudgingly, John honored the students' requests, while thinking to himself, "The middle of the session is boring. And the end is the end, what's the big deal?"

So now we pose the question to you: "Which phase of the interview do you like best?" Stop and answer that question, then continue reading.

After teaching interviewing courses a few years, John began to wonder why he liked the beginning phase so much, and so much *more* than most of his students did. He came to the conclusion that his preference for the opening interview phases was a reflection of his personality. First, he likes beginnings. He likes the excitement, the hopes and expectations, and the purity of beginnings. Second, he has a strong intuitive or impressionistic tendency. Rather than dive into facts and concrete details, he would rather speculate, guess, and make wagers. John sometimes deceives himself into believing that his intuitive skills are more accurate than factual information. Third, John could usually impress his students with a few surprisingly accurate predictions based on analyzing a client's particular vocal qualities and word choice. This provided his ego with infinite gratification, as he is the kind of person who really enjoys impressing people with the wonders of psychology. Students would sometimes leave classes murmuring to one another, "How did he figure that out based on the first sentence that person said?" Unfortunately, other students were muttering to themselves, "Why did we just spend twenty minutes analyzing one sentence of tape?"

The point is that often an interviewer's natural preferences reflect the interviewer's personality traits. Upon inquiring further, John discovered that some students loved the middle portion of the interview. These students were most often detail-oriented individuals who loved getting their hands on all that information. Some students hate the end of interviews because it involves saying good-bye. Usually these students hate good-byes in their own lives, and many either have been traumatized by good-byes before or simply tend to avoid being separated from others with whom they have emotional ties. And some students hate the opening phase of interviews. Perhaps they feel they make poor first impressions, or perhaps they distrust their intuition. They prefer getting on with the interview so they can prove themselves with more substantial interviewing activities.

An interviewer growth activity that we have often thought about, but never tried, involves having interviewers complete the Myers-Briggs Type Indicator and then tell which phase of therapeutic interviewing they prefer and at which they believe they are most proficient. One hypothesis is that interviewers who score as highly intuitive will prefer the opening, while those who score as "sensing" will prefer the body.

TABLE 8-3 Checklist for Body Phase

Interviewer Task	Tools
___ 1. Transition from nondirective to more directive listening	Role induction. Explain this shift of style to the client, if necessary.
___ 2. Gather information	Open and closed questions (see chapter 9)
___ 3. Obtain diagnostic information	Use DSM-III-R, ICD-9, or the four guiding principles discussed in this chapter to formulate useful questions
___ 4. Shift from information gathering to preparation for closing	Acknowledge that time is passing. Explain and discuss the need to summarize major issues.

tional, or recreational functioning? Is it rationally unjustifiable? You should not rely solely upon any one of these criteria to determine that an individual you interview has a psychological disorder. Each criterion has its shortcomings. Instead, examine your client's thoughts, feelings, and behavior with respect to all of these standards in order to obtain a clearer sense of whether or not psychopathology is present in an individual case.

The Closing

As time passes during the interview, both the interviewer and client may begin to feel pressure. Usually the interviewer begins to feel pressured to fire a few more pertinent questions at the client; it becomes a race to see if you can fit all you would like into the fifty-minute span of a typical interview. We would like to reassure beginning and advanced interviewers that there will always be more information that can be obtained. Nonetheless, interviewers need to stop obtaining information because a key to a smooth closing is to consciously make a decision, about five to ten minutes before your interviewing time is expired, to stop questioning and obtaining additional information. Shea (1988) notes that "one of the most frequent problems I see in supervision remains the over-extension of the main body of the interview, thus forcing the clinician to rush through the closing phase" (p. 130).

Clients also begin to feel pressure as time passes in the interview. Generally, they may begin to wonder about whether they've been able to express themselves adequately and whether or not the interviewer will be able to provide help or adequate recommendations. Clients also may feel worse than they did at the outset of the interview because they have discussed their problems too graphically or simply because as they discuss their problems, they begin to feel worse and worse. Because clients are likely to feel such pressures and think such thoughts, interviewers should be sure to leave ample time to do the following during closing: reassure and support the client, summarize crucial themes and issues, instill hope, guide and empower the client, and tie up any loose ends.

Reassuring and Supporting Your Client

Clients need to be reassured and supported in two major areas. First, clients need to have their expressive capabilities praised. Nearly all clients who voluntarily seek professional assistance "do the best they can" during an initial interview. An initial interview is a challenging and stressful experience. Therefore, during the closing, interviewers should make comments like:

- "You sure covered lots of material today."
- "I appreciate your efforts in telling me about yourself."
- "First sessions are always difficult because there's so much to cover and so little time."
- "I feel I know you quite well given the fact that we've had such little time together."
- "Thanks for being so open and sharing so much about yourself with me."

These comments are designed to acknowledge the difficulty of an interview situation and to commend clients for their expressive efforts.

Second, most clients come to their first interview session with feelings of ambivalence; they both hope and fear the interview and the therapeutic experience. Therefore, the interviewer should try to support the healthy part of the client—the part that made the decision to seek professional services. For example:

- "You made a good decision when you decided to come for an appointment here."
- "I want to congratulate you for coming here today. Coming to someone for help can be hard. I know some people think otherwise, but I believe that seeking help is a sign of strength."

The purpose of this type of statement is to acknowledge the reality of how difficult it sometimes is to seek professional help. Clients should be supported for making such a difficult decision. Providing support may help clients indeed feel that their decision to seek help was a good one.

In some cases clients will have seemed defensive and nondisclosing during the interview hour. Nonetheless, as a professional interviewer you should recognize and acknowledge that clients are generally doing their best to interact with you on any given day. It is fair to note the difficulty of the task or to comment on how the client seemed to have some reluctance to be open with you. However, care should be taken to refrain from expressing anger or disappointment toward clients who are resistant, defensive, or nondisclosing; such reactions will probably make it less likely that they will seek professional help again in the future. Instead, if your client is defensive, try to remain optimistic:

> "I know it was hard for you to talk with me today. . . . That's not surprising, after all, we're basically strangers. Usually it gets easier over time

and as we get to know one another (or as you get to know your therapist) and you'll probably find you're able to talk more freely than you were able to talk today."

Summarizing Crucial Themes and Issues

As Shea (1988) points out, perhaps the most important task of the closing is "solidifying the patient's desire to return for a second appointment or to follow the clinician's referral" (p. 125). One of the best methods for enhancing the likelihood of a client returning for therapy is to clearly identify, during the closing phase, precisely why the client has come for professional assistance. This particular method can be difficult because often clients themselves are not exactly sure why they have come for assistance. Variations on the following statement may be useful:

> "Based on what you've said to me today, it seems that you're here because you recognize some ways in which your life could be going more smoothly. Specifically, you'd like to feel less self-conscious when you're in social situations; you'd like to feel more positive about yourself, or as you said, 'I want to believe in myself'; and you also talked about how difficult it is for you to figure out what you're feeling inside and to share your emotions with others you care about."

Most clients come to professionals at least partly because they have hopes that their lives can improve. If you can summarize to your clients how they would like to improve their lives, then it is much more likely they will choose to return to see you or follow your recommendations; they will see you as a credible authority with useful information and skills.

Instilling Hope

If appropriate, after you have accurately summarized why your client has sought professional assistance, you should make a statement about how counseling or psychotherapy may help address the client's personal issues and concerns. A supervisor of ours used to recommend the following very brief, but positive, statement: "I think therapy can help" (Spitzform, 1982).

In a sense, if we believe in our best clinical judgment that therapy can be helpful to a particular client, part of our task is to "sell" counseling or psychotherapy to that client. After all, most clients are somewhat naive about the potential benefits (and detriments) of psychotherapy. It is our job to inform them of the potential effects:

> "You've said very clearly that you want to feel better. I'm sure it is possible for you to feel better, and therapy is one of the best ways for you to move in that direction. I'd be lying if I told you that everyone who comes for therapy benefits from therapy. But, I can tell you that most people who use therapy in an effort to improve their lives are successful, and I believe that you're the type of person who is very likely to reap benefits from this process."

Guiding and Empowering Your Client

You've just spent thirty-five or forty minutes with someone you'd never met before, listening to her deepest fears, pain, confusion, and problems. You hope you've listened well, summarized along the way, and, when necessary, guided the direction of the talk. In a sense, regardless of how accepting you may have been, you have sat in judgment of the client, her problems, and her life. No matter how well you've functioned as an interviewer, your client may still feel that the experience was overwhelmingly one-sided; you know a huge amount about her, while she knows next to nothing about you. Therefore, it is often useful to consciously shift the focus and give the opportunity for your client to have a bit more power and control at the close of the interview. Some potential methods for such a shift follow:

- "You know, I've done all the questioning here. I wonder if you have any questions of me?"
- "Has this interview been as you expected it to be?"
- "Are there any areas that you feel we've missed or that you would like to discuss at greater length?"
- "I wonder if you felt there was anything I could have done in this interview that would have helped you feel more comfortable (or helped you talk more freely)?"

These queries help give power and control back to the client. Although, as Foley and Sharf (1981) point out, it is important to maintain control toward the end of an interview, it is also important to share that control with the client. In most cases clients do not take the opportunity to ask questions or comment on the interviewer's style; however, we have found that clients like to at least be offered such an opportunity. In addition, we have found that comments solicited from clients augment our own professional growth.

TABLE 8-4 Checklist for Closing Phase

Interviewer Task	Tools
___ 1. Reassure and support the client.	Feeling reflection, validation. Openly appreciate your client's efforts at expression
___ 2. Summarize crucial themes and issues.	Summarization. Use interpretation to determine client's insight and ability to integrate themes and issues
___ 3. Instill hope.	Suggestion, explanation of counseling process and how it is usually helpful
___ 4. Guide and empower your client.	Questions (Ask client for comments or questions of you)
___ 5. Tie up loose ends.	Clarify the nature of further contact, if any. Schedule next appointment.

Tying Up Loose Ends

The final formal task of the interviewer is to clarify what will happen in terms of further professional contact. This involves specific and concrete steps such as scheduling additional appointments, dealing with fee payment, and handling any other administrative issues associated with working in your particular setting.

Termination

Some clinicians and counselors believe that each termination we face is a mini-death (Maholick & Turner, 1979). Although comparing the termination of an interview session with death is a bit dramatic, it does point out how important endings are in our lives. For many people, saying good-bye is difficult. Some bolt away, avoiding the issue all together. Others linger, hoping it won't have to happen. Still others have strong emotional responses such as anger, sadness, or relief. Certainly, the way clients cope with the end of an initial session may foreshadow the way therapy will terminate. It may also represent some of our own or our client's unresolved feelings or conflicts in the areas of separation and individuation. In our opinion, termination is an essential and often overlooked component of therapeutic interviewing.

Watching the Clock

Of course interviewers should not literally watch the clock, but instead take note of the importance of ending each session on time. A key issue with regard to termination is to begin the closing phase early enough so that enough time remains to terminate the session at the prearranged time. If there is not adequate time and the client and interviewer are rushed through closing, then termination is affected. The ideal is to finish with all clinical business on time so that the client's termination behavior can be observed and evaluated. When it is time to end the session, clients often begin thinking, feeling, and behaving in ways that give the sensitive clinician clues regarding therapeutic issues, level of psychopathology, and diagnostic category (see Box 8-3).

BOX 8-3 ──────────────────────────────────────

Significant Termination Statements and Actions (Doorknob Statements)

Examine some of the following client termination statements and actions, and discuss their potential clinical significance.

1. "Thank you." (accompanied by a handshake at the end of every session)
2. "By the way, my thoughts about killing myself have really intensified these past few days." (Clients often wait until the final minute of a session to mention suicidal thoughts.)
3. "Maybe sometime we could get together for coffee or something."
4. "That was great! I feel lots better now."
5. "So when am I gonna start feeling better?"

Guiding or Controlling Termination

Following the closing phase, interviewers need to have some control over the act of termination. This may involve escorting the client out of the office with a comfortable farewell gesture or ritual. One of our colleagues always says, "Take care," in a kind voice but with a tone of finality. Some interviewers like to set up the next session as a final ritual and finish by saying, "See you then." Author John can also recall a colleague who would peek her head out of her office as the client was leaving and say, "Hang in there!" You should examine whatever particular parting statement or activity you feel most comfortable with to determine how it might affect your clients. For example, some clients might be put off by being told to "hang in there," taking it to suggest that the interviewer believes the client is in a situation in which the best option is simply to "hang in" rather than constructively deal with it. It is important to find a comfortable method of bringing about final closure and to do it firmly.

In some cases clients don't let interviewers have control over termination. A client may keep an eye on the clock and then two, five, or fifteen minutes before time is officially up, state something like, "Well, I'm done talking for today." It may be important to explore what is underlying the client's desire to terminate the session early. As a general rule, interview sessions have a designated ending time, and clients should not be excused early. Clients' desire to leave early often signals that important but anxiety-provoking material is near the surface; the desire to leave may be a defense—conscious or otherwise—designed to avoid experiencing and talking about their anxiety. As an interviewer you should be prepared for the client who wants to leave early. Below are several strategies that may be used alone or in combination when you encounter a client who wants to terminate an interview early.

1. Inquire the reasons why the client wants to leave early.
2. Ask the client to talk about his thoughts or feelings in reaction to the interview process or in reaction to you.
3. Find out whether your client usually ends relationships or says good-bye quickly.
4. Gently ask the client to simply "say whatever comes to mind."
5. Consult a detailed outline you've prepared before the session to evaluate whether or not you've covered all the potential issues that you wanted to cover during the interview.
6. Let the client know that there's no hurry by saying something like, "We still have plenty of time left," and then continue to go about the business of closure (see The Closing, this chapter).

In rare cases your client may desperately want to leave the interview room. In such cases you should not engage in a power struggle aimed at keeping the client in the room. Instead, make again, sometime in the future, visit a professional. For example:

> "I can see that you really want to leave right now, even though we still have some time remaining. Your desire to leave could simply mean that

you've really talked about everything you wanted to talk about today or it could mean that you're not ready to go deeper into personal issues for any of a number of reasons. Obviously, I'm not going to force you to stay when you want to go. But I hope you can come back and meet with me, or perhaps someone else again in the future if there are deeper or personal issues that some part of you would like to discuss or address more completely."

Facing Termination

Often, our own issues creep out and affect the way we terminate with clients. Author John recalls his final session with a twenty-five-year-old college student. She was attractive, intelligent, and physically active and had shown a good sense of humor throughout their sessions. At one point in therapy there had been an intense transference wherein she viewed John as similar to her father and then as similar as her boyfriend. Therapy was ending prematurely; John was finishing his internship and moving away. When the final session came, John felt that he would miss the client. He did not want therapy to end. When the hour came to an end and they rose, he intended to say "Good-bye and good luck," but instead the words "See you later" slipped out of his mouth. It was as if John, very briefly, lost conscious control over what he was saying. In retrospect, John believes this episode was indicative of his own unresolved dependency needs and his fantasies of continuing a social relationship with the client.

Time limits are important from both a practical and an interpretive perspective. For your own professional survival, you need to stay in bounds with regard to beginning and ending on time. At a deeper level, you need to model for your clients that therapy, too, is bound in time, place, and the demands of the real world. You are not omniscient. You are not the all-good parent. You *can* withstand the clients' efforts to push the limits. In our experience, students sometimes feel guilty for being firm and ending a session on time. They allow

TABLE 8-5 Checklist for Termination Phase

Interviewer Task	Methods
____ 1. Watch the clock.	Place a clock where you can see it without straining. Explain that time is nearly up.
____ 2. Observe for clients' significant doorknob statements.	Paraphrase. Make feeling reflections.
____ 3. Guide or control termination.	Use a standardized ending. Make a warm and comfortable termination statement. Discuss termination and time boundaries with your client.
____ 4. Face termination.	Evaluate your own response to ending sessions. Stay within time boundaries.

clients to go on and collude with the client in breaking the rules a little. We feel this does not serve clients well in the end, even though they may feel special or that they got a little extra for their money. In fact, their excessive need to feel special may be what they most need to face and work on. Reality is not always easy, and neither is closing an interview or therapy session, but by doing so in a kind, timely, professional manner, the message you give your client is: "I play by the rules, and I believe you can, too. I will be here next week. I hold you in positive regard and am interested in your getting better, but I cannot work magic or change reality for you."

Chapter Summary

Although the preceding therapeutic interview structure is designed primarily as a means of describing how typical assessment interviews proceed, it also has implications pertaining to the temporal structure of psychotherapy or counseling sessions. Specifically, sessions normally proceed in a similar manner; however, the body of a therapy interview consists of implementation of therapeutic interventions rather than information gathering.

Although therapeutic interviewing never involves following a prescribed path from point A to point B, examination and analysis of general phases within a typical interview are useful and important. Researchers and clinicians have developed many models to describe the temporal structure of what occurs during a therapeutic interview. The model described by Shea (1988) is used in this chapter as a means of highlighting the events and tasks that have a place in the typical interview.

The introduction phase of an interview begins with the client's first contact with the interviewer. This contact occurs over the telephone or during the first face-to-face meeting in the waiting room. It is important that as an interviewer you plan ahead how you will handle your first contact with a potential client. Some interviewers try to follow a standard procedure when first meeting clients. Although standardization is useful, it may be perceived by clients as artificial or sterile. Consequently, a balance between standardization and flexibility is recommended.

Some amount of small talk usually occurs during the introduction phase. Again, interviewers should plan ahead what kind of issues they will feel comfortable discussing with new clients. Conversation and small talk should be limited to impersonal and relatively emotion-free issues.

Toward the end of the introduction, interviewers should seek to educate clients on key issues such as confidentiality and the purpose of the interview. It is also important to check that the client's perception of the interview's purpose is consistent with the interviewer's stated purpose.

The opening phase of an interview begins when the interviewer first makes an open-ended inquiry into the client's condition. According to Shea (1988), this phase lasts only five to eight minutes and is normally a nondirective period during which the interviewer allows clients to express themselves freely. The opening phase typically consists of several activities, including the interviewer's opening statement, the client's opening response, and the interviewer's silent evaluation of the client's expressive abilities.

The opening phase ends when the interviewer has listened adequately to the client's efforts to express, without much direction from the interviewer, the main reasons he has sought professional assistance. Clients vary in their abilities to express themselves; the opening phase provides an excellent opportunity to assess how well clients can independently express personal concerns. In some cases interviewers will need to assist clients to express themselves by providing additional structure, direction, or support.

The body of an interview focuses primarily on information gathering. The particular information to be gathered during an interview depends in part upon the purpose of the interview and in part upon what clinical material is revealed during the course of an interview. After a therapeutic interview the interviewer will usually be required to make some statements about the client's level of functioning and specific problems and concerns, recommended treatment approaches, and therapy goals. Consequently, interviewers need to be capable of making inferences based on their clinical sensitivity and judgment.

An important component of therapeutic interviewing involves diagnosis and assessment of mental and emotional problems or disorders. The two most commonly used references for diagnosing mental disorders are the Diagnostic and Statistical Manual of Mental Disorders, third edition, revised (DSM-III-R) and the International Classification of Diseases, ninth edition (ICD-9). These two references provide specific criteria for the diagnosis of mental disorders.

Interviewers need to obtain a sense of whether a client is engaging in ways of thinking, feeling, or behaving that can be classified as disordered. In general, if clients engage in ways of thinking, feeling or behaving that are statistically infrequent, disturbing to themselves or others, maladaptive, and rationally unjustifiable, then there may be grounds for rendering a specific diagnosis or for recommending psychological treatment.

The closing phase of an interview consists of a shift from information gathering to activities that prepare clients for interview termination. Often both clients and interviewers feel pressured during this part of the interview because time is running short and there is usually more information that could be obtained or additional feelings that could be discussed. Clients may feel insecure and vulnerable because they have just disclosed so much information to a virtual stranger. Consequently, it is appropriate for the interviewer to be supportive and reassuring to clients during the closing phase. Interviewers should also take time to summarize key issues discussed in the session, instill hope for positive change, and empower clients by asking them if they have questions or feedback for the interviewer.

Interview termination sometimes brings important separation or loss issues to the surface in both clients and interviewers. Clients may express anger, disappointment, relief, or a number of other strong emotions at the end of an interview. These emotions may reflect unresolved feelings that the client has concerning previous separations from significant figures in his life. Similarly, client behavior may become especially significant. For example, there may be a dawdling at the door or a surge in talk about suicide.

It is important that interviewers plan ahead how they can most effectively end an interview. Some standardization is useful, but often clients will not let interviewers completely control what happens at the end of an interview. Rather than engage clients in a power struggle regarding how (and sometimes when) an interview should end, competent interviewers remain somewhat flexible and deviate from planned endings depending upon the individual client's needs. The interviewer may also experience thoughts, feelings, or behavioral reactions that are related to termination.

The temporal structure for therapeutic interviews modeled in this chapter serves as a means of describing how typical assessment interviews proceed. Psychotherapy interviews may proceed in a similar manner; however, the body of a psychotherapy interview often consists of implementation of therapeutic interventions rather than information gathering.

Suggested Readings

American Psychiatric Association. (1987). *Diagnostic and statistical manual of mental disorders* (3rd ed., revised). Washington, DC: Author. All professional interviewers should be at least familiar with this standard for diagnostic classification of mental disorders.

Foley, R., & Sharf, B. F. (1981). The five interviewing techniques most frequently overlooked by primary care physicians. *Behavioral Medicine, 8,* 26–31. This is a brief article outlining one view of the temporal structure of a therapeutic interview. The authors discuss the criteria they view as basic for effective client interviewing.

Mezzich, J. E., & Shea, S. C. (1990). Interviewing and diagnosis. In M. E. Thase, B. A. Edelstein, & M. Hersen (Eds.), *Handbook of outpatient treatment of adults: Nonpsychotic mental disorders.* New York: Plenum.

Shea, S. C. (1988). *Psychiatric interviewing: The art of understanding.* Philadelphia: W. B. Saunders. Shea's second chapter, entitled The Dynamic Structure of the Interview, is a thorough and practical discussion of the temporal structure typical of most diagnostic clinical interviews.

9

THE INTAKE INTERVIEW

Using Questions
    Types of Questions
    Benefits and Liabilities of Questions
    Guidelines in Using Questions

Objectives of Intake Interviewing
    Identifying, Evaluating, and Exploring Client Problems
    Obtaining Background and Historical Information
    Evaluating Interpersonal Style
    Current Functioning
    Identifying Goals and Monitoring Change

Factors Affecting Intake Interview Procedures
    Client Registration Forms
    Institutional Setting
    Theoretical Orientation
    Professional Background and Professional Affiliation

Chapter Summary

Suggested Readings

Interviewing is the foundation from which all of the outpatient's psychiatric care proceeds. It demands psychopathological knowledge, interpersonal skills, and intuitive abilities. Thus, it is a true blending of science, craft, and art.
                    —*MEZZICH & SHEA, "Interviewing and Diagnosis"*

The intake interview, by its nature, is primarily an assessment interview. It is required prior to initiating psychological or psychiatric treatment. Whether the setting is a social service agency, hospital, mental health center, college counseling center, or a private office, some form of an intake interview precedes treatment or disposition of each case. Similarly, it matters not whether the practitioner is a social worker, psychiatrist, psychologist, or counselor: all practitioners must have the ability to conduct an adequate intake interview. Of course, the nature and focus of an intake interview varies depending upon the type of practitioner, setting, and the interview's purpose, but even so, there usually is, or should be, more consistency than variation. This chapter provides a broad outline and discussion of major content areas and special issues of which intake interviewers should be aware.

In most practical settings the intake interview is referred to simply as an "intake." "Intake" is defined as "a taking in" or "input" (*Webster's*, *1985*), reflecting the fact that an "intake" is needed to get something into a system. The intake interview is the entry point for clients seeking professional mental health assistance. Although some interviews are simultaneously helping and assessment-oriented, the intake is not designed to provide treatment or help, but is almost purely assessment-oriented.

Using Questions

Grown-ups love figures. When you tell them that you have made a new friend, they never ask you any questions about essential matters. They never say to you, "What does his voice sound like? What games does he love best? Does he collect butterflies?" Instead, they demand: "How old is he? How many brothers has he? How much does he weigh? How much money does his father make?" Only from these figures do they think they have learned anything about him. (Saint-Exupery, *The Little Prince*, 1971, pp. 16-17)

To this point we have emphasized the importance and utility of nondirective interviewing techniques. In contrast, this chapter emphasizes a crucial directive technique: the question.

It can be argued that questions are one of the most commonly used and abused clinical interviewing techniques. Virtually everyone asks questions at some point during their interviews; asking questions, especially when you are interested in a particular bit of information, is hard to resist. Unfortunately, as with the case of the little prince in the excerpt above, there is no guarantee that the questions of interest to the questioner are also of interest to the one who is questioned.

Despite controversy over the potential benefits and liabilities associated with using questions with clients, questions are an essential aspect of intake interviewing. This chapter focuses on using questions to obtain information. However, we recommend that before you read using questions you engage in the interviewing activity described in Box 9-1. It will enable you to experience personally the benefits and liabilities of questions before learning, in an intellectual sense, about their potential use and abuse.

Types of Questions

There are many types of questions at an interviewer's disposal. It is important to be able to differentiate among types of questions because different types of questions tend to produce different response patterns. The categories of questions utilized by therapeutic interviewers are open, closed, swing, indirect or implied, and projective.

Open Questions Open questions are questions that facilitate talk. By definition, they are questions that require a response of more than one word; they cannot be answered with a simple yes or no. Most commonly, open questions begin with the word "how" or "what." Writers have often classified questions that begin with the words "where," or "when," or "why," and "who" as open questions, but such questions are really only partially open in that they do not facilitate talk nearly as effectively as do "how" and "what" questions (Cormier & Cormier, 1985; Hutchins & Cole, 1986). Examine the following hypothetical dialogue that uses questions generally classified as open.

> I: "*When* did you first begin having panic attacks?"
>
> C: "In 1986, I believe."
>
> I: "*Where* were you the first time?"
>
> C: "I was just getting on the subway in New York City."
>
> I: "*What* happened?"

BOX 9-1 ━━━━━━━━━━━━━━━━━━━━━━━━━━━━━━━━━━━━━━

Gathering Information with Questions

To participate in this activity, the class should divide into groups of three. In each group, one individual functions as an interviewer, another as a client, and the third as an observer. The interviewer's assignment is to spend five minutes obtaining information from the client about himself. The only restriction is that the interviewer can use *only* questions to obtain the information; summary, reflection of feeling, paraphrase, advice, and other techniques cannot be used. The client's assignment is to respond as directly as possible to the questions posed by the interviewer, while noting any internal feelings, thoughts, or reactions that seem associated with this brief interview experience. The observer's assignment is to identify patterns exhibited by either the interviewer or the client. For example, the observer should note the type of questions asked by the interviewer and the quality of response produced by the client. The observer also should pay attention to any perceived links between a particular type of question asked by the interviewer and the type of response produced by the client. Questions for discussion following this activity are listed in Box 9-2.

C: "When I stepped inside the train, I felt my heart begin to pound. I thought I was going to die. I just held onto the metal post next to my seat as hard as I could because I was afraid I would fall over and be humiliated. Then I got off the train at my stop and I've never been back on the subway again."

I: "*Who* was with you?"

C: "No one."

I: "*Why* haven't you tried to ride the subway again?"

C: "Because I'm afraid I'll have another panic attack."

I: "*How* are you handling the fact that your fear of panic attacks are so restrictive for you?"

C: "Well, frankly, not so good. I've been slowly restricting myself more and more. Pretty soon I'm afraid I'll be too scared to leave my house."

As you can see from this example (and Table 9-1), even questions generally considered open vary in their degree of openness. That is, they do not uniformly facilitate talk.

Although questions beginning with what or how usually elicit the most elaborate responses from clients, such is not always the case. The way a particular "what" or "how" question is phrased may produce a very specific response. For example; "What time did you get home after your appointment?" and "How are you feeling?" are questions that are usually answered very succinctly. The openness of a particular question is best judged by the response it elicits.

Questions beginning with "why" are unique in that they commonly elicit defensive explanations. Meier (1989) states, "Questions, particularly 'why?' questions put clients on the defensive and ask them to explain their behavior" (p. 22). Why questions usually produce one of three types of responses. Some clients respond with a defensive "Because!" Others defend themselves with a "Why not!" Still others they wax intellectual and explain, sometimes in great detail, exactly why they did what they did, said what they said, and thought what they thought. Usually clinicians avoid using why questions because of their tendency to facilitate defensiveness and diminish rapport. On the other hand, in cases in which rapport is good and you want the clients to speculate or intellectualize regarding a particular aspect of their lives, "why" questions may be appropriate.

Questions that begin with who, where, or when direct clients toward very specific information. These questions do not invite elaboration or speculation; they invite precise answers. Therefore, in many cases they should be considered equivalent to closed questions, which are discussed below.

Closed Questions Closed questions are usually defined as "questions that could . . . be answered with a yes or no response" (Hutchins & Cole, 1986, p. 39).

Many open questions can be rephrased in a manner that produces a closed question. Compare the four sets of questions below:

1. "How are you feeling about being in psychotherapy?"
2. "Are you feeling alright about being in psychotherapy?"

1. "What happened next, after you walked onto the subway and you felt your heart begin to pound?"
2. "Did you feel lightheaded or dizzy after you walked onto the subway?"

1. "What was it like for you to confront your father after having been angry with him for so many years?"
2. "Was it gratifying for you to confront your father after having been angry with him for so many years?"

1. "How do you feel?"
2. "Do you feel angry?"

Closed questions restrict verbalization. Therefore, they can be viewed as a technique of reducing or controlling how much clients talk during a session. Restricting verbalization is useful when interviewing a client who is excessively verbal and who overelaborates to every query made by the interviewer.

Sometimes interviewers will transform an open question into a closed question in midsentence. For example, we often hear students formulate questions like, "What was it like for you to confront your father after all these years—was it gratifying?" As you can see, transforming open questions into closed questions greatly limits how much a client can elaborate when giving a response. Unless the client faced with such a question is exceptionally expressive or assertive, or perhaps oppositional, she will answer only the question of whether or not she felt gratification when confronting her father; she may or may not elaborate on feelings of fear, relief, or resentment that she may have experienced and which may be every bit as significant as her feelings of gratification.

Closed questions usually begin with words such as "do," or "is," or "are."They are most useful when the interviewer wants to solicit specific information. Closed questions are often used more frequently toward the end of an interview. This is because late in the interview rapport should already have been established and time is running low, so efficient questioning and answering is more justifiable.

Swing Questions Swing questions are questions that can be answered with a yes or no, but usually produce elaborative discussion of feelings, thoughts, or issues (Shea, 1988). In a sense, swing questions inquire as to whether the client wants to respond. Such questions usually begin with "could," or "would," "can," or "will." For example:

- "*Could* you talk about how it was when you first discovered you had AIDS?"
- "*Would* you describe how you feel your parents might react to finding out you're gay?"

- *"Can* you tell me more about that?"
- *"Will* you tell me what happened in the argument between you and your husband last night?

Ivey (1988) considers swing questions the most open of all forms of questions: "Could questions are considered maximally open and contain some of the advantages of closed questions in that the client is free to say 'No, I don't want to talk about that.' Could questions reflect less control and command than others" (p. 51).

For swing questions to function effectively, the interviewer should observe two basic rules. First, avoid using swing questions unless an adequate rapport has been established (Shea, 1988). If rapport has not been adequately established, then a swing question may backfire and function as a closed question (i.e., the client will respond with yes or no, and rapport may be hampered). Second, avoid using swing questions with children or adolescents. This is because children and adolescents often will interpret swing questions concretely or oppositionally. For example, if you ask child clients "Will you come back to my office now?", they will likely respond, "No!," putting you in a difficult predicament.

Indirect or Implied Questions   Indirect or implied questions often begin with the phrase "I wonder" or "You must" (Benjamin, 1981, p. 75). They are asked when interviewers are curious about what clients are thinking or feeling but don't want to cause clients to feel forced to respond. Below are some examples of indirect or implied questions:

- "I wonder how you're feeling about your upcoming wedding."
- "I wonder what your plans are after graduation."
- "I wonder if you've given any thought to searching for a job."
- "You must have some thoughts or feelings about your parents' divorce."
- "It must be hard for you to cope with the loss of your health."

Indirect questions can seem sneaky or manipulative. Therefore, they should be used only occasionally and when adequate rapport has been established.

Projective Questions   Projective questions are designed to help clients identify, articulate, and explore unconscious or partially conscious conflicts, values, thoughts, and feelings. Projective questions usually begin with some form of "What if?" and invite client speculation. Often projective questions can be used in combination with mental imagery in an effort to help clients explore *what* thoughts, feelings, and behavioral impulses they might have *if* they found themselves in a particular situation. Common projective questions include:

- "What would you do if you suddenly won or inherited a million dollars?"
- "If you had three wishes granted to you, what would you wish for?"
- "If you could be an animal, what would you choose to be?"
- "What if you could go back and change how you acted during that party (or other significant life event); what would you do differently?"

TABLE 9-1 Question Classification

Word Question Begins With	Type of Question	Usual Client Responses
What	Open	Produces factual and descriptive information
How	Open	Produces process or sequential information
Why	Partially open	Elicits explanations and defensiveness
Where	Minimally open	Produces information pertaining to location
When	Minimally open	Produces information pertaining to time
Who	Minimally open	Produces information pertaining to a person
Do/Did	Closed	Pinpoints specific information related to any variety of content areas
Could/Would/Can/Will	Swing	Can produce a large amount of information, but can be rejected
I wonder/You must	Indirect	Gently explores or pinpoints thoughts of feelings. Can be viewed as sneaky or manipulative
What if	Projective	Invites speculation. Helps evaluate client judgment and values

Projective questions are commonly used to evaluate client values and judgment. After the interview, the interviewer can examine a client's response to "What would you do if you won a million dollars?" to determine who and what a client considers valuable in life. The interviewer can also evaluate whether or not the client used good judgment in choosing how to spend the money (i.e., the interviewer can perform an evaluation of judgment and reasoning; see chapter 10).

Benefits and Liabilities of Questions

After participating as an interviewer in the activity described in Box 9-1, therapeutic interviewing students have made these statements:

- "I felt more powerful as an interviewer."
- "I felt more in control."
- "I felt more pressure."
- "I had to think more. It was hard to think of questions while I was trying to listen to the client."
- "I seemed to have less patience. I had an impulse to cut in and ask questions all the time."
- "I felt less pressure. I like asking questions."

BOX 9-2

Discussion Questions for Box 9-1

The purpose of the activity was to heighten your sense of how questions can affect clients. Some interviewers and clients may have enjoyed the activity more than others. Perhaps how much you feel comfortable with questions is related to how much control and structure you like to have in your own life. Reflect on and discuss the following questions in your groups or with the entire class. See if you can identify, from your experience with this activity, the positive and negative effects of questions.

Questions for the Interviewer:

1. How did it feel only to ask questions as an interviewer?
2. As you proceeded in the interview, what thoughts did you have about your performance and about the client's response to you?
3. Did you notice that you relied mostly upon certain types of questions? If so, which types?
4. How did asking questions seem to affect the relationship between you and the client?

Questions for the Client:

1. How did it feel only to be asked questions by the interviewer?
2. What thoughts did you have about your performance and about the interviewer's behavior as the interview progressed?
3. Did you notice the interviewer relying on any particular question type?
4. How did the question-asking format seem to affect your relationship with the interviewer?

Questions for the Observer:

1. Did the interviewer and client seem comfortable with this interviewing approach?
2. What types of questions did the interviewer utilize most?
3. Was there a link between types of questions asked by the interviewer and the quality of response produced by the client?
4. How did the question-asking format seem to affect the client-interviewer relationship?

The variety of reactions to the experience of only being allowed to ask questions illustrates that questions are anything but a neutral interviewing techniques. Questions produce reactions—reactions within interviewers as well as clients. It is important to sort out these reactions. Some are unique to an individual; others are more standard or universal. As professional interviewers it is crucial that our choice to employ questions is based on their usefulness, both for ourselves and our clients. Unfortunately, it is often difficult to balance our own needs to ask, or not ask, questions, with clients' needs to be asked, or not asked, questions.

Asking questions commonly produces several positive results. Open questions can direct clients to discuss their thoughts and feelings about issues the interviewer deems important. Closed questions can help interviewers pinpoint specific information that would not be available if questions were completely avoided. When interviewers control the interview with questions, thus assuming an authoritative role, some clients feel relief. Questions can clarify specific aspects of what clients are discussing. And questions can elicit specific, concrete examples of client behavior.

Using questions may also produce negative results. Questioning emphasizes what the interviewer considers interesting and important. Consequently, clients may react by feeling that their viewpoint is unimportant. Of course, effective interviewers who use questions liberally can avoid this problem by asking the client, "What have we not yet discussed that you feel is important?" (Meier, 1991). Questioning also sets up the interviewer as an expert who is responsible for asking the right questions and, sometimes, for coming up with the right answers. Consequently a differential of power, responsibility, and authority is established. Questioning may also make clients feel defensive, especially if they are asked several questions in succession. Questioning tends to make clients less spontaneous. They may begin to sit back and wait for their interviewer to ask the *right* question. This produces a paradox. You began asking questions because you wanted information, but the process of questioning decreases client spontaneity, increases defensiveness, and results in less information being obtained. Excessive questioning may also foster dependency. Clients may come to rely too heavily on the interviewer or therapist for questions and answers to the important problems in their lives.

Guidelines in Using Questions

As noted, both clients and interviewers sometimes have strong reactions to questions. Therefore, it is useful to keep in mind the following guidelines in order to increase the likelihood that your use of questions is maximally facilitative.

Prepare Your Clients for Questions Clients should be forewarned and have a chance to prepare when the interviewer is about to embark upon a series of questions. Informing clients that you will be asking questions can help decrease the potentially threatening nature of questions and help clients be less defensive and more cooperative in response to your questions. You can forewarn your clients by stating something like the following:

> "There is some specific information I need to obtain, so for the next few minutes I'll primarily be asking you specific questions designed to help me get that information. Some of the questions may seem odd or may not make much sense to you. If you want, afterward I can explain why I asked the types of questions I asked."

Do Not Use Questions as Your Primary Listening or Action Response Questions should always be used in combination with other listening responses, especially nondirective listening responses. For example, it is important to follow your client's response to your question at least occasionally, with a listening response:

I: "What happened when you first stepped onto the subway?"

C: "When I stepped inside the train I felt my heart begin to pound. I thought I was going to die. I just held onto the metal post next to my seat as hard as I could because I was afraid I would fall over and be humiliated. Then I got off the train at my stop and I've never been back on the subway again."

I: "So that was a pretty frightening experience for you. You were doing about everything you could to stay in control. Was anyone with you when you went through this panicky experience?"

Unless some sensitive listening responses are used in combination with an interviewing strategy emphasizing questioning, clients are likely to feel "bombarded" or "interrogated" by repeated questions (Benjamin, 1981; Cormier & Cormier, 1991).

Make Your Questions Relevant to Clients' Concerns   Clients are more likely to view their interviewer as competent and credible if the interviewer focuses directly on their major concerns. Therefore, for the most part, questions should be closely connected to major client issues. In cases where your questions are designed to provide you with diagnostic or mental status information, clients may not clearly understand the relevance of your questions. For example, when interviewing a depressed client you may want to closely evaluate eating patterns, sleeping patterns, and concentration ability. Consequently, you will want to ask questions such as:

- "How has your appetite been?"
- "Have you been sleeping through the night?"
- "Has it been hard for you to focus on a single activity? (e.g., for a client who usually likes to read, "Have you found yourself reading a single paragraph over several times because you couldn't concentrate on it very well the first time?")

Imagine how a depressed client who is irritable and psychologically naive and who believes, somewhat accurately, that her bad mood is related to ten years of abuse by her husband might perceive such a series of questions. She might think something like, "I couldn't believe that counselor. What do my appetite and reading habits have to do with why I came to see her?"

Of course, the counselor is trying to evaluate the extent of the client's depression. Unfortunately, unless the client can see the relevance of the counselor's questions, the questions will diminish rapport and the likelihood that the client will return for counseling.

Use Questions to Elicit Concrete Behavioral Examples   Perhaps the most productive use of questions is to obtain clear concrete examples of what is and has been happening in the client's life. Instead of relying upon abstract reports of what a client's life is like, use questions—especially swing questions—to obtain specific behavioral examples:

C: "I have so much trouble with social situations. I guess I'm just an anxious and insecure person."

I: "Could you give me an example of a recent social situation when you felt anxious and thought you were insecure?"

C: "Yeah, let me think. Well, there was the party at the frat the other night. Everyone else seemed to be having a great time and I just felt left out and like no one wanted to talk with me."

In this interchange, the client needs even more assistance from the interviewer to produce a clear and concrete behavioral example. Some open and closed questions could help the client become more specific and concrete in describing his anxiety and insecurity:

- "What exactly was happening when you felt anxious and insecure at the party?"
- "Who was standing near you when you had these feelings?"
- "What thoughts were going through your mind?"
- "What ways would you rather have acted in this situation if you could do it all over again?"

Even when tracking clients' concrete experiences, be sure to intersperse paraphrases and feeling reflections in order to assure your clients that you are listening and that you understand their experience.

Moursund (1990) provides a helpful suggestion for obtaining additional information when tracking a client's experience: "If there are major gaps in the client's story, ask for information to fill them; do so with open-ended questions. Say 'What did you do next?' rather than 'Did you talk to her about it?'" (p. 23).

Approach Sensitive Areas Cautiously Be especially careful when questioning sensitive areas. As Wolberg (1988) has noted, it is important not to question new clients in sensitive areas (e.g., appearance, status, sexual difficulties, and life failures). Wolberg suggests instead that clients be allowed to talk freely about such topics, but if blocking occurs, questioning should be avoided until such time that the relationship has been established. Wolberg believes that relationship building should be given higher priority than information gathering.

This is not a simple issue. Despite Wolberg's generally good advice, we feel that at times the therapeutic relationship must take a back seat to information gathering. This is especially the case when you are conducting an intake interview or when your client is in crisis. For example, if a client is potentially suicidal or homicidal, gathering assessment data to make a competent clinical decision is top priority. Similarly, if you are a designated intake worker and you will not be seeing the client for counseling, once again, information gathering is probably of greater importance than relationship building (However, you should make this clear to the client by stating something like, "This

BOX 9-3

Review Questions

Without looking back through the chapter, respond to the following queries.

1. Give two examples of an open question.
2. Give three examples of a closed question.
3. Give an example of a swing question.
4. Give an example of an indirect question.
5. Give an example of a projective question.

After you are clear on the particular types of questions available to you during an interview, try the following practice activities.

1. Find a partner and practice using the various types of questions.
2. Sit down, relax, and imagine how and when you might use the different types of questions. Visualize yourself asking questions in an interview setting.
3. Practice asking different types of questions into a video- or audiotape recorder.

interview is not really much like counseling. Mostly I'll be gathering information about you to pass on to your counselor. So if sometimes it seems like I'm firing a lot of questions your way, that's probably because I am").

Sometimes, because of eagerness, unrealistic expectations, or sadistic tendencies, interviewers make the mistake of leaping into sensitive areas despite signals from the client that such areas are off limits. As Wolberg (1988) advises, if you have plans to continue with a client in counseling, be sure to approach sensitive areas cautiously. See Box 9-3 to review this section on questions.

Objectives of Intake Interviewing

There are three basic objectives associated with intake interviewing:

1. Identifying, evaluating, and exploring the chief complaint.
2. Obtaining a sense of the client's interpersonal style, interpersonal skills, and personal history.
3. Evaluating the client's current life situation.

Put another way, the intake involves getting to know the problem, the person, and the situation as presented to you by the client. We recommend you go about accomplishing these objectives in this order: problem, person, situation.

These objectives are very general and may sound deceptively simple. In fact, achieving these three objectives during the usually brief period of time associated with an intake interview is quite a challenge. This section is designed to help prepare you to meet the challenge of the intake.

Identifying, Evaluating, and Exploring Client Problems

Most clients come to a professional because they are in distress. It follows that your first, and perhaps primary, objective is to find out about their distress. As an interviewer you begin your exploration of a client's chief complaint with your opening statement (e.g., "What brings you here?" or "How can I be of help?," see chapter 8). After the opening statement, you spend at least five to eight minutes tracking the client and trying to understand exactly why, the client has come to see you, from the client's perspective. (Shea, 1988)

In some cases clients will clearly identify why they have sought professional assistance; in other cases, perhaps most often, they will be vague as to the precise reasons they are in your office. As your clients begin to articulate their problems, utilize primarily nondirective listening responses. Then, as you begin to get a sense of the primary concerns, shift to more directive listening responses, including questions.

The types of client problems an interviewer encounters depend upon the clinical population the interviewer works with. Common problems presented by clients include: anxiety, depression, and relationship conflicts. Other problems for which clients frequently seek professional assistance include eating disorders, alcoholism or drug addiction, social skill deficits, physical or sexual abuse, stress reactions, vocational confusion, and sexual dysfunction. Because of the wide range of symptoms or problems clients can present, it is crucial that interviewers have at least a general knowledge of psychopathology.

Prioritizing and Selecting a Problem Most clients do not come to an interview with a single defined problem, but instead present a number of concerns, some of which may be interconnected. Consequently, toward the end of the opening phase and the beginning of the body, interviewers should seek to establish a range of primary problems of concern to the client. This transition from opening to body has a dual purpose in the intake. First, it allows interviewers to check for any additional problems that the client has not yet talked about. Second, the transition begins the process of problem prioritization and selection.

> *I:* "So far you've talked mostly about how you've been feeling so down lately, how it's so hard for you to get up in the morning, and how most things that are usually fun for you haven't been fun lately. I'm wondering if you have any other major concerns or distress in your life right now."

> *C:* "As a matter of fact, yes, I do. I get these awful butterflies, a strong feeling of apprehension sometimes. Mostly these feelings seem connected to my career, or maybe I should say lack of career."

At the beginning of the body of an intake, interviewers need to help clients identify a range of problems or concerns. Problem identification is an exploratory process during which interviewers listen closely to problems that clients discuss and then inquire about the existence of any other significant concerns.

In the preceding exchange, the interviewer used an indirect question to continue exploring for problems. After the range of problems is identified, the interviewer then moves to the task of prioritization or selection. Because all problems cannot be addressed simultaneously, interviewer and client must choose together which problem or problems are to receive most attention during an intake.

> *I:* "I guess so far we could summarize your major concerns as your low mood, your anxiety over your career, and some social inhibition or shyness that you talked about. Which of these would you say is currently most troubling to you?"

> *C:* "Well, they all bother me, but I guess the low mood is worst. If I don't want to get out of bed all day, then I never have to face those other issues anyway."

This client has signaled that depression is his biggest concern. Of course, an alternative formulation of the problem is that social inhibition and anxiety are producing the low mood and therefore should be dealt with directly; otherwise, the client will never get out of bed because he is afraid of life. However, it is usually best to follow client leads and explore *their* biggest concerns first. (Psychiatrists refer to what the client considers the main problem as the chief complaint.) In this example, all three symptoms may eventually be linked together anyway. Exploring depression probably will allow you eventually to integrate anxiety and shyness symptoms into the picture as well.

If as a professional interviewer you believe a different issue than the one the client identifies should be explored instead (e.g., alcoholism or psychotic thinking), it is best to wait and try to explore your own priority concern after at least a cursory examination of what the client thinks is the main problem (chief complaint). This is because you need to respect the client's perspective and pace. If you do not, you may offend the client and make it less likely that you or any other mental health professional will ever see the client again.

Analyzing a Symptom   Once you have identified and selected a symptom in collaboration with your client, you should turn your attention to a thorough analysis of that symptom. Whatever the symptom, a behavioral and symptom analysis is warranted. You should seek answers to a list of questions similar to the following:

1. When did the symptom first occur (in some cases the symptom will be one that the client has experienced before. If so, you should explore its original *and* more recent development and maintenance)?
2. Where were you and what exactly was happening when you first noticed this symptom (what was the setting, who was there, etc.)?
3. How have you tried to cope with or eliminate this symptom?
4. Of all the efforts you've made to cope with or eliminate this problem, which has been most effective?

5. Can you identify any situations, people, or events that it seems usually precede your experience of this symptom?
6. What exactly happens when the symptom begins?
7. What thoughts or images go through your mind when the symptom is occurring?
8. Do you have any physical sensations before, during, or after the symptom occurs?
9. Where and what do you feel in your body? Describe it as precisely as possible.
10. How frequently do you experience this symptom?
11. How long does the symptom usually last?
12. Does the symptom affect or interfere with your usual ability to function at work, at home, or at play?
13. In what ways does the symptom interfere with your work, relationships, school, or recreational pursuits?
14. Describe the worst experience you have had with this particular symptom. When the symptom is at its worst, what are your thoughts, images, and feelings like then?
15. Have you ever expected the symptom to occur and had it not occur, or had it occur only for a few moments and then disappear?
16. If you were to rate the severity of your problem, with 1 indicating it is not distressful at all and 100 indicating it is so distressful that it is going to cause you to kill yourself or die, how would you rate it today?
17. What rating would you have given your symptom on its worst day ever?
18. What is the lowest rating you would ever have given it? In other words, has the symptom ever been completely absent?
19. As we have discussed your symptom during this interview, have you noticed any changes (i.e., has it gotten any worse or better as we have discussed it)?
20. If you were to give this symptom and its effects on you a title, like the title of a book or play, what title would you give?

These questions are listed in an order that we have found makes them flow smoothly in many interviews. However, these particular questions and their order should not be viewed as standard. Before an interview, take time to read through a list of questions such as these. Reword them to fit your style, add new questions, and delete others until you believe you have a set of questions that meets your intake interviewing symptom analysis needs. Then, after implementing your set of questions, continually revise them so you can become increasingly efficient and sensitive when questioning clients. Practice with different amounts of questions during various intake interviews so that you can determine an estimate of how many specific questions you can fit reasonably into a single interviewing session.

We should note that sometimes even the best-laid plans fail. Some clients are very skillful at drawing interviewers off track. Sometimes it is important for interviewers to let themselves be drawn off track; diverging from one's planned menu of questions can lead to a different and perhaps more significant area, such as reports of sexual or physical abuse or suicidal ideation. Therefore, lists of questions and content areas that you find or formulate are not to be followed in a rigid manner. You should make efforts to stick with your planned task, but at the same time remain flexible so you will not inadvertently overlook important clues clients may be giving you regarding potentially fruitful or significant problem areas.

Using Problem Conceptualization Systems   Some authors recommend that interviewers use organized systems of problem conceptualization when analyzing client problems (Cormier & Cormier, 1991; Seay, 1978). Usually these systems are theory-based, but several systems reflect a growing trend toward eclecticism (Cormier & Cormier, 1991; Lazarus, 1976). Most conceptualization systems recommend that problems be analyzed and conceptualized with strict attention to prespecified domains of functioning. Lazarus's (1976; 1981) approach is termed "multi-modal." He suggests that problems be assessed and treated via seven specific modalities. Lazarus (1976) developed the acronym BASIC ID to represent his seven-modality system:

- B: Behavior. Specific and concrete behavioral responses are analyzed in Lazarus's system. He particularly attends to behaviors that clients seem to engage in too often or too infrequently.
- A: Affect. Although affect is traditionally defined as emotions identified and observed by another individual, Lazarus's definition includes feelings (self-reported and self-described emotions).
- S: Sensation. This modality refers to the sensory processing of information. For example, clients often report physical symptoms associated with high levels of anxiety (e.g., choking, elevated temperature, heart palpitations, etc.).
- I: Imagery. Imagery consists of internal visual cognitive processes. Clients often experience pictures or images of themselves that influence their overall functioning.
- C: Cognition. Lazarus believes in closely evaluating client thinking patterns and beliefs. This process usually includes an evaluation of distorted or irrational thinking patterns that seem to occur almost automatically and that lead to emotional distress.
- I: Interpersonal Relationships. This modality concerns interpersonal variables such as communication skills, relationship patterns, and assertive capabilities as manifested during role-play and as observed in the client-interviewer relationship.
- D: Drugs. This modality refers to biochemical and neurological factors that often affect behavior, emotions, and thinking patterns. It includes physical illnesses and nutritional patterns.

Lazarus's (1976) model is broad based, popular, and useful to interviewers of different theoretical orientations. However, it slightly overemphasizes cognitive processes (two separate cognitive modalities exist within his seven modality system—cognition and imaging) while neglecting or deemphasizing spiritual, cultural, and recreational domains. As we suggested previously, every system designed to aid in problem identification, exploration, and conceptualization is imperfect. It is important to be familiar with a number of systems so that as a competent professional interviewer you can be flexible in your questioning and conceptualizing and adapt to your setting and the individual problems and needs of your clients.

Behavioral and cognitive psychologists have emphasized the importance of antecedents and consequences in the development and maintenance of problems. Such psychologists strongly believe that analysis of clients' environments and interpretation of environmental stimuli allows counselors to explain, predict, and control specific symptoms. This model of conceptualizing problem behavior has been called by behaviorists the ABC model (Thoresen & Mahoney, 1974). A refers to behavioral Antecedents, B to the Behavior or problem itself, and C to behavioral Consequences. Although this model has been criticized by writers and psychotherapists of opposing orientations (Goldfried, 1990), it is useful for all interviewers to be aware of three crucial questions it implies:

- What events, thoughts, and experiences, precede the identified problem?
- What is the precise operational definition of the problem (i.e., what behaviors constitute the problem)?.
- What events, thoughts, and experiences, etc., follow the identified problem?

When following the ABC model, interviewers can be meticulous in their search for potential behavioral antecedents and consequences. For example, an interviewer could assess for behavioral antecedents and consequences through all modalities identified by Lazarus (1976):

- What behaviors precede and follow symptom occurrence?
- What affective experiences precede and follow symptom occurrence?
- What physical sensations precede and follow symptom occurrence?
- What images precede and follow symptom occurrence?
- What specific thoughts precede and follow symptom occurrence?
- What relationship events or experiences precede or follow symptom occurrence?
- What biochemical, physiological, or drug-use experiences precede or follow symptom occurrence?

The Diagnostic Look: Search for a Syndrome A syndrome is a set of symptoms that usually occur together. After you have identified a symptom, such as low mood, your next task is to explore it in greater depth. A client's reported "low mood" may represent nothing more than a single symptom (i.e., sadness) caused by the natural ups and downs of life. On the other hand, low mood may represent the tip of the iceberg. Once a primary symptom has been identified and the client has acknowledged it as a significant concern, a search for accompanying symptoms is warranted. It is important for interviewers to determine if a particular symptom is accompanied by an associated set of symptoms that constitute a syndrome, or mental disorder (see Box 9-4):

DSM-III-R (American Psychiatric Association, 1987) provides standards for diagnostic classification. Numerous structured diagnostic interview systems are also used by clinicians to reliably identify a client's DSM-III-R diagnosis. Structured diagnostic interviewing is a particular type of interviewing specifically designed to rule out and rule in psychiatric diagnoses. In order to maximize the reliability of such procedures, extremely standardized approaches have been developed. These approaches are essentially menu-driven; if a client responds to a particular question with a yes, then there is a specific question the evaluator must subsequently ask. Obviously, rigid adherence to standardized diagnostic interviewing protocols can have an adverse impact on rapport. On the other hand, if clients are adequately informed by their interviewers of the nature and purpose of the structured diagnostic interview, such approaches can be utilized effectively and efficiently, with little adverse client

---

BOX 9-4 ━━

Does the Symptom Represent Sadness or Dysthymia?

If a client reports being "sad," it is important to explore whether or not the sadness is of diagnostic significance. Criteria for diagnosis of Dysthymia (one type of clinical depression; from DSM-III-R) follows.

Dysthymia
   A. Depressed mood (or can be irritable mood in children and adolescents). The depressive symptoms have been present at least two years in adults and at least one year in children.
   B. At least two of the following symptoms have been present:
      (1) appetite problems
      (2) insomnia or excessive sleep
      (3) general fatigue
      (4) low self-esteem
      (5) difficulty concentrating or making decisions
      (6) feelings of hopelessness
   C. During a two-year period (one year for children and adolescents) the person has never been free of symptoms in A for more than two months at a time.
   D. No evidence that a different mental disorder such as bipolar disorder, schizophrenia, or an organic process is present or caused the depressive symptoms.

Note: These criteria are adapted from DSM-III-R; they are not the exact diagnostic criteria.

As you can see from this example of diagnostic criteria, diagnosing mental disorders is not a simple process. Not only are there specific criteria that *must* be present to support the diagnosis, there are also specific factors that *must not* be present in order for a diagnosis of dysthymia to be given.

━━

reaction. Several specific diagnostic interviewing procedures are included in the Suggested Readings at the end of this chapter.

Obtaining Background and Historical Information

In an intake interview three sources of information are used to assess the client's personality and mental condition. These include:

- The client's personal history
- The client's manner of interacting with others
- Formal evaluation of the client's mental status

The remainder of this section discusses methods and issues related to obtaining a client's personal history and evaluating a client's interpersonal style. (A method for evaluating mental status is the focus of chapter 10.)

Shifting to the Personal History   After you have spent perhaps fifteen to twenty-five minutes exploring the presenting complaint, it becomes time to consider shifting the focus of the interview. At that point you should know reasonably well the primary reasons your client is consulting a professional. A useful bridge from problem exploration to personal history is the "Why now?" question. Say to the client something like, "You know, I think I'm pretty clear on the nature of your main concerns, but one thing I'd like to know is why exactly you chose to come for counseling now."

The purpose of this question is to determine what specific factors convinced the client to make the decision to seek professional help. This question helps determine whether a specific precipitating event produced the referral. The client's response can also shed light on whether or not the client is a willing participant in the interview; perhaps he has been coerced by friends or family to come for assistance. If the client balks or scoffs at your question of "Why now?" simply continue to pursue the question, perhaps through alternative approaches such as:

- "Why didn't you come in a few weeks ago when you were first jilted by your girlfriend?"
- "You've had these symptoms so long, I'm still a little puzzled over exactly what prompted you to seek counseling now. Why not before? And why didn't you choose to wait and 'tough it out' as you have in the past?"

After your client has responded to the "Why now?" question (and after you have summarized or made a reflection of that response), it is time to formally shift the focus of the interview from the problem to the person. This shift can be made with a statement similar to the following:

"So far we've spent most of our time discussing the symptoms that cause you distress. Now I'd like to try and get a more complete sense of how you've become the person you are today. One of the best ways for me to do that is to shift the focus to your personal history."

Nondirective Historical Leads Immediately following your shift to personal history, you should become very nondirective. Lead the client into her past and then give control over to her. Some effective historical leads include:

- "How about if you begin by telling me some about your growing-up years?"
- "Maybe it would be easiest if you started with where you were born and raised and then talk about whatever significant details come to mind."
- "Tell me about some of your childhood memories."

The shift to personal history is crucial; clients reveal significant material by what they choose to focus on or by what they choose to avoid. It is important to remain nondirective for at least a brief period following the transition to personal history taking because as professional interviewers we are interested in what clients feel is personally significant. After a brief nondirective period (perhaps two to five minutes), you can provide clients with more structure and guidance and begin asking specific questions about their past.

As discussed in chapter 8, many clients balk when asked to free associate to their childhood experiences. They may ask for structure and guidance. For a few minutes during the personal history it is your main job to avoid giving structure and guidance. If you provide structure and ask specific questions, you may never know what the client truly views as significant past material. If your client presses you on this issue, you can state directly, "I'll ask you some specific questions about your childhood in a few minutes, but right now I'm interested in the past experiences and memories that you spontaneously recall. Just tell me a few memories that seem important to you." After making such a statement, simply sit back and lend an interested ear. Clients may feel anxious and uncomfortable, but if you appear genuinely interested in hearing about what *they* think is important about their past, it will help ease their discomfort.

Still, many clients will resist delving into their personal history. Often the personal histories of people who go to counselors have been traumatic and distressing. In other cases historical experiences may be repressed. In our experience, clients frequently claim, "I really can't remember much of my past" or "My childhood is mostly a blank." If this is the case, try to be supportive and reassuring:

> "You know, memory is a funny thing. Sometimes bits of it will come back to you as we discuss it. Of course, most of us have memories we would rather not recall because they are painful or traumatic. My job isn't to force you into talking about difficult past experiences. On the other hand, I hope you feel free to discuss whatever past events you want to discuss."

Obtaining a personal history is a delicate and sensitive process. We shouldn't see our job as being to reinforce clients to report traumatic experiences. On the other hand, to discuss old pains can be a therapeutic and emotionally ventilating experience (Greenberg & Safran, 1987; Pennebaker, Keicolt-Glaser, & Glaser, 1988; Pennebaker & O'Heeron, 1984). Effective therapeutic interviewers give their clients the opportunity to disclose past traumatic events, but they do *not* require their clients to do so.

Perhaps more than any other time during the intake, the interviewer must be ready during the personal history to shift back into a nondirective listening mode. Many times our students have asked, "What if my client has been sexually abused?" or "What if my client's parents died when she was a young child, what do I do then?" The fact is, when you delve into a client's personal history you run the risk of stumbling onto emotionally charged or "hot" material. Be prepared; expect that you will likely come across at least a few warm, if not hot, memories. And when you do run across such memories, do nothing more than listen well. You cannot fix the memories or change the past. When clients first disclose a traumatic experience to an interviewer, they need most of all a supportive and empathic ear. Comments that track your client's experience, such as "Sounds like that was an especially difficult time" or "That was a time when you were really down (or angry, or anxious,)" might be all that your client needs when disclosing personally traumatic experiences.

Some clients may have trouble pulling themselves out of their emotionally distressing memories. In such cases, make clear distinctions between what happened then and what is happening now. Explore with clients how they managed to handle the trying times in their lives. Exploring, identifying, and emphasizing how clients coped and survived during a difficult past situation is helpful and appropriate. In fact, you may find it is easy to point out ways in which your clients were strong during their most difficult times. It is also helpful to lead your clients back to the present as you gather historical information. As you move into the present, your clients may be able to once again gain distance from painful past experiences. Of course, there is always the possibility that a client will remain consumed with negative emotions. Sometimes this will happen because of the powerful nature of traumatic memories. Other times clients will get stuck because they do not view the present as an improvement over the bad times in the past. We will discuss methods for dealing with such situations in chapter 11, Suicide Assessment.

Directive Historical Leads After the brief period in which you allow your client to freely discuss what he feels is significant in his past, you should initiate another transition in the interview and become a directive explorer of your client's past. Of course, there is a huge amount of historical material you can potentially obtain from a client. In a typical intake you have a limited amount of time and therefore must decide on which historical areas to focus. A good place to begin your directive exploration of a client's past is with an early memory (Adler, 1958).

> *I:* "What is your earliest memory ... the first thing you can remember from your childhood?"
>
> *C:* "I remember my brothers trying to get me to get into my dad's pickup. They wanted me to pretend I was driving it. They were laughing. I got into the cab and somehow got the truck's brake off, because it started

to roll. My dad got pretty mad, but my brothers were always trying to get me to do these outrageous things."

I: "How old were you?"

C: "I suppose about four, maybe five."

Often memories reported by clients have significance in terms of their present lives; (that is, the memories represent major themes or issues the client is currently struggling with (Adler, 1958; Mosak, 1989; Parrot, 1992). For example, the actual client who revealed the memory above reported that his life was characterized by performances that he put on for others. He admitted to having strong urges to do "outrageous" things in order to get the attention of others.

In cases when clients reveal memories that are either strikingly positive or strikingly negative, it is useful to follow up with questions that seek an opposite type of memory. Virtually everyone has both positive and negative memories of childhood. It is a good practice to assess whether your client can produce a balanced report of positive and negative childhood experiences. Clients who remember mostly negative childhood experiences may be suffering from a depressive disorder, while clients who never mention negative experiences may be utilizing defense mechanisms of denial, repression, or dissociation (Mosak, 1989).

C: "I remember breaking a pipe down in the basement of my house. I had gotten into my dad's tools and was striking an exposed pipe with a hammer. It started leaking and flooding the basement. I was in big trouble."

I: "It sounds like that memory was mostly of a negative time when you got in trouble. Can you think of an early memory of something with a more positive flavor?"

C: "Oh yeah, my memories of playing with my next door neighbor are great. My mom used to have him over and we would play with every game and toy in the house."

I: "Do you remember a specific time when he came over and you played?"

C: "Uh . . . yeah. He always wanted to play army, but I liked dinosaurs better. We got in a fight, and I ended up throwing all the army men out into the front yard. Then we stayed in and played dinosaurs."

Sometimes even when you ask for a positive memory you will get a response with negative and conflicted tones. On the other hand, some clients will deny that they've had any negative memories. There's probably no use in pointing out to the client, unless he notes it himself, the fact that he reported another largely negative (or positive) event. Instead, merely take note of the quality of his memories and move on.

Another standard method for exploring childhood, or, more specifically, parent-child relationships, is to ask your client to describe his parents with three words.

I: "Give me three words to describe your mother."

C: "What do you mean?"

I: "When you think of your mother and what she is like, what three words best describe her?"

C: "I suppose . . . clean, . . . and proper, and uh, intense. That's it, intense."

As we have noted above, there is a high likelihood of stumbling into strong, affectively charged memories when exploring your clients' personal histories. This is especially true when exploring parent-child relationships. The words used by clients to describe their parents may be just the tip of the iceberg. Further exploration may be conducted by asking clients to provide examples of their descriptions: "You said your mother was intense. Can you give me an example of her behavior that fits that word?"

A natural flow for a personal history is from first memories, to memories of parents, siblings (if any), school and peer relations, work or employment, and so on. Areas of personal history commonly covered in a very thorough intake interview are listed in Table 9-2. Note that this is a fairly comprehensive list of potentially significant historical domains. In a typical clinical intake you will need to decide as you proceed which of these areas demand most of your attention. It is a gross understatement to say that in most cases you cannot cover everything in the fifteen to twenty minutes you have to devote to personal history taking. In fact, even in a fifty-minute interview designed for obtaining historical background information only, judicious selection from the areas listed in Table 9-2 is necessary.

Table 9-2 should not be takens as a rigid outline for structured historical interviewing. Other, more specific interviewing guides are available for many of the content areas (or domains) listed in the table. (see the Suggested Readings at the end of the chapter).

Because it is often difficult to choose which of the many domains to explore during the limited time available in an interview, agencies and individual clinicians often use registration forms or intake questionnaires for new clients. These forms are designed to provide interviewers with client information before they see the client for the first time. On the basis of such information, interviewers can select domains that may be important to cover with a new client. Recently a considerable amount of research has been carried out on computer administration of intake interviews and mental status examinations. Although this type of approach is impersonal, it has some advantages: com-

TABLE 9-2 Potentially Significant Domains in the Personal History: Sample Questions

Content Areas	Questions
1. First memories	What is your first memory? How old were you then? Do you have any very positive (or negative) early memories?
2. Descriptions and memories of parents	Give me three words to describe your mother (or father). Who did you spend more time with, Mom or Dad? What methods of discipline did your parents use with you? What recreational or fun activities did you do with your parents?
3. Descriptions and memories of siblings	Did you have any brothers or sisters? (If so, how many?) What memories do you have of time spent with your siblings? Who was your closest sibling and why? Who were you most similar to in your family? Who were you most dissimilar to in your family?
4. Elementary school experiences	Do you remember your first day of school? How was school for you? (Did you like school?) What was your favorite (or best) subject in school? What subject did you like least (or were you worst at)? Do you have any vivid school memories? Who was your favorite (or least favorite) teacher? What made you like (or dislike) this teacher so much? Were you ever suspended or expelled from school? Describe the worst trouble you were ever in when in school. Were you in any special or remedial classes in school?
5. Peer relationships (in and out of school)	Do you remember having many friends in school? What kinds of things did you do for fun with your friends? Did you get along better with boys or girls? What positive (or negative) memories do you have from relationships you had with peers in elementary school?
6. Junior high school, high school, and college school experiences	Do you remember having many friends in high school? What kinds of things did you do for fun with your friends? Did you get along better with boys or girls? What positive (or negative) memories do you have from high school? Do you remember your first day of high school? How was high school for you (did you like high school? What was your favorite (or best) subject in high school? What subject did you like least (or were you worst at)?

TABLE 9-2 *Continued*

Content Areas	Questions
6. Junior high school, high school, and college school experiences *(continued)*	Do you have any vivid high school memories? Who was your favorite (or least favorite) high school teacher? What made you like (or dislike) this teacher so much? Were you ever suspended or expelled from high school? Describe the worst trouble you were ever in when in high school. What was your greatest high school achievement (or award)? Did you go to college? What were your reasons for going (or not going) to college? What was your major field of study in college? What is the highest degree you obtained?
7. First employment and work experience	What was your first job or the first way you ever earned money? How did you get along with your coworkers? What kinds of positive and negative job memories do you have? Have you ever been fired from a job? What is your ultimate career goal? How much money would you like to make annually?
8. Military history and experiences	Were you ever in the military? Did you volunteer, or were you drafted? Tell me about your most positive (or most negative) experience in the military. What was your final rank? Were you ever disciplined? What was your offense?
9. Romantic relationship history	Have you ever had romantic feelings for someone? Do you remember your first date? What do you think makes a good romantic or loving relationship? What do you look for in a romantic (or marital) partner? What first attracted you to your spouse (or significant other)?
10. Sexual history (including first sexual experience)	Describe your first sexual or sensual experience. What did you learn about sex from your parents (or school, siblings, peers, television, or movies)? What do you think is most important in a sexual relationship? Have you had any traumatic sexual experiences (e.g., rape or incest)?
11. Aggressive history	What is the most angry you have ever been? Have you ever been in a fight? Have you ever been hit by someone else?

(continued)

TABLE 9-2 *Continued*

Content Areas	Questions
11. Aggressive history *(continued)*	What did you learn about anger and how to deal with it from your parents (or siblings, friends, or television)? What do you usually do when you get angry? Tell me about a time when you got too angry and regretted it later.
12. Medical and health history	Did you have any childhood diseases? Any medical hospitalizations? Any surgeries? Do you have any current medical concerns or problems? Are you taking any prescription medications? When was your last physical examination? Do you have any problems with eating or sleeping or weight loss or gain? Have you ever been unconscious? Are there any major diseases that seem to run in your family (e.g., heart disease or cancer)? Tell me about your usual diet. What kinds of foods do you eat most often? Do you have any allergies to foods, medicines, or anything else? What are your exercise patterns? How often do you engage in aerobic exercise?
13. Psychiatric or counseling history	Have you ever been in counseling before? If so, with whom and for what problems, and how long did the counseling last? Do you remember anything your previous counselor did that was particularly helpful (or particularly unhelpful)? Did counseling help with the problem? If not, what did help? Why did you end counseling? Have you ever been hospitalized for psychological reasons? What was the problem then? Have you ever taken medication for psychiatric problems? Has anyone in your family been hospitalized for psychological reasons? Has anyone in your family had significant mental disturbances? Can your remember exactly what that person's problem or diagnosis was?
14. Alcohol and drug history. These questions can be modified to address any substance use problem.	When did you have your first drink of alcohol? About how much alcohol do you consume each day (or week or month)? What is your "drink of choice?" Have you ever had any medical, legal, familial, or vocational problems related to alcohol? Under what circumstances are you most likely to drink? What benefits do you believe you get from drinking?

(continued)

TABLE 9-2 *Continued*

Content Areas	Questions
15. Legal history	Have you ever been arrested or ticketed for an illegal activity? Have you been issued any tickets for driving under the influence? Have you been given any tickets for speeding? How many or how often? Have you ever declared bankruptcy?
16. Recreational history	What is your favorite recreational activity? What recreational activities do you hate or avoid? What sport, hobby, or leisure time pursuit are you best at? How often do you engage in your favorite (or best) activity? What prevents you from engaging in this activity more often? Who do you do this activity with? Are there any recreational activities that you'd like to do, but you've never had the time or opportunity to try?
17. Developmental history	Do you know the circumstances surrounding your conception? Was your mother's pregnancy normal? What was your birth weight? Do you know whether you were nursed or bottlefed? When did you sit, stand, and walk? What have your parents told you about your toilet-training experience? When did you menses begin? (for females)
18. Spiritual or religious history	What is your religious background? What are your current religious or spiritual beliefs? Do you have a religious affiliation? Do you attend church, pray, meditate, or otherwise participate in religious activities? What other spiritual activities have you been involved in previously?

puters do not forget to ask particular questions, and some clients will feel more comfortable disclosing their drug abuse history, sexual history, or other delicate facts (e.g., HIV status) to a computer than to an interviewer (Erdman, Klein, & Greist, 1985; Meier, 1991).

Evaluating Interpersonal Style
The claim that individuals have personality traits resulting in consistent or predictable patterns of behavior is more or less controversial, depending upon one's theoretical orientation, (Bem & Allen, 1974). Psychoanalytic and interpersonal psychotherapists base their therapy approaches on the assumption that individuals behave in highly consistent ways, depending upon their personality or interpersonal style (Fairbairn, 1952; Kelly, 1955; Sullivan, 1970). In con-

trast, cognitive and behavioral psychotherapists are more likely to reject the concept of personality and claim that behavior is a function of the situation or one's cognitions about the situation (Beck, 1976; Mischel, 1968; Ullmann & Krasner, 1965).

For the purposes of this section, we are assuming that people *do* engage in consistent behavior patterns, while recognizing that these patterns may vary greatly depending upon particular persons and situations. Of course, some theorists and therapists may object to this assumption, but generally speaking, even behaviorists (and even some radical behaviorists) are becoming more open to acknowledging the existence of consistent behavior patterns that may reflect something similar to what has been traditionally referred to as personality (Burns, 1990; Goldfried, 1990; Staats, 1990).

Interpersonal Styles   People tend to assume specific roles in their interpersonal relationships. Some people behave in dominant ways, while others are more submissive and self-effacing. Other individuals adopt a hostile or aggressive stance in interpersonal relationships; still others prefer to function in a warm and affiliative manner when relating to others. Some people seem to stay consistently in one role, while others behave much differently depending upon the situation and people involved. This interplay between consistency and variance can be informative and useful in assessing clients' interpersonal problem areas.

During an intake interview, there are three primary sources of data to help interviewers evaluate client interpersonal style. First, you may examine ways in which a client has related to others in the past (e.g., during childhood, adolescence, and young adulthood). Second, you may assess how clients relate to others in their contemporary relationships. Third, you can examine client behavioral interactions with you during the interview session.

Leary's Interpersonal Circumplex   Leary's (1957) interpersonal circumplex is a useful model for identifying patterns of client interpersonal style. Simply put, Leary's model postulates that individuals relate to others on a continuum along two different dimensions: affiliation versus hostility and dominance versus submission. The utility of this conceptualization of interpersonal behavior is that it allows interviewers to identify quickly clients' recurrent interpersonal behavior styles.

Interviewers can use Leary's circumplex model to evaluate client behavior in the context of past relationships, contemporary relationships, and the in-session client-interviewer relationship. During and after an interview, interviewers should ask themselves questions similar to the following:

1. How can the client's description of past relationships be characterized? Has she been dominant or submissive in interpersonal relationships? Have her needs for affection and affiliation guided most of her interpersonal behavior, or has she tended to be aggressive and hostile with others? Put another way, does the client control others, or is she controlled by others? Does she pull others toward her and into relationships, or does she distance them with aggressive acts? How does she behave differently toward different peo-

ple, depending on whether they are family members, older or younger people, males, or females. What is her behavior in various settings?

2. How can the client's description of contemporary relationships be best characterized? Does she describe herself as the bossy or managerial type? Does she see others as looking to her for advice and direction? Or does she look to others for direction? How does she manage her love life? Is she interested in developing love relationships? What is top priority, work, love, or play? Does she wait for others to initiate relationships, or does she seek out relationships? Are her relationships warm and loving or ambivalent and hostile? Again, how does her behavior vary with regard to different individuals and settings?

3. How does the client relate to you during the interview? Is she constantly fighting with you for control (e.g., asking you pointed questions, putting you on the spot)? Or does she quickly let you know that she wants you to take care of her? Does she seem to wait for your lead in every area of questioning, or does she spontaneously pursue issues important to her? Is she aggressive, critical, and hostile or warm and overly cooperative?

Many contemporary forms of psychotherapy place great importance on evaluating a client's interpersonal style. Luborsky (1984) refers to a client's "core conflictual relationship theme" (p. 98). He believes the purpose of psychotherapy is to allow clients greater conscious choice regarding their interpersonal behavior. Similarly, Schact, Binder, and Strupp (1984) consider the appropriate focus of psychotherapy to be: "human actions, embedded in a context of interpersonal transactions, organized in a cyclical psychodynamic pattern, that have been a recurrent source of problems in living and are also currently a source of difficulty" (p. 70).

It is not necessary, and perhaps not appropriate, to have a clear sense of a client's interpersonal style after only a single brief interview. What is necessary and appropriate is to have a few working hypotheses about how a client generally relates to others. Further, as noted by Teyber (1988), interviewers should "attend to the feelings and reactions that the client tends to elicit" in others (p.137). In other words, clients will affect others through their usual interpersonal behaviors by eliciting specific responses from them. As you may already have noticed, this conceptualization is related to countertransference and suggests how important it is for interviewers to examine what thoughts, feelings, and behaviors each client elicits in them.

Exploring Underlying Dynamics   When interviewers begin to have a grasp of a client's interpersonal style, it is sometimes appropriate to explore for dynamics that might underlie the pattern. One way of exploring underlying dynamics is to examine the nature of the client's early significant relationships. This process is fairly straightforward, but unfortunately, clients tend to reconstruct or distort their early interpersonal relationships. Strupp and Binder (1984) comment on this issue:

> A patient's memories of personally relevant events, particularly those referring to early childhood, are often subject to a variety of reconstruc-

tions. While such information may be useful for gaining a better understanding of a patient's emotional life, it is hazardous to rely on it as a
primary source for formulating the patient's current problem. (p. 53)

A more effective way of exploring a client's underlying dynamics involves direct questioning about a client's thoughts, feelings, and memories
associated with deviation from a particular pattern of behavior. This is an
advanced form of interviewing involving questioning, trial interpretation of
life patterns, and checking the client's ability to respond to this type of approach. Although this approach is not always advisable, it can certainly provide important information when the situation is appropriate. For example:

> I: "It seems that many of your relationships have been and are character-
> ized by your tendency to wait for others to meet your emotional and
> sometimes physical needs."
>
> C: "Yeah, that's right . . . and I always end up waiting a long time too,
> don't I?"
>
> I: "I wonder what would happen if you were to take a different, more
> active approach to having your needs met."
>
> C: "I don't know, I suppose it would be better, but I just can't seem able
> to pull it off when the time is right."
>
> I: "Well, let's try something. Imagine your relationship with Anne. What
> if instead of waiting for her to call you, you took the initiative and called
> her first and even made a suggestion about what you could do together?
> Imagine doing that and then describe to me what thoughts, feelings, and
> images come to mind."
>
> C: "Well . . . its hard for me to even imagine doing that, but, well, she
> probably wouldn't want to do something I suggested. Or maybe she'd do
> it, but not enjoy it and then it would be my fault."

Notice the interviewer traced the client's interpersonal pattern to
thoughts and feelings related to fear of rejection and responsibility.

This type of exploration can provide useful information to psychotherapists of virtually any theoretical orientation. Behaviorists could consider it an
evaluation of a client's behavioral repertoire. Cognitive therapists could use
this approach to examine a client's underlying irrational beliefs. Psychoanalytic therapists might focus on what underlies the client's irrational fears;
perhaps traumatic events that occurred early in the context of significant
interpersonal relationships (e.g., dependency issues related to repressed memories of being rejected when one asks directly to have one's needs met).

As noted above, the previous client interviewer exchange uses what
psychoanalytic psychotherapist refer to as a trial interpretation. Some clinicians suggest that trial interpretations be used in initial sessions to determine
whether or not a client is a good candidate for psychoanalytic forms of psycho-

therapy (Sifneos, 1987; Strupp & Binder, 1984). In the previous example, the client responds positively to the trial interpretation and, therefore, evidence to support his ability to engage in insight-oriented therapy is provided. However, it is also possible for clients to respond very negatively to trial interpretations:

> *I:* "It seems that many of your relationships have been and are character-ized by your tendency to wait for others to meet your emotional and sometimes physical needs."
>
> *C:* "I don't know what you mean."
>
> *I:* "In lots of the examples you've talked about in here, you've been waiting for someone to provide you with financial support, fix your car, or supply you with recreational entertainment. Seems like kind of a pattern in terms of how you relate to others."
>
> *C:* "That's ridiculous! Just because my parents are a couple of scrooges doesn't have the least bit to do with me."

This exchange not only provides important information about the client's capacity for insight, it also suggests he is unable to take feedback or criticism well and that he may have a tendency to blame others for his personal situations. In some ways, there is no better vehicle than the interviewer-client relationship for examining a client's interpersonal behavioral tendencies.

Evaluating a client's personal history and interpersonal style are formida-ble tasks that can easily take several sessions. The purpose of exploring these issues in an intake is to formulate hypotheses, not to provide definitive case formulations. Further information regarding these assessment areas may be obtained through review of the suggested readings at the end of this chapter.

Current Functioning

After focusing on historical and interpersonal issues, interviewers should make one more major shift and focus on current functioning. Not only is it important to assess current functioning, it is equally important not to end an interview while focusing on the past. The shift to current functioning provides both a symbolic and a concrete return to the present. The end of the interview should also be a time when interviewers encourage clients to focus on personal strengths and environmental resources, not on past problems.

Questions during this last portion of the intake should focus on current client involvements. Below are some statements and questions interviewers can use to transition to and focus on current functioning:

1. "We've talked about your major concerns and a bit about your past. I'd like to shift to what's happening in your life right now."
2. "What kinds of activities fill up your usual day?"
3. "Describe what a typical day in your life is like?
4. "How much time do you spend at work?"
5. "About how much time do you spend with your partner (spouse)?"

6. "What kinds of things do you and your partner do together? How often do you do these activities?"
7. "Do you spend much time alone?"
8. "What do you most enjoy doing all by yourself?"

Identifying Goals and Monitoring Change

Another key issue toward the end of the interview is the future. Clients supposedly come to professionals because they would like to see some sort of change in their lives. Change implies the future. Consequently, it is appropriate to focus not only on the present but also on the future when discussing current functioning. Many interviewers pose what has been referred to as "the question" to clients at this point in the interview: "Let's say that therapy is successful and in two months you notice some major changes. What will have changed?" Of course, other future-oriented questions may also be appropriate, including "How do you see yourself changing in the next several years?" or "What kind of personal goals (or career goals) are you striving toward?"

Discussion of therapy goals during an intake interview, or in early therapy sessions provides a foundation for termination (Zaro, Barach, Nedelman, & Dreiblatt, 1977). Corey (1991) suggests that initial interview assessments include a question like, "What are the prospects for meaningful change, and how will we know when that change has occurred?" (p. 13). Through establishing clear definitions of desired change, clients and interviewers can jointly monitor the progress of therapy and jointly determine when the end of therapy is approaching.

Factors Affecting Intake Interview Procedures

To conduct an intake interview that thoroughly covers each of the areas described in this chapter within a fifty-minute period is virtually impossible. As a professional interviewer, you must make choices regarding which areas to emphasize, which to deemphasize, and which to ignore. Several factors affect your decisions regarding what to cover during an intake.

Client Registration Forms

Some agencies and practitioners rely heavily on client registration forms or intake questionnaires as sources of information about clients. Our position is that this practice is acceptable in moderation, but when used excessively, it may offend potential clients and referral sources. For example, one agency we have had contact with used a twelve-page intake questionnaire to screen potential clients. The questionnaire contained a number of extremely personal questions such as "Have you experienced sexual abuse?" and "Describe how you were punished as a child." This questionnaire offended many potential clients and frequently produced brief and trite answers to some of the most significant questions. On the other hand, brief and tactful intake questionnaires and registration forms can be immensely helpful in guiding interviewers' selection of especially significant areas to explore with particular clients prior to meeting with them.

Institutional Setting

Often the information to be obtained in an initial interview is partly a function of agency or interviewer policy. Some institutions, such as many psychiatric hospitals, demand a great emphasis on diagnostic or historical information, while other settings, such as health maintenance organizations, focus almost exclusively on problem or symptom analysis, goal setting, and treatment planning. Consequently, interviewers should keep in mind the needs of their institution when conducting intake interviews.

Theoretical Orientation

Perhaps the main factor influencing what information is obtained during an intake session is the interviewer's theoretical orientation. Specifically, behavioral and cognitively oriented interviewers tend to focus on current problems, while psychoanalytically oriented interviewers downplay current problem analysis in favor of historical data. Person-centered therapists focus on the current situation and how clients feel about themselves (e.g., whether any discrepancies exist between clients' real and ideal selves). Psychoanalytic and person-centered interviewers are also less likely to make use of detailed client registration forms or computerized interviewing procedures.

Professional Background and Professional Affiliation

Finally, one's professional background and professional affiliation may have a strong influence on what information is obtained in an intake interview. Before we wrote this book, we asked professionals with different backgrounds for their opinions about what was most needed in an interviewing textbook. The correlation between response content and respondents' area of professional training was strikingly high. Psychiatrists emphasized the importance of mental status exam and diagnostic interviewing, based on DSM-III-R. Clinical psychologists were interested in assessment and diagnosis as well, but they also emphasized problem assessment and behavioral and cognitive analysis. Counseling psychologists focused less on assessment and more on listening skills and helping strategies, while social workers expressed primary interest in developmental history taking, treatment planning, and listening skills.

Chapter Summary

The intake interview is probably the most basic type of interview conducted by mental health professionals. It usually involves obtaining information about a new client in order to identify what type of treatment, if any, is most appropriate. The intake is primarily an assessment interview. Consequently, it usually involves the liberal use of questions.

Many types of questions are available to therapeutic interviewers. Different types of questions produce different types of client response. Most questions beginning with "what?" or "how?" are considered open because they are less likely to restrict client talk and must be answered with more than a yes or a no. Questions beginning with "why" are partially open in that they facilitate talk but sometimes also elicit intellectual explanations or defensiveness. In contrast, "where," "when," and "who" questions are minimally open because they ordinarily produce limited information pertaining to location, time, and people. Closed questions usually begin with "do" or "did" and are defined as questions that can be answered with a yes or no response. Swing questions, which normally begin with "could," "would," "can," or "will", may be answered with yes or no, but, if rapport is adequate, they facilitate talk and open elaboration by clients. Indirect questions are statements made by interviewers beginning with phrases such as "I wonder" and "you must." These statements are implied questions to which clients may or may not choose to respond. Finally, projective questions usually begin with "what if" and invite client speculation about hypothetical situations.

Questions are associated with a wide range of potential benefits and liabilities. In some cases, questions can cause a pattern to form wherein the client simply waits for the interviewer to ask the "right" question. This may result in client passivity or dependency. Excessive questioning can also result in rapport problems. On the other hand, questions constitute an efficient method of obtaining important information about clients.

Competent interviewers do not rely exclusively on questioning as an interviewing tool. They also take steps to prepare their clients for questions, make their questions relevant to client concerns, use questions to effectively elicit concrete behavioral examples and are cautious and sensitive when asking questions directed at very personal information.

The three major objectives of intake interviewing are evaluating the client's problem, the client's personality and mental condition, and the client's current situation.

Evaluating clients' problems requires that interviewers identify their clients' main source of personal distress as well the range of other problems that may be contributing to discomfort. Problems need to be prioritized and selected for potential therapeutic intervention. Many systems are available to help interviewers analyze and conceptualize client symptoms. Usually these processes involve identifying the factors or events that precede and follow occurrence of client symptoms.

Sometimes client symptoms cluster together in such a way as to constitute a diagnostic syndrome. Consequently, client symptomatology should be explored in order to determine whether a particular mental disorder is present. This requires reference to DSM-III-R, ICD-9, or any one of a number of diagnostic interviewing schedules (some of which are listed in the Suggested Readings).

Three main sources of information pertaining to client personality and mental condition can be obtained in an interview: client personal history, client manner of interacting with others, and formal evaluation of client mental status (covered in chapter 10).

Obtaining information about client personal history is a sensitive and challenging process. Many clients will claim they recall little of their childhood. Others will not want to discuss their childhood because it was emotionally or physically painful.

Interviewers should begin by exploring their client's personal histories nondirectively. This allows clients to freely discuss memories that they consider significant. A natural flow of personal history is from earliest memories, to descriptions of parents and family experiences, to school and peer relationships, to employment. Interviewers must be selective and flexible regarding the historical information they choose to obtain from their clients; there is too much information to cover in a typical interview, and clients may have strong ideas of their own regarding what information they want to discuss.

Although there is some controversy regarding whether or not personality (or interpersonal style) exists as a stable and concrete construct, interviewers should be sensitive to this concept and know how to evaluate for its presence. Three sources of information pertaining to client interpersonal style are available to interviewers: the client's historically consistent patterns of relating to others, the client's contemporary patterns of relating to others, and the client's pattern of relating to the interviewer during the interviewing session. Because the first two of these sources may be distorted by clients, many clinicians consider the interaction between client and interviewer as the best source of information about client interpersonal style.

Leary (1957) established a system for identifying client interpersonal style that involves identifying whether clients are more affiliative or hostile and more dominant or submissive. Clients may be more or less consistent in terms of how they relate to others along these dimensions. Leary's system can be used to identify client interpersonal style in the context of a client's personal history, contemporary relationships, and therapeutic relationship.

Advanced interviewing techniques such as trial interpretation and projective questioning can help interviewers explore underlying client dynamics (i.e., what thoughts and experiences underlie particular personal styles). Trial interpretations may be used to determine if a client is capable of engaging effectively in insight-oriented psychotherapy.

The last major area of focus in an intake interview is client current functioning. Interviewers should focus on current functioning last so as to bring clients back in touch with their current situation, both liabilities and assets. The end of the interview should slightly emphasize client personal strengths and environmental resources and should focus on the future and on setting goals.

It is impossible to cover thoroughly all of the areas discussed in this chapter in a single intake interview. Client registration forms and intake questionnaires can help interviewers determine in advance some of the areas to cover in a given intake. The interviewer's theoretical orientation, therapeutic setting, and professional background and affiliation also help guide the focus of intake interviews.

Suggested Readings

Benjamin, A. (1981). *The helping interview*. (3rd ed.). Boston: Houghton-Mifflin. Chapter 5 of Benjamin's classic work is devoted to a discussion and analysis of the uses and abuses of questions.

Bornstein, P. H., & Bornstein, M. T. (1986). *Marital therapy: A behavioral-communications approach*. New York: Pergamon. This text contains useful information pertaining to interviewing couples.

Gunderson, J. G., Ronningstam, E., & Bodkin, A. (1990). The diagnostic interview for narcissistic patients. *Archives of General Psychiatry, 47*, 676-680. This article describes an approach for diagnosing narcissistic patients through an interview format.

Gustafson, J. P. (1986). *The complex secret of brief psychotherapy*. New York: W. W. Norton. Chapters 19 and 20 of this text focus on preliminary interviews and trial therapy from a brief psychoanalytic perspective.

Hersen, M., & Turner, S. M. (1985). *Diagnostic interviewing*. New York: Plenum. This edited volume focuses on diagnostic interviewing with a number of clinical populations (i.e., populations classified by specific disorder), including those experiencing alcoholism, sexual dysfunction, and anxiety disorders. Most of the expert contributors specialize in psychiatry or clinical behavior therapy.

Lazarus, A. A. (1976). *Multimodal behavior therapy*. New York: Springer. This is Lazarus's classic text on multimodal behavior therapy. In it he describes his BASIC ID model in great detail.

Riskind, J. H., Beck, A. T., Brown, G., & Steer, R. A. (1987). Taking the measure of anxiety and depression: Validity of the reconstructed Hamilton Scales. *Journal of Nervous and Mental Disease, 175*, 474-479. This article evaluates the validity of a newly constructed diagnostic interview schedule for anxiety and depression. The newly constructed scales are derived from Hamilton's (1967) original anxiety and depression scales.

Teyber, E. (1988). *Interpersonal process in psychotherapy: A guide for clinical training*. Chicago: The Dorsey Press. This book focuses on assessment from the interpersonal perspective in chapters 6 through 8. It is a good source for beginning graduate students who want to employ interpersonal psychotherapeutic approaches.

Zaro, J. S., Barach, R., Nedelman, D. J., & Dreiblatt, I. S. (1977). A guide for beginning psychotherapists. New York: Cambridge University Press. Chapters 3 through 6 of this text focus on first contact and assessment. Written from an eclectic perspective, this work is a good source for beginning psychotherapists.

10

THE MENTAL STATUS EXAMINATION

What is a Mental Status Exam?

A Generic Approach to Mental Status Examination
    Appearance
    Behavior or Psychomotor Activity
    Attitude Toward Examiner (Interviewer)
    Affect and Mood
    Speech and Thought
    Perceptual Disturbances
    Orientation and Consciousness
    Memory and Intelligence
    Reliability, Judgment, and Insight

When to Use Mental Status Examinations

Chapter Summary

Suggested Readings

There are some who make a point of trying to investigate the world we live in with full scientific rigour without becoming estranged from it. This is never easy: is it possible?
        —R. D. LAING, The Voice of Experience

Objectivity is like a wet bar of soap and may clean up people and things, but it also slips easily out of hand, and if you try to stand on it you're likely to fall and break your neck.
        —JOHN R. MEANS

When it comes to objectivity and clinical interviewing there are two major questions to ask ourselves: First, is complete objectivity possible? Second, even if it were possible, is complete objectivity desirable?

It is important to be careful when being objective. Good interviewers need to be able to make an emotional connection with their clients. Good *evaluators* may or may not establish an emotional connection with their clients. This is because emotional connection can interfere with objectivity; for the sake of objectivity, many evaluators minimize rapport and emotional involvement. Our position is that one need not sacrifice human connection for objectivity. We believe the cost of being too objective is greater than the cost of having an emotional connection that lets a little subjectivity into an evaluation.

Total objectivity requires complete emotional distance. Of course, it may be that neither total objectivity nor complete emotional distance exists in any human endeavor. This issue is eloquently addressed by Fritjof Capra in *The Tao of Physics* (1975):

> A careful analysis of the process of observation in atomic physics has shown that the subatomic particles have no meaning as isolated entities, but can only be understood as interconnections between the preparation of an experiment and the subsequent measurement. . . . In atomic physics, we can never speak about nature without at the same time speaking about ourselves. (p. 19)

Attempting to be emotionally distant or uninvested may be desirable when studying microbes or physical objects, but, even in such hard-science enterprises, one is well advised to recognize the human element. When studying humans, excessive emotional distance is neither desirable nor useful. Instead, interviewers must use their own emotional reactions to help them understand the human in question. The critical challenge of mental status evaluations is to combine emotional sensitivity with objective detachment.

What Is a Mental Status Exam?

The mental status examination is a method of organizing and evaluating clinical observations pertaining to mental status. The primary purpose of the mental status examination is to evaluate accurately *current* cognitive processes (Strub & Black, 1977). However, in recent years mental status exams have become increasingly comprehensive, and some now include sections on historical information, treatment planning, and diagnostic impressions (Siassi, 1984). The mental status exam we will describe is considered a generic model that emphasizes, in the tradition of Strub and Black (1977), assessment of current cognitive functions. Other sections of this chapter and text are devoted to historical and psychodiagnostic interviewing, and to treatment planning.

The mental status exam is popular in medical settings. "In the psychiatric evaluation the mental status examination is considered to be analogous to the physical examination in general medicine" (Siassi, 1984, p. 267).

In hospitals and medical centers, it is not unusual for admitting psychiatrists to request administration of daily mental status examinations on acutely disturbed patients. The results are reported in clear, concise descriptions of about one medium-length paragraph per patient. Communication of mental status is basic procedure within medical settings. Anyone who seeks employment in the medical system's mental health domain should be fluent in the language of mental status.

A Generic Approach to Mental Status Examination

The main categories covered in a basic mental status examination are listed below.

- Appearance
- Behavior/Psychomotor activity
- Attitude toward examiner (interviewer)
- Affect and mood
- Speech and thought
- Perceptual disturbances
- Orientation and consciousness
- Memory and intelligence
- Reliability, judgment, and insight

During a mental status examination, observations are compiled and organized in an effort to establish hypotheses about the client's mental functioning. The examiner does not at this time interpret specific phenomena (e.g., sad affect, psychomotor retardation, or tangential speech) as signs of a particular mental state or psychiatric condition. Although a clear and objective mental status examination usually provides important diagnostic information, administration of the exam is not primarily a diagnostic procedure.

Each assessment domain covered during a traditional mental status examination is defined and described below.

Appearance

In the mental status examination, the interviewer takes note of a client's general appearance. Appearance observation is limited primarily to physical characteristics, but some demographic information is also included within this domain.

Physical characteristics commonly noted on a mental status exam include grooming, dress, pupil dilation/contraction, facial expression, perspiration, use of makeup, presence of tatoos, height, weight, and nutritional status. A client's physical appearance may be a manifestation of mental state. Similarly, physical appearance may be indicative of particular psychiatric diagnoses. For example, dilated pupils are sometimes associated with drug intoxication and pinpoint pupils with drug withdrawal. However, as noted above, the presence of dilated pupils should not be considered as conclusive evidence of drug intoxication but as one bit of evidence that might lead an examiner to eventually conclude that drug intoxication has produced a particular mental state.

Client sex, age, race, and ethnic background are also concrete variables noted during a mental status exam. Each of these factors is sometimes related to psychiatric diagnosis and treatment planning. For example, males are more likely to be diagnosed as having antisocial personality disorder and as being alcohol abusers, while females receive diagnoses of eating disorders and depression more often. As Othmer and Othmer (1989) note, the relationship between appearance and biological age may have significance: "A patient who appears older than his stated age may have a history of drug or alcohol abuse, organic mental disorder, depression, or physical illness" (p. 114).

Behavior or Psychomotor Activity

This category is concerned with physical movement. A client's level of activity throughout the evaluation should be noted.

Examiners look for excessive or limited bodily movements as well as particular physical movements, such as eye contact, excessive eye movement (scanning), odd or repeated gestures, and posture. Clients may deny experiencing particular thoughts or emotions (e.g., paranoia or depression), while their body movements suggest otherwise (e.g., vigilant posturing and scanning or slowed psychomotor activity and lack of facial expression).

Excessive bodily movements may be associated with anxiety or affective disorders, while a paucity of movement may represent depression, organicity, catatonic schizophrenia, or drug-induced stupor. Sometimes paranoid clients will constantly scan their visual field in an effort to be on guard against external threat. Repeated motor movements (such as dusting off one's shoes) may signal the presence of obsessive-compulsive disorder. Similarly, repeated picking of imagined lint or dirt off of one's clothing or skin is sometimes associated with delirium or toxic conditions.

Attitude toward Examiner (Interviewer)

The word attitude is often overused by parents, teachers, and mental health professionals. When someone claims a student or client has an "attitude problem" or a "bad attitude," it is difficult to precisely determine what is meant by such a statement. "Attitude" is often used in a vague manner.

In the mental health field, "attitude toward the interviewer" refers to how clients behave in relation to the interviewer; that is attitude is defined as behavior that occurs in an interpersonal context. The observation of concrete physical characteristics and physical movement provides a foundation for evaluating client attitude toward the interviewer.

Judging a client's manner of relating to an examiner requires inference. This portion of the mental status exam *requires* emotional subjectivity. Interviewers must allow themselves to respond honestly to their clients and then turn their attention to scrutinizing their own reactions for clues to the clients. Such judgments are based on interviewers' internal cognitive processes and consequently are subject to personal biases. For example, a male interviewer may infer seductiveness from the behavior of an attractive female because of his own wish that she behave seductively, rather than any actual seductive behavior. Furthermore, what is considered seductive by the examiner may not be considered seductive by the client. The difference may be based on individual or cultural differences. It is the interviewer's responsibility to make great efforts not to overinterpret client behavior by attributing it to a general client attitude or, in some cases, a personality trait. When making judgments or attributions about client behavior, interviewers should recall the criteria for disordered behavior presented in chapter 8 and ask themselves:

- Is the behavior unusual, or statistically infrequent?
- Is the behavior disturbing to the client or to others within the client's environment at home or work?
- Is the behavior maladaptive, that is, does it contribute to the client's difficulty?
- Is the client's behavior justifiable based on present environmental contingencies?

There are many ways a client can relate to an interviewer. Words commonly used to describe client attitude toward the interview or interviewer are in Table 10-1.

Affect and Mood

Affect is defined as the prevailing emotional tone as observed by the interviewer during mental status examination. Under ordinary conditions affect varies slightly depending upon the client's current situation and the subject under discussion. Access to a wide variety of emotional experiences tends to be associated with mental health. However, in some cases affect may be too variable.

Affect Affect may be described in terms of its content or type, range and duration (also known as variability and duration), appropriateness, and depth or intensity. For example, a depressed client may be described with the following terms referring to affect:

- Sad (content or type). Referring to behavior suggesting depression (e.g., tears, expressions of hopelessness, slowed or retarded psychomotor activity).
- Constricted (range and duration). Referring to a narrow band of affective expression maintained over time (i.e., virtually only sadness is expressed).
- Appropriate with respect to speech content and life situation (appropriateness). Referring to the fact that the client has recently experienced a number of losses in his life.
- Profound (depth or intensity). Referring to the "deep" quality of the client's affect (e.g., the client sobs powerfully during the session).

TABLE 10-1 Descriptors of Client Attitude toward the Examiner

1. Aggressive: The client attacks the examiner physically or verbally or through grimaces and gestures. The client may "flip off" the examiner or simply say in reply to an examiner response, "That's a stupid question" or "Of course I'm feeling angry, can't you do anything but mimic back to me what I've already said?!!"

2. Cooperative: The client responds directly to interviewer comments or questions. He may openly try to work with the interviewer in an effort to gather data or solve problems. Frequent head nods and receptive body posture are common.

3. Hostile: Clients who are indirectly nasty or biting. Sarcasm, rolling back one's eyes in apparent disgust over an interviewer comment or question, or staring off with a sour grimace may represent subtle, or not so subtle, hostility.

4. Impatient: The client is on the edge of her seat. She is not very tolerant of pauses or of times when interviewer speech becomes deliberate. She may make statements about wanting an answer to her concerns immediately. There may be associated hostility and competitiveness in the case of Type A personality styles.

5. Indifferent: The client's appearance and movements suggest he is unconcerned or uninterested in the interview. He may yawn, drum his fingers, or become distracted by irrelevant issues or details. The client could also be described as apathetic.

6. Ingratiating: The client is obsequious and overly solicitous of approval and interviewer reinforcement. She may try to present herself in an overly positive manner. She may agree with everything and anything the interviewer says. There may be excessive head nodding, eye contact, and smiles.

7. Intense: The client's eye contact is constant, or almost so, his body leans forward, and he listens intensely to the interviewer's every word. Client voice volume may be loud and voice tone forceful. The client is the opposite of indifferent.

8. Manipulative: The client tries to use the examiner for her own purpose or edification. She may interpret examiner statements to represent her own best interests. Statements like, "His behavior isn't fair, is it Doctor?" are efforts to solicit agreement and may represent manipulation.

9. Negativistic: The client opposes virtually everything the examiner says. The client may disagree with reflections, paraphrases, or summaries that are clearly accurate. The client may refuse to answer questions or be completely silent throughout an interview. This behavior is also called oppositional.

10. Open: The client openly and straightforwardly discusses his problems and concerns. He may also be open to examiner suggestions or interpretations.

11. Passive: The client offers little or no active opposition or participation in the interview. She may say things like, "Whatever you think." She may simply sit passively until told what to do or say.

12. Seductive: The client may touch himself in seductive or suggestive ways (e.g., rubbing body parts). He may expose skin or make efforts to be "too close" to or to touch the examiner. He may make flirtatious and suggestive verbal comments.

13. Suspicious: The client may look around the room suspiciously (some even actively check for hidden microphones). Squinting or looking out of the corner of one's eyes also may be interpreted as suspiciousness. Questions about what the examiner is writing down or about why such information is needed may also signal suspiciousness.

This client might be described as "exhibiting profoundly sad and constricted affect that is appropriate with respect to his life situation."

In contrast, a client who presents with symptoms of mania might have much different affective descriptors:

- Euphoric (content or type). Referring to behavior suggestive of mania (e.g., claims of omnipotence, agitation or increased psychomotor activity, exaggerated gestures).
- Labile (range and duration). Referring to a wide band of affective expression over a short time period (e.g., the client shifts quickly from tears to laughter).
- Inappropriate with respect to speech content and life situation (appropriateness). Referring to the client's euphoria over job loss and marital separation.
- Shallow (depth or intensity). Referring to little depth or maintenance of emotion (e.g., client claims to be "happy" because "I smile" and "smiling always takes care of everything").

This client might be described as having a "labile but primarily euphoric affect that is inappropriate and shallow."

Mood   In the mental status exam, mood is different than affect. Mood is defined simply as the client's self-report regarding her prevailing emotional state. Mood should be evaluated through a simple nonleading, open-ended question such as, "How are you feeling today?", rather than a leading question that suggests an answer to the client: "Are you depressed?"

Most often it is desirable to record a client's response to your "mood" question verbatim. This makes it easier to compare a client's self-reported mood with your evaluation of affect. Also, it is important to compare self-reported mood with self-reported thought content, because the thought content may account for the predominance of a particular mood.

Mood can be distinguished from affect on the basis of several features. Mood tends to last longer than affect. Mood changes more spontaneously than affect. Mood constitutes the emotional background. And, mood is reported by the client, while affect is observed by the interviewer (from Othmer & Othmer, 1989). Put another way, mood is to climate as affect is to weather.

Speech and Thought

Speech   Speech is ordinarily described in terms of its rate and volume. Rate refers to the observed speed of a client's speech. Volume refers to how loud a client talks. Both rate and volume can be categorized as

- High (fast or loud)
- Medium (normal of average)
- Low (slow or soft)

Client speech is usually described as pressured (high speed), loud (high volume), slow or halting (low speed), or soft or inaudible (low volume). Special speech qualities should also be noted. These may include stuttering, an accent, high and screeching or low and gravelly pitch, and poor or distorted enunciation. In many cases, the examiner may simply comment, "The patient's speech was of normal rate and volume."

Forms of disturbed speech include dysarthria (problems with articulation or slurring of speech) and dysprosody (problems with rhythm, such as mumbling or long pauses or latencies between syllables of words). These speech disturbances are usually caused by specific brain disturbances. For example, mumbling may occur in patients with Huntington's chorea and slurring of speech in intoxicated patients.

Speech, or verbal expression, constitutes the most direct "road" to thought process and content. It is primarily through speech that mental status examiners are able to observe and evaluate thought. There are, however, other modalities for observing and evaluating thought processes. Nonverbal behavior, sign language (in deaf clients), and writing are also good sources of information pertaining to thinking processes.

Thought Process Observation and evaluation of thought is usually broken into two broad categories: thought process and thought content. Thought processes refer to "how" a client expresses herself. In other words, does thinking proceed in a systematic, organized, and logical manner? Can the client "get to the point" when expressing herself? In many cases it is useful to obtain a verbatim sample of client speech in order to capture any psychopathological processes. The following sample was taken from a client's letter to his therapist, who was relocating to seek further professional education.

> Dear Bill:
> My success finally came around and I finally made plenty of good common sense with my attitude and I hope your sister will come along just fine really now and learn maybe at her elementary school whatever she may ask will not really develop to bad a complication of any kind I don't know for sure whether you're married or not yet but I hope you come along just fine with yourself and your plans on being a doctor somewhere or whatever or however too maybe well now so. I suppose I'll be at one of those inside sanitariums where I'll work out . . . and it'll come around okay really,
> Bye for now Bill

The client who wrote this letter clearly had a thinking process dysfunction. His expression is disorganized and only minimally coherent. Initially his communication is characterized by a loosening of association; then, after writing the word "doctor," the client decompensates into complete incoherence (i.e., "word salad"; see Table 10-2).

There are many ways to describe speech or thought processes. Some of the most common thought-process descriptors are listed and defined in Table 10.2.

TABLE 10-2 Thought Process Descriptors

1. Blocking: Sudden cessation of speech in the midst of a stream of talk. There is no clear external reason for the client to stop talking, and the client cannot explain why she stopped talking. Blocking may indicate that the client was about to associate to an extremely anxiety-laden topic. It also can indicate intrusion of delusional thoughts or disturbed perceptual experiences.

2. Circumstantiality: Excessive and unnecessary detail provided by the client. Sometimes very intellectual people (e.g., scientists or even college professors) can become circumstantial; they eventually make their point, but they do not do so directly and efficiently. Circumstantiality or overelaboration also may be a sign of defensiveness and can be associated with paranoid thinking styles. (It can also simply be a sign the professor was not well-prepared for the lecture.)

3. Clang Associations: Combining unrelated words or phrases simply because they have similar sounds. Usually this is manifest through rhyming or alliteration. For example: "I'm slime, dime, do some mime," or "When I think of my dad, rad, mad, pad, lad, sad." Some clients who clang are also perseverating (see below). Clanging usually occurs among very disturbed clients (e.g., schizophrenics). Of course, with all psychiatric symptoms, sometimes a specific situation or subculture encourages the behavior in which cases it should not be considered abnormal (e.g., clanging behavior of rap group members is not abnormal).

4. Flight of Ideas: Continuous and overproductive speech in which the client's ideas are fragmented. Usually an idea is stimulated by either a previous idea or an external event, but the relationship among ideas or ideas and events may be weak. In contrast to loose associations (see below), there are some perceivable connections in the client's thinking. However, unlike circumstantiality, the client never gets to the original point or never really answers the original question. Clients who exhibit flight of ideas often appear overenergized or overstimulated (e.g., manic or hypomanic clients). Of course, many normal people exhibit flight of ideas after excessive caffeine or stimulant intake.

5. Loose Associations: A lack of logical relationship between thoughts and ideas. Sometimes interviewers can perceive the connections but must strain to do so. For example: "I love you. Bread is the staff of life. Haven't I seen you in church? I think incest is horrible." In this example the client thinks of attraction and love, then of God's love as expressed through communion, then of church, and then of a presentation he heard in church about incest. The associations are loose but not completely nonexistent. Such communication may be an indicator of schizotypal personality disorder, schizophrenia, or other psychotic or pre- or postpsychotic disorders. Of course, some extremely creative people regularly exhibit loosening of associations, but most are able to find a socially acceptable vehicle through which they express their ideas.

6. Mutism: Virtually total unexpressiveness. There may be some signs that the client is in contact with others, but these are usually limited. Mutism can indicate autism or schizophrenia, catatonic subtype.

7. Neologisms: Client-invented words. They are more than mispronunciations and are also rather spontaneously created; in other words, they are products of the moment rather than of a thoughtful creative process. We have heard words such as "slibber" and "temperaturific." It is important to check with the client with regard to word meaning and origin. Unusual words may be real words, or they may be taken from popular songs, television shows, or other sources. Neologisms are usually intentionally created. They are associated with psychotic disorders.

8. Perseveration: Involuntary repetition of a single response or idea. The concept of perseveration may apply to speech or movement. Perseveration is often associated with brain damage or disease and with psychotic disorders. After being told no, teenagers often engage in this behavior, although normal teenagers are being persistent

(continued)

TABLE 10-2 *Continued*

than perseverative—that is, if properly motivated, they are able to stop themselves voluntarily.

9. Tangentiality: Similar to circumstantiality, but the client never returns to her central point; she never answers the original question. Tangential speech represents greater thought disturbance and disorganization than circumstantial speech, but less thought disturbance than loose association. Tangential speech is discriminated from flight of ideas because flight of ideas involves greater overproductivity of speech.

10. Word Salad: Client says a series of words that seem completely unrelated. Word salad represents probably the highest level of thinking disorganization. Clients who exhibit word salad are grossly incoherent. (For an example of word salad, see the client letter on page 224.)

When describing client speech and thought process, a mental status examiner might state, "The client's speech was loud and pressured. Her communication was somewhat incoherent; she exhibited flight of ideas and neologisms."

Thought Content   Thought content refers to specific meaning expressed in client communication. While thought process constitutes the "how" of client thinking, thought content constitutes the "what" of client thinking. What clients talk about can give interviewers a sense of their mental status.

Clients can talk about a virtually unlimited array of subjects during an interview. There are several specific content areas, which, if discussed, should be noted and explored in a mental status exam. These include delusions, obsessions, suicidal or homicidal thoughts or plans, specific phobias, and preoccupation with any emotion, particularly guilt. In this section discussion will focus on delusions and obsessions.

Delusions are defined as false beliefs. They represent a break from reality in that they are not based on facts or real events. Examiners may find it useful to record client reports of delusions verbatim. Examiners must take care not to dispute clients' beliefs.

Clients may refer to many different types of delusions. Delusions of grandeur are false beliefs pertaining to one's own ability or status. Most frequently clients with delusions of grandeur believe they have extraordinary mental powers, physical strength, wealth, or sexual potency. They are usually unaffected by discrepancies between their beliefs and objective reality. In some cases grandiose clients begin to believe they are a specific historical or contemporary figure (Napoleon, Jesus Christ, and Joan of Arc are particularly common).

Clients with delusions of persecution or paranoid delusions often hold false beliefs that others are "out to get them" or are spying on them. Clients with such delusions may falsely believe that their home or telephone is bugged or that they are under surveillance by a neighbor who they believe to be an FBI agent. Clients with paranoid delusions often have "ideas of reference," which are beliefs that one is an object of attention or focus in situations that actually have nothing whatsoever to do with one. Many paranoid clients believe the television, newspaper, or radio is talking to or about them. Author John worked with a hospitalized man who complained that the television news was broadcasting his "life story" every night and thereby humiliating him in front of the rest of the patients and community.

Delusions of alien control are characterized by feelings and beliefs that one is under the control or influence of some outside force or power. Symptoms such as alien control usually involve a "disowning" of one's own volition and personal responsibility. Clients will report feeling as if they are puppets, passive and unable to assert personal control. In years past it was popular to report being controlled by the "Russians" or "Communists," while in recent years the delusion of being possessed or controlled by supernatural forces has increased in popularity.

Somatic delusions usually involve false beliefs about having a medical condition or disease, such as cancer, a heart condition, or obstructed bowels. Not surprisingly, AIDS has become a frequent preoccupation for clients who have somatic delusions. It is not uncommon for very disturbed clients to believe they have AIDS despite the fact they have never used intravenous drugs or had sexual relations. Similarly, clients may believe they are pregnant when they have not had intercourse. Anorexic clients may falsely believe they are grossly overweight when, in fact, they are dying of malnutrition.

Depressed clients often manifest delusions of self-deprecation. They may believe they are the "worst case ever" or that their skills and abilities are grossly impaired. Common self-deprecating comments include statements about sinfulness, ugliness, and stupidity. In some cases clients will have engaged in a behavior or thought that causes them to feel negative about themselves. During mental status exams interviewers should explore the roots of self-deprecating delusions.

It is always important to seek factual evidence to determine whether or not a client is truly delusional, especially in cases of suspected somatic delusions. These clients should be examined by a physician to rule out the possibility that a medical condition really does exist. Exploring delusional beliefs can also provide examiners with insights into client thought processes and personal experiences. The client who claims the "body snatchers" are making him shout profanities at his parents may feel overly controlled by his parents. He may also feel extremely angry toward them and find it less threatening to disown his impulses to shout at his parents by ascribing the shouted profanities to some peculiar evil force. Similarly, the grandiose client may feel unimportant or neglected, while the paranoid client cannot trust anyone and therefore projects his feelings of distrust onto others and then comes to believe he is being constantly watched by others.

Obsessions   Obsessions are recurrent and persistent ideas, thoughts, and images. True obsessions are involuntary and viewed as senseless or irrational by those who are experiencing them. Clients may intentionally ruminate about a wide variety of issues, but only if they lose voluntary control over whether or not they think a particular thought are they obsessing. One obsessive-compulsive client had obsessions about being contaminated by "worms" and "germs" (Sommers, 1986). He reported that once as he rode his bicycle down the street, he noticed an open garbage dumpster on the opposite side of the street and immediately became overwhelmed with the thought that perhaps he had "gotten some of the garbage on [his] lips." Intense obsessions are often followed by compulsive behaviors. In the same case, the client felt compelled to ride back and forth down the street past the garbage dumpster to determine whether he possibly could have reached his head across the street and into the garbage. Such a case illustrates the irrational and sometimes even delusional nature of obsessions.

Most individuals who present with clinically significant compulsions exhibit either washing or checking behavior. In other words, they continually feel the need to wash or clean something, or they constantly need to check whether a particular event has occurred or is going to occur. The most common examples are compulsions to wash one's hands, clean one's house, check the locks, and check to see if an intruder has gained entry into a bedroom or house. Clinically significant compulsions are virtually always preceded by clinically significant obsessions. Obsessions are characterized primarily by a sense of doubt. Commonly, obsessive-compulsive clients will wonder:

- Are my hands clean?
- Have I been contaminated?
- Did I remember to lock the front door?
- Did I remember to turn off the oven (lights, stereo, etc.)?
- Is anyone under my bed?

Although everyone experiences obsessive thoughts on occasion, such thoughts may or may not be clinically or diagnostically significant. We should clarify the difference between clinical and diagnostic significance: Information is of clinical significance if it contributes to the treatment process; information is of diagnostic significance if it contributes to the diagnostic process. During a mental status exam, it is always important to evaluate obsessions because they reveal to an examiner what the client spends time thinking about. Such information may be clinically significant; that is, it may enhance empathy and treatment planning. However, the same obsessions may or may not be diagnostically significant. For example, if a client describes obsessions that do not interfere with his ability to function at work, school, home, or play, they may not be diagnostically significant.

Perceptual Disturbances

There are two major types of perceptual disturbances: hallucinations and illusions. Hallucinations are defined as false sensory impressions or experiences. Illusions are defined as perceptual distortions.

Hallucinations may occur in any of the five major sensory modalities: visual, auditory, olfactory, gustatory, and tactile.

Auditory hallucinations are the most common type reported by clients. Clients who report hearing things (usually voices) that others do not hear usually suffer from either an affective disorder or schizophrenia. However, on occasion such experiences may be produced by states of chemical intoxication or as a consequence of acute traumatic stress. In other instances clients may report "especially good hearing" or listening to their own "inner voice." While such reports are worth exploring, they are not in and of themselves signs of perceptual disturbance. In addition, people often report odd perceptual experiences, similar to hallucinations, that occur as they fall off to sleep or when they are just waking up. Such perceptual disturbances are normal and are a consistent part of most people's sleep patterns. Therefore, when evaluating for hallucinations, interviewers should always determine *when* such experiences usually occur. If they occur exclusively when a client is in a stage of sleep, then they are of less significance.

Due to the psychotic nature of delusions and hallucinations, and the bizarre nature of some obsessive-compulsive symptoms, interviewers should approach questioning in these areas with an especially gentle and explorative manner. The following sample interview dialogue illustrates how interviewers can help clients admit their unusual or bizarre experiences:

I: "I'm going to ask you some questions about personal experiences you may have had or may be having. Some of the questions may seem odd or unusual, while others may fit some personal experiences you've had but haven't yet spoken about."

C: "Okay."

I: "Sometimes radio broadcasts or television newscasts or programming can feel very personal, as if the people in them were speaking directly to you. Have you ever thought a particular program was talking about you or to you on a personal basis?"

C: "That program the other night was about my life. It was about me and Cybil Shepard."

I: "You know Cybil Shepard?"

C: "I sure do, she's my woman."

I: "And how did you and she meet?"

C: "We met cause I was her director in about five or six movies she filmed."

The next dialogue models a way you might evaluate for auditory perceptual disturbances:

I: "I've noticed you seem to be a pretty sensitive person. Is your hearing especially good?"

C: "Yes, as a matter of fact, I have better hearing than most people."

I: "Really. What kinds of things do you hear that most people can't hear."

C: "I can hear people talking through walls, in the next room."

I: "Right now?"

C: "Yeah."

I: "What are the voices saying?"

C: "They're talking about me and Cybil . . . about our sex life."

I: "How about your vision? Is it especially keen too? Can you see things that others can't?"

The next dialogue models an evaluation for obsessions:

I: "You know how sometimes people get a song or tune stuck in their head and they can't stop thinking about it? Have you ever had that kind of experience?"

C: "Sure, doesn't everybody?"

I: "Yeah, that's true. I'm wondering if you have some particular thoughts, kind of like a musical tune, that you wish you could get rid of, but can't?"

C: "Maybe sometimes, but it's no big deal."

I: "How about images. Do you have any images that seem to intrude into your mind and that you can't get rid of?"

Notice how the interviewer in these examples normalizes each type of pathology and then inquires as to its presence.

Visual or tactile hallucinations are often associated with organic conditions. These conditions may include drug intoxication or withdrawal, brain trauma, or brain disease. Clients in acute delirious states may pick at their clothes or skin in an effort to remove objects or organisms (e.g., insects) that they believe are producing their sensory experiences. Similarly, clients may reach out or call out for people or objects that do not exist. Obviously, when clients report such experiences or you observe clients as they experience such perceptual disturbances, the disorder is usually of a very serious nature. Acute therapeutic medical intervention is warranted in most cases.

Orientation and Consciousness

Mental status examiners routinely evaluate clients' orientations to a current situation. The question of whether or not a client is oriented involves evaluating very basic cognitive functions. Typically, the examiner simply asks a client three simple questions:

- What is your name?
- Where are you? (i.e., what city or where within a particular building)
- What is today's date?

When a client answers these queries correctly, the examiner simply notes the client was "O × 3" which is stated as "oriented times three" and refers to the fact that the client is aware of who he is, where he is, and what day it is. Evaluating a client's orientation is a direct way to assess his level of confusion or disorientation. Extremely disturbed clients may not be able to respond accurately to one or more of these seemingly simple questions.

Level of orientation can be pursued in greater depth. For example, clients can be asked what county they are in, who the governor of the state is, and the name of the mayor or local newspaper. They also can be asked if they recognize hospital personnel, visitors, and family. However, these additional questions may be confounded by factors such as the client's level of intelligence, social awareness, or cultural background, and therefore they are not always accurate measures of orientation.

Clients can become disoriented for a number of reasons. Common causes include drug intoxication, recent brain trauma, and dementia (e.g., Alzheimer's). It is not necessarily the task of the mental status examiner to determine the cause of a client's disorientation.

In cases of delirium, acutely disoriented clients may experience a gradual clearing of consciousness. When clients become disoriented they usually lose their sense of time first, then of place and finally of person. Orientation is recovered in reverse order (first person, then place, and lastly time).

Questioning for orientation can be viewed as offensive by fully oriented clients. They may feel belittled by the examiner asking such simple questions. Therefore questioning for orientation should be approached gently and used primarily with clients who stand a good possibility of being disoriented (e.g., hospitalized schizophrenics, clients who are intoxicated, or clients with head injuries). The client's orientation to self should be checked at the beginning of an interview. The effective examiner uses questions such as those in the following list in combination with more chatty or social questions or statements in an effort to appear curious about the person when obtaining information pertaining to orientation and consciousness.

1. Self/Person   What is your name?
                  Where are you from?
                  Where do you currently live?
                  What kinds of activities do you engage in during your free time?
                  Are you employed? If so, what do you do for a living?
                  Are you married? If so, what is your spouse's name?
                  Do you have any children?

2. Place		There's been a lot happening these past few days (or hours); I wonder if you can describe for me where you are?
		Do you recall what city we're in?
		What is the name of the building we're in right now?
		Do you know what part of the hospital we're in?
3. Time		Have you been keeping track of the time lately?
		What is the date today? (If client claims not to recall ask for an estimate; estimates can help assess level of disorientation.)
		What month (or year) is it?
		How long have you been here?

Consciousness is usually evaluated by assigning a point along a continuum from alert to comatose. Examiners evaluate level of consciousness as well as degree of orientation, because although the two concepts are related, they are not identical. As examiners observe clients' responses and behaviors during an interview, they select a descriptor of consciousness. Descriptors include:

- Alert
- Confused
- Clouded
- Stuporous
- Unconscious
- Comatose

After evaluating a relatively intact client a mental examiner might state, "The client was alert and oriented to person, place, and time." An acutely delirious client might be described with "The client's consciousness was clouded; she was oriented to person (oriented times one)."

Memory and Intelligence

Mental status examinations include at least a cursory assessment of client thinking abilities. These assessments usually focus on memory and general intelligence.

Memory A mental status exam can provide a quick screening of potential memory problems, but not a definitive answer as to whether or not a specific impairment exists. Neuropsychological assessment is required to specify the nature and extent of memory impairment.

Memory is broadly defined as the ability to recall past experiences. Three types of memory are typically assessed in a mental status examination: remote, recent, and immediate. Remote memory refers to recall of events, information, and people from the distant past. Recent memory refers to recall of events, information, and people from past week or so. Immediate memory refers to retention of information or data to which one was exposed only minutes previously.

Recall of remote events involves reviewing chronologic information from the client's history. Some clinicians simply weave an evaluation of remote memory into the history-taking portion of the intake interview. This type of assessment would involve questions about time and place of birth, names of schools attended, date of marriage, age differences between client and siblings, and so forth. The problem with basing an assessment of remote memory on self-report of historical information is that the examiner is unable to tell if the client is recalling historical experiences and information accurately. This problem reflects the main dilemma in assessment of remote memory impairment: the possibility of confabulation.

The word confabulation refers to spontaneous fabrication or distortion of memories. Confabulation occurs during recall. Everyone confabulates to some extent. In fact, we have found that intense marital disputes can occur when memories of key events fail to jibe. Our memories are imperfect and subject to reinterpretation. This is especially the case if an individual feels pressured into responding to questions about the past. A client may be able to recall only a portion of a specific memory, and when the client is exposed to pressure to elaborate on that memory, confabulation occurs. When clients respond to questions about their history, the answers will always contain some degree of inaccuracy or confabulation. It becomes the examiner's responsibility to determine the accuracy of a client's historical reports. The pursuit of elusive truth can be a challenging experience.

When confabulation or memory impairment is suspected, it may be helpful to ask clients about objective events that occurred during their childhood or early adulthood. This usually involves inquiring about significant and memorable social or political events (e.g., who was president when you were growing up? What countries were involved in World War II? What were some popular recreational activities during your high school years?). Of course, using social and political questions may be unfair to cultural minorities, so exercise caution when you use such strategies.

If the accuracy of a client's historical report is questionable, then it may be useful to call upon friends or family of the client to confirm historical information. Such a procedure can be complicated because releases of information must be signed by all parties in order to ensure legal protection. Also, friends and family members may not be honest with you or may have impaired memory capacities or confabulated memories. Consequently, although verification of client personal history is in some cases essential, it is by no means problem-free.

Some clients may directly admit to memory problems. However, such an admission does not necessarily constitute evidence of memory impairment. In addition, client's admission to actual memory problems does not indicate that the impairment has a neurological or organic component. In fact, clients with actual brain injury or damage are sometimes more likely to deny memory problems and try to cover them up through confabulation. Conversely, clients who are depressed commonly and sometimes incorrectly view all of their cognitive skills as having diminished (Othmer & Othmer, 1989), complaining to great lengths that something is wrong with their brain.

Depressed clients' cognitive skills are, in fact, sometimes impaired. This phenomenon has been referred to as pseudodementia (Othmer & Othmer, 1989). In other words, these clients may have no organic impairment but still suffer from emotionally based memory problems. In many cases, once the depression is alleviated, the memory problems are also resolved.

Evaluating clients' recent and immediate memories is simpler than evaluating remote memory because experiences of the recent past are more easily verified. If the client has been hospitalized, questions can be asked pertaining to reasons for hospitalization, treatments received, and hospital personnel with whom the client has had contact. Clients may be asked what they ate for breakfast, what clothes they wore the day before, and whether they recall the weather from the day before.

Immediate memory requires sustained attention, the ability to concentrate on cognitive input. There are several formal ways of evaluating client immediate memory. The most common of these are serial sevens, recall of brief stories, and digit span (Folstein, Folstein, & McHugh, 1975; Wechsler & Stone, 1945).

Serial sevens are administered by simply asking the client to "begin with 100 and count backwards by 7" (Folstein, Folstein, & McHugh, 1975, p. 197). Clients who are able to sustain attention (and who have adequate cognitive abilities) should be able to perform serial sevens without difficulty. However, excessive anxiety may interfere with concentration and impair performance. Consequently, anxiety level, educational background, and distractibility should all be considered when evaluating a client's memory with serial sevens.

Digit span is administered by saying something like, "I am going to say a series of numbers. When I am finished, repeat them to me in the same order." A series of numbers should then be read clearly to the client, with about one second intervals between numbers. Examiners should begin with a short series of numbers they believe the client can accurately repeat and then proceed to longer and longer lists. For example:

> *I:* "I want to do a simple test with you to check your ability to concentrate. First I'll say a series of numbers. Then when I'm finished, you repeat them to me. Okay?
>
> *C:* "Okay."
>
> *I:* "Here's the first series of numbers: 6–1–7–4."
>
> *C:* "6 . . . 1 . . . 7 . . . 4."
>
> *I:* "Okay, good. Now try this one: 8–5–9–3–7."
>
> *C:* "Um . . . 8 . . . 5 . . . 9 . . . 7 . . . 3."

I: "Okay, here's another set: 2–6–1–3–9" (Notice that the examiner does not point out the client's incorrect response but simply provides another set of five numbers to give the client another opportunity to respond correctly.)

After completing digit span forward, you may want to administer digit span backward. To do so, simply state:

I: "Now I'm going to have you do something slightly different. Once again I'll read a short list of numbers, but this time when I'm finished I'd like you to repeat them to me in reverse order. For example, if I said: 7–2–8, what would you say?"

C: "Uh . . . 8 . . . 2 . . . 7. That's pretty hard. These better be real short lists of numbers."

I: "That's right, I think you've got it. Now try this: 4–2–5–8."

Clients may become especially sensitive about their performance on specific cognitive tasks. Their responses may range from overconfidence (not acknowledging the need to guess or their fears of poor performance), to excuse making (e.g., "Today's just not a good day for me!"), to open acknowledgment of concern over their performance (e.g., "I'm afraid I got that one wrong, too. I'm just horrible at this.") The way clients respond to cognitive performance tests may reveal important client clinical information, such as an inability to admit weaknesses, a style of rationalizing or making excuses for poor performance, or a tendency toward negative self-evaluation.

Intelligence Evaluation of intellectual functioning is traditionally a controversial subject, perhaps especially so when the evaluation takes place in the context of a brief clinical interview. Despite the potential of evaluation misuse, general statements about intellectual functioning are usually made following administration of a mental status exam. However, we would like to emphasize the importance of exercising caution when judging intelligence after the brief and limited contact typical of a mental status examination. Statements about intellectual functioning should be phrased in a tentative manner.

Few people agree on a single definition of intelligence. Wechsler (1958) defined it as a person's "global capacity . . . to act purposefully, to think rationally, and to deal effectively with his environment" (p. 35).

While general, this definition is still of some use to the clinical interviewer. As a question it might be put, "Is there evidence that the client is resourceful and consequently functions adequately in a number of life domains?" Or "Does the client make mistakes in life that appear to be a function of limited 'brain power' rather than clinical psychopathology?" While this type of question is difficult to answer, an answer should nonetheless be attempted by the interviewer at the conclusion of a mental status exam.

Recent research suggests that it may be more reasonable to view intelligence as a composite of several specific abilities than as a general adaptive tendency (Gardner, 1983; Sternberg, 1985; Sternberg & Wagner, 1986). Using this construct, a single individual might be evaluated as having strong intellectual skills in one area but as having deficiencies in another.

Sternberg and Wagner (1987) have referred to a triarchic theory of intelligence that has relevance for the mental status examiner. They identify three forms of intelligence:

- Academic problem solving
- Practical intelligence
- Creative intelligence

Using this concept of triarchic intelligence, a mental status examiner might conclude that a client has excellent practical and creative intellectual skills as exemplified by social competence, good street survival skills, and the ability to come up with creative solutions to mechanical problems. However, the same individual might lack formal education and appear unintelligent if evaluated strictly from the perspective of academic problem-solving abilities.

During a mental status exam, intelligence is usually measured with several methods. First, native intelligence is inferred from a client's level of education. Obviously, this method is biased in terms of academic intelligence (Gould, 1981). Second, intelligence is assessed by observing a client's use and comprehension of language (i.e., vocabulary or verbal comprehension). It has been shown that vocabulary is the strongest single predictor of IQ score on traditional intelligence tests (Sattler, 1988). Again, this method is biased in favor of the formally educated against cultural minorities (Elliot, 1988). Third, intelligence is inferred from client responses to questions designed to determine fund of knowledge. Once again, fund of knowledge is often a by-product of a stimulating educational background, and questions used to assess knowledge are generally culturally biased. Fourth, intelligence is measured through client responses to questions designed to evaluate abstract thinking abilities. Fifth, questions designed to measure social judgment are used to evaluate intellectual functioning. (See Table 10-3 for sample questions that test fund of knowledge, abstract thinking, and social judgment.) Sixth, intelligence is inferred from observations of responses to tests of orientation, consciousness, and memory.

Reliability, Judgment, and Insight

Reliability Reliability refers to a client's credibility and trustworthiness in terms of honest and accurate reporting of life events and circumstances. A reliable informant is one who takes care to present information accurately. In contrast, some clients may be highly unreliable; they may for one reason or another distort, confabulate, or blatantly lie about their life circumstances and personal history.

TABLE 10-3 Sample Mental Status Exam Questions Used
to Assess Intelligence

Many questions used to assess intelligence during a mental status exam are taken
from standardized tests or are otherwise copyrighted, and therefore it is inappropriate
to reproduce them here. The following questions are similar in content to typical questions used by mental status examiners.

Fund of Knowledge

Name six large U.S. cities.

What is the direction you go when travelling from New York to Rome?

Who was president of the United States during the Vietnam War? Which president
"freed the slaves"?

What poisonous chemical substance is in automobile emissions?

What is Stevie Wonder's profession?

Abstract Thinking

In what way are a pencil and a typewriter alike?

In what way are a whale and a dolphin alike?

What does this saying mean: People who live in glass houses shouldn't throw stones?

What does this saying mean: A bird in the hand is worth two in the bush?

Judgment

What would you do if you discovered a gun hidden in the bushes of a local park?

If you won ten thousand dollars, how would you spend it?

How far would you say it is from Los Angeles to Chicago?

If you were stuck in a desert for twenty-four hours, what measures might you take in
order to survive?

How would you handle it if you discovered that your best friend was having an affair
with your boss's spouse?

Note: These items were developed for illustrative purposes. Interviewers should consult published, standardized testing materials when conducting formal evaluations of
intelligence.

It is often difficult to determine when a client is being untruthful during
an interview. Even the best and most experienced interviewers occasionally
have the "wool pulled over their eyes" by a client. Author John recalls interviewing a very depressed male client who had recently been admitted to a
psychiatric hospital. When asked if he would like to participate in the
hospital's recreational program, the client replied, "I'm too depressed to
move." The next day this same client managed to find the energy to run away
from the hospital without medical approval. His report regarding his ability to
move had been extremely unreliable.

Reliability may be related to a number of observable factors. Clients with
good attention to detail and who spontaneously elaborate regarding personal
issues are likely to be reliable informants. In contrast, clients who answer
questions in a vague or defensive manner have a greater probability of being

unreliable. In some cases you will have a clear sense that the client is intentionally omitting or minimizing parts of his history.

When you suspect a client is unreliable, it is useful to contact family, employers, or other associates of the client in an effort to corroborate the client's story. This step can be problematic, but it is necessary. If no one is available with whom you can discuss the client's story, it is advisable to proceed cautiously with the client's care while observing his behavior closely. You should also note your reservations about the client's reliability in your mental status report.

Judgment Judgment involves making decisions that are constructive and adaptive. Client judgment can be evaluated during an intake interview by exploring a client's involvement in activities, relationships, and vocational choices. Ask for example, if the client regularly involves himself in illegal activities or in relationships that seem destructive. Does he flirt with danger by engaging in potentially life-threatening activities? Obviously, consistent participation in illegal activities, destructive relationships, and life-threatening activities constitutes evidence that an individual is exercising poor judgment regarding choice of activities or relationships.

Adolescent clients frequently have poor judgment. They may grossly overestimate or underestimate their physical, mental, and social attributes. Author Rita Sommers-Flanagan once worked with a fifteen-year-old who impulsively quit his job as a busboy at an expensive restaurant simply because he found out an hour before his shift that he would be working that shift with a fellow employee whom he didn't like and viewed as lazy. Six months later, still complaining about lack of money and looking for a job, he continued to defend his impulsive move, despite the fact that it obviously was an excellent example of shortsightedness and poor judgment.

Judgment is frequently assessed by having clients respond to hypothetical scenarios. Some samples scenarios are given in Table 10-3.

Insight Insight refers to the client's understanding of the nature of his illness. Author Rita once treated a male client who presented with symptoms of exhaustion. During the interview she inquired as to whether he sometimes experienced anxiety and tension. He insisted, despite shallow breathing, flushing on the neck, and clenched fists, that he did not have a problem with tension and that therefore learning to relax would be of no use to him. She further inquired whether or not there might be, in some cases, a connection between chronically high levels of tension and exhaustion. His response was a terse "No, and anyway I told you I don't have a problem with tension." This client displayed absolutely no insight into the nature of one of his primary problems.

Toward the end of the mental status examination it is useful to ask the client to speculate on the cause or causes of his symptoms. Some clients will respond with powerfully insightful responses, others will immediately begin discussing a number of physical illnesses they may have contracted (e.g., "I don't know, maybe I have mono?"), while still others will simply have no clue as to potential underlying causes or dynamics. Generally speaking, clients with high levels of insight are able to intelligently discuss the possibility of emotional or psychosocial factors contributing to the illness; they are, at least, open to considering and addressing nonbiological factors. In contrast, clients with little or no insight become defensive when faced with possible psychosocial or emotional explanations for their condition.

Interviewers usually describe degree of client insight by reference to one of four descriptors:

- Absent. The client shows no evidence of grasping a reasonable explanation for her illness. If an interviewer suggests a plausible contributing factor, the client denies its possibility.
- Poor. The client tends to rely exclusively on physical or medical explanations for his illness. There is some resistance to accepting the fact that life situations or emotional states can contribute to personal problems or illnesses. However, the client does *not* completely deny the possibility of nonphysical contributing factors.
- Partial. The client occasionally can articulate how situational or emotional factors might be contributing to her condition. She is reluctant to focus on such factors, but gentle reminders serve to motivate her to work with nonphysical treatment approaches.
- Good. The client can articulate and utilize nonphysical treatment approaches with minimal help from the therapists. The client may even be exceptionally creative in formulating ways he might address his illness through nonphysical methods.

BOX 10-1 ━━━

Following is a sample mental status report. A good report is brief, clear, concise and includes information addressing all the areas noted in this chapter.

A Sample Mental Status Report

Warren Guffin, a forty-two-year-old Caucasian male, was disheveled and unkempt upon presentation to the hospital emergency room. During the interview, he was agitated and restless, frequently changing seats. He was impatient and sometimes rude in his interactions with this examiner. Mr. Guffin reported that today was the "best day" of his life, because he had decided to join the professional golf circuit. His affect was labile, but appropriate to the content of his speech (i.e., he became tearful when reporting he had "bogeyed number 18"). His speech was loud, pressured, and overelaborative. He exhibited loosening of associations and flight of ideas. Mr. Guffin described grandiose delusions regarding his sexual and athletic performance. He reported auditory hallucinations (God had told him to quit his job and become a professional golfer) and was preoccupied with his athletic and sexual accomplishments. He was oriented to time and place, but claimed he was the son of Ben Hogan. He denied suicidal and homicidal ideation. He refused to participate in intellectual or memory-related portions of the examination. Mr. Guffin was unreliable and exhibited poor judgment. Insight was absent.

━━━

When to Use Mental Status Examinations

Formal mental status examinations are not appropriate for all clients. A good basic guideline is that mental status examinations become more necessary as suspected level of client psychopathology increases. If clients appear well adjusted and you are not working in a medical setting, it is unlikely you will need to conduct a full mental status evaluation. However, if you have questions about diagnosis or extent of client psychopathology and you are working in a medical setting, then administration of a formal mental status examination is appropriate and likely. Rosenthal and Akiskal (1985) state:

> Some individuals who present for outpatient psychotherapy or counseling can be viewed as having 'problems of living.' In such cases, the relevant mental status information can be largely gleaned from a well-conducted history-taking or intake interview. . . . On the other hand, if the patient appears to be suffering from significant disturbance of mood, perception, thinking, or memory, a formal Mental Status Examination is in order. (p. 25)

Chapter Summary

Two major problems are associated with objective clinical assessment. First, it is extremely difficult to be objective and dispassionate when working with human beings. Second, even if complete objectivity were possible, it would probably be undesirable because of its adverse effects on clients. Clinical interviewers should be cautious when implementing objective assessment procedures such as the mental status examination.

Mental status examinations organize clinical observations in such a way so as to maximize evaluation of current mental status. Administration of an examination is an extremely popular approach in medical settings. Although mental status information is useful in the diagnostic process, mental status examinations are not primarily diagnostic procedures.

Complete mental status examinations require that interviewers observe and query client functioning in nine areas: appearance; behavior or psychomotor activity; attitude toward examiner (interviewer); affect and mood; speech and thought; perceptual disturbances; orientation and consciousness; memory and intelligence; and reliability, judgment, and insight.

Appearance refers to client physical and demographic characteristics (such as sex, age, and race). Appearance variables may have a direct bearing on diagnosis or treatment and therefore should be noted.

Behavior or psychomotor activity refers to physical movements made by clients during an interview. Movements may be excessive, limited, absent, or bizarre. Documentation of client movement during an interview is important evidence that may support your conclusions about a client mental status.

Client attitude toward the evaluator should be assessed as behavior occurring within an interpersonal context. Determination of client attitude may be affected by an interviewer's emotional reactions during an interview, so interviewers should exercise caution before labeling client attitude.

Affect refers to clients' prevailing emotional tone as observed by an interviewer, while mood refers to clients' self-reported emotional state. Affect may be described in terms of its content or type, range or variability and duration, appropriateness, and depth or intensity. In contrast, mood consists simply of clients' response to the question, "How are you feeling?"

Evaluation of speech and thought are intertwined because speech constitutes one of the main vehicles for evaluating thought. Speech may be categorized in terms of its concrete qualities (i.e., rate and volume). It also may be described in terms of its functional qualities (e.g., articulation disturbances in speech, also known as dysarthria, may be identified). Evaluation of thought is divided into two categories: thought process and thought content. Thought process refers to how a person thinks, while thought content refers to what a person is thinking about. Thought process is identified by a number of descriptors such as "flight of ideas" and "word salad." Thought content generally refers to the quality of clients' delusions or obsessions. Suicidal or homicidal thought content is also noted on a mental status examination.

Hallucinations and illusions constitute the two major forms of perceptual disturbances. They may occur via any of the five sensory modalities. Hallucinations are false or inaccurate perceptual experiences, while illusions are distorted perceptual disturbances.

Client orientation and level of consciousness are routinely evaluated during a mental status exam. An orientation evaluation determines whether or not a client is oriented to his current situation. Clients may or may not be oriented to person, place, and time. Consciousness is evaluated along a continuum, from alert to comatose.

Mental status exams provide a cursory assessment of client memory and intellectual functioning. Client memory for remote, recent, and immediate information is assessed. Evaluation of remote and recent memory may be difficult because interviewers cannot always verify the accuracy of client claims. Intellectual functioning is evaluated by determining client level of education, language use and comprehension, fund of knowledge, abstract reasoning ability, and social judgment. Intellectual and memory assessments involve only surface evaluations during a mental status exam; more formalized assessments should follow if potential problems are identified. Interviewers should take care to avoid cultural biases when making such assessments.

Reliability, judgment, and insight are grouped together in a final category in the mental status exam. Reliability refers to the degree to which a client's reports about self and situation can be trusted as accurate. Judgment refers to the presence or absence of impulsive activities and poor decision making. Insight refers to the degree to which a client is aware of the emotional or psychological nature of his problems.

Mental status examinations are usually administered in cases in which psychopathology is suspected. If clients are being seen on an outpatient basis for problems associated with daily living, then mental status evaluation is of less importance.

Suggested Readings

Folstein, M. F., Folstein, S. E., & McHugh, P. R. (1975). "Mini-mental state": A practical method for grading the cognitive state of patients for the clinician. *Journal of Psychiatric Research, 12,* 189–198. This article presents a quick method for evaluating client mental state. The "mini-mental state" is a popular technique in psychiatric and geriatric settings.

Othmer, E., & Othmer, S. C. (1989). *The clinical interview using DSM-III-R.* Washington, DC: American Psychiatric Press. Chapter 4 of this text, Four Methods to Assess Mental Status, is strongly recommended.

Strub, R. L., & Black, W. (1977). *The mental status examination in neurology.* Philadelphia: F. A. Davis. This text provides excellent practical and sensitive methods for determining client mental status.

11

SUICIDE ASSESSMENT

Written with Holly K. Krueger
and Janet P. Wollersheim

Suicide Statistics
  Considering Suicide Myths
  Risk Factors Associated with Suicide

Conducting a Thorough Suicide Assessment
  Assessing Level of Depression
  Exploring Suicidal Ideation
  Assessing Suicide Plans
  Assessing Client Self-Control
  Assessing Intent

Crisis Intervention with Suicidal Clients
  Listening and Being Empathic
  Establishing a Therapeutic Relationship
  Identifying Alternatives to Suicide
  Establishing Suicide-Prevention Contracts
  Becoming Directive and Responsible
  Making Decisions about Hospitalization and Referral

Professional Issues
  Can You Work with Suicidal Clients?
  Consultation
  Documentation
  Dealing with Completed Suicides

Chapter Summary

Suggested Readings

There was no answer.
The door of the lighthouse was ajar. They pushed it open and walked into a shuttered twilight. Through an archway on the further side of the room they could see the bottom of the staircase that led up to the higher floors. Just under the crown of the arch dangled a pair of feet.   *—ALDOUS HUXLEY, Brave New World*

There are two basic, albeit contradictory, truths about suicide: (A) Suicide should never be committed when one is depressed (or disturbed or constricted); and (B) almost every suicide is committed for reasons that make sense to the person who does it.   *—SHNEIDMAN, "Aphorisms of Suicide and Some Implications*
for Psychotherapy"

Nearly all of us think about suicide at some point in our lives. For some, it is merely a fleeting thought countered by thoughts about all the positive reasons for living. For others, suicide is a very serious consideration, and for a few, it becomes a preoccupation. In some cases, repeated suicide gestures may be interpreted more as cries for help and attention than as a serious wish to die. In other cases, the opposite is true: Life has become so full of dissatisfaction, disappointment, or pain that a quiet, unobserved death has become a more attractive option than life.

Suicide is a relatively common topic during therapeutic interviews. As a consequence, it is our policy to lecture about suicide assessment prior to assigning practicum cases to students. We believe that an interviewer should not sit down in a room with a client unless that interviewer understands how to competently conduct a suicide assessment. Dealing with suicidal clients is nearly always anxiety-provoking. Dealing with suicidal clients without adequate preparation is not only anxiety-provoking, but risky and unprofessional as well.

Suicide Statistics

Approximately 22,000 recorded suicides occur annually in the United States. This number constitutes an average rate of 11 deaths per 100,000 people and ranks suicide as the ninth leading cause of death in the United States (Resnik, 1980). These statistics indicate that suicide is a significant preventable cause of death. They also illustrate that suicide is a relatively rare event. If suicide is, statistically speaking, rare, then how are interviewers to evaluate, predict, and potentially control its occurrence?

Certainly interviewers are in a difficult position when they seek to assess suicidality. Despite the difficulty of prediction and the infrequency of suicide,

BOX 11-1 ━━━

A Suicide Quiz

Before you read this chapter, take the following true-false quiz to test your knowledge about suicide. Answers and explanations are in Box 11-2.

_____ 1. Twenty-five to 50 percent of people who kill themselves have previously attempted to do so.

_____ 2. People who talk about suicide won't commit suicide.

_____ 3. Suicide happens without warning.

_____ 4. If a parent of a child under five years of age commits suicide, the surviving child is many more times likely to grow up and commit suicide than a child who did not have that experience.

_____ 5. Suicide attempters are more likely than other psychiatric patients to use substances in the twenty-four hours prior to admission to a hospital.

_____ 6. Patients under a doctor's care are not at risk of suicide.

_____ 7. Life stress factors are good predictors of suicide.

_____ 8. More men commit suicide than women.

_____ 9. In the United States, suicide is more prominent among Protestants than Catholics.

_____ 10. A person who is very ill, perhaps even terminally ill, is not likely to commit suicide.

_____ 11. When a suicidal patient begins to improve, it's usually a sign that the "danger is over."

_____ 12. A great deal of regional variation in suicide can be accounted for by weather variables such as temperature and precipitation.

_____ 13. Improved standard of living is associated with higher rates of suicide and lower rates of homicide.

_____ 14. The appearance of Halley's Comet is associated with historical increases in the number of suicides.

_____ 15. The most common means of suicide among women is a gun.

therapeutic interviewers must make efforts to assess for suicide potential, because assessment constitutes one of the first steps in suicide prevention. Unless efforts are made to predict suicide, there will be less opportunity to prevent suicide attempts.

Efforts to predict suicide risk are justifiable on many grounds. First, suicide occurs much more frequently in a clinical population than in the general population (e.g., clients with clinical depression, panic disorder, alcoholism, and schizophrenia are at greater risk; Johnson, Weissman, & Klerman, 1990; Murphy & Wetzel, 1990; Roy, 1989). Second, suicide attempts occur ten to twenty times more frequently than completed suicides; the clinical interviewer's task is not only to try to reduce the incidence of completed suicides but also of suicide attempts. Finally, clinically and ethically speaking, it is better to err by assuming a client may be suicidal than to err by assuming wrongly a suicidal client is not suicidal.

Considering Suicide Myths

There are many unfounded myths about suicide. Perhaps the most dangerous is the belief that asking a person about suicide may cause that person to commit suicide. Pipes and Davenport (1990) offer the following reassurance:

> You can take solace in the fact that there is, as far as we know, consensus among experienced therapists that asking about suicide does not cause suicide. It is entirely possible that by not asking a client about suicidal thoughts you will lose an opportunity to help prevent suicide. (p. 113)

Therefore, if you have any reason to believe your client might be thinking about suicide, go ahead and inquire.

With regard to other suicide myths, stop and think of what you believe about this topic and consider the sources of those beliefs. If someone tries a dramatic and obviously nonlethal method (e.g., lying down in front of a brigade of mountain bikes), is she just playing games? Is the third time a charm? Is suicide ultimately manipulative? Is suicide an act of anger? Do females merely threaten suicide whereas males really mean it? Do old people do it more often? Disabled people? People of particular religious groups? If a person talks about his thoughts of suicide, is he more or less likely to attempt or complete suicide? And what about full moons? Seasons? The weather?

Clearly, there are many misconceptions and fears associated with suicide. Rather than systematically listing and dispelling all the myths, this chapter offers a section on risk factors associated with suicide. To prepare yourself adequately to conduct suicide assessments, we encourage you, at the very least, to read this chapter. We also recommend strongly that you explore the suggested readings to further expand your knowledge about suicide and its assessment. Proceeding with knowledge and caution, obtaining good supervision, developing a norm of consulting with colleagues, and documenting factors contributing to your clinical decision are the basic rules for handling this area of mental health care.

Risk Factors Associated with Suicide

Many specific risk factors are associated with suicide, but there are no outstanding predictors of suicide behavior. Therefore, although we offer a brief discussion of factors associated with increased suicide risk, the absence of these factors in an individual client should not reassure you as an interviewer that there is no likelihood of that client attempting or committing suicide. An important rule of conducting suicide assessment is to avoid overestimating your ability to predict suicide.

Depression The relationship between depression and suicide potential is well documented (Miles, 1977; Roy, 1989). Some experts feel that some form of depression prior to suicide is probably universal (Silverman, 1968). Among the evidence for this belief is a 1987 study by Westefeld and Furr reporting that every member of a sample of college students who had attempted suicide reported experiencing at least some depressive symptoms.

The risk of suicide in a depressed population is about thirty times greater than the risk in the general population. In fact, it has been estimated that 10 to 15 percent of all clinically depressed individuals will commit suicide (Georgotas, 1985). Although not all depressed people are suicidal, depression is probably one of the best predictors and is the predictor that can be most reliably evaluated in a clinical interview (Resnik, 1980).

Research has determined six variables that are most often associated with suicidal behavior among depressed clients (Fawcett et al, 1990):

1. Severe psychic anxiety (general thoughts and feelings of anxiety).
2. Panic attacks (specific bouts of anxiety, including physical symptoms of panic).
3. Anhedonia (loss of pleasure when engaging in usually pleasurable activities).
4. Alcohol abuse (increased alcohol consumption during the depressive episode).
5. Decreased ability to concentrate (high distractibility).
6. Global insomnia (difficulty falling asleep, intermittent awakening, and early morning awakening).

In addition, feelings of hopelessness and helplessness are important predictors of suicide (Beck, Brown, & Steer, 1989). These symptoms are experienced by most depressed, and some nondepressed, clients.

Age During the past thirty years, the suicide rate in the U.S. population overall has risen only 20 percent (Giffen & Felsenthal, 1983). Among adolescents in the fifteen to nineteen years old, however, the suicide rate increased 300 percent for males and 200 percent for females (Sudak, Ford, & Rushforth, 1984; this percentage increase, however, has leveled off recently and is expected to decline slowly through the mid-1990s, Holinger, Offer, & Zola, 1988). In addition, it is likely that many of the lethal "accidents" that compose the second leading cause of adolescent death may actually be suicides that are concealed by friends, relatives, and attending physicians because of the stigma associated with suicide. Based on age alone, the adolescent should be considered high risk.

College students compose another high-risk category. Suicide is the second leading cause of death among college students (McIntosh, 1991), and their suicide rate is 50 percent higher than that of the general population. Also, older Americans are at high risk for suicide; at least 10,000 people over the age of sixty kill themselves each year (Miller, 1979); even that figure may be conservative given underreporting of suicides. Older Americans tend to use lethal weapons more frequently and tend to be more successful in killing themselves than the young. They also tend to communicate their suicidal intent less often. Finally, it should be noted that suicide numbers rise after age forty-five for men and after age fifty-five for women (Resnik, 1980).

Sex Statistics on suicide generally indicate that three times more women than men *attempt* suicide, but three times more men than women successfully *complete* suicide (Shneidman, 1980). In later life, the disparity of male/female rates becomes even more marked. During ages sixty-five to sixty-nine, men complete suicide at a rate four times greater than females and by age eighty-five, this ratio increases to approximately twelve to one (Miller, 1979). One explanation for the discrepancy between male and female successful suicides is that men usually choose more lethal methods, such as guns, while women choose less lethal methods, such as poison or pills. Regardless of the sex of the user, guns are more lethal and lead to a greater ratio of completions to attempts (Sudak, Ford, & Rushforth, 1984). It also should be noted that adolescent females complete suicide using guns more frequently than any other method (Evans & Farberow, 1988).

Race and Ethnic Background Whites are approximately two times more likely to complete suicide than African-Americans. Suicide rates for white Americans in general are higher than for nonwhites, and only among white males does the suicide rate increase throughout the life cycle. An exception to this tendency for whites to commit suicide at higher rates than nonwhites occurs within the fifteen to twenty-nine age bracket; Native Americans and African-Americans have higher suicide rates than whites at those ages (Miller, 1979). Among certain Native American and Alaskan tribes, the suicide rate greatly exceeds the rate of the general U.S. population (Resnik, 1980).

Religion Among the three major religious groups in the United States, rates for Catholics have historically been slightly lower than the rates among Protestants and Jews. However, rather than religious denomination, degree of religious affiliation appears to be the more decisive factor (Resnik, 1980). However, there are currently no data available that identify religion as a major variable in predicting an individual's suicide potential.

Marital Status Divorced, widowed, and separated people are in a high-risk category for suicide (Tuckman & Youngman, 1968). Single, never-married individuals have a suicide rate of nearly double the rate of married individuals. Among divorced people, men have a suicide rate of 69 deaths per 100,000 compared to 18 per 100,000 for women. Marriage, especially when reinforced by children, acts as a buffer against suicide. However, as we noted earlier, rates climb as people age, and this is true even of married people. Being unmarried may be one reason that single males over seventy years old have the highest per-capita suicide rate of any group.

Employment Status Unemployed and retired individuals are in a high-risk category for suicide. Loss of employment can be a blow to anyone and can contribute to depression and a sense of meaninglessness. Those who have retired are removed from a significant source of identity and esteem, which seems to be related to the increase in suicide after the age of sixty (Miller, 1979).

Socioeconomic Status Higher rates of suicide exist at both socioeconomic extremes, with lower rates for middle-class people. Although physicians have traditionally been considered at high risk, they show no higher rates than the general population when the rates are adjusted for age and education (Resnik, 1980). As noted in Box 11-2, low standard of living is associated with higher rates of homicide, while higher standard of living is associated with suicide.

Physical Health The majority of research on suicide rates among hospital patients has focused on psychiatric patients. However, suicide occurs among patients in medical and surgical sections as well. Researchers have linked the following factors to increased risk: frequent major surgery, depression related to chronic pain and altered body functions, fears of death and suffering, incapacitation, stroke, rheumatoid arthritis, and loss of social support. Hemodialysis patients have been identified as a special risk group as well (DiBianco, 1979). One problem with studying the relationship between physical illness and suicide is the overlap between depressive symptoms and other symptoms. Research by Brown, Henteleff, Barakat, and Rowe (1986) indicates that suicidal thoughts and the desire for death were linked exclusively to the presence of depression. These authors suggest that physicians may fail to recognize and treat the depression, which points again to the importance of the depression factor in suicide. Physical infirmity in itself may not present a higher risk for suicide. However, individuals who are unable to cope with their illness and become depressed are clearly at high risk.

Social and Personal Factors The role of social and personal resources in suicide potential should not be underestimated. Such factors include availability of food, shelter, clothing, and transportation; adequate health care; physical and mental strength; availability of productive and meaningful activities to pursue; and finally, significant and supportive relationships with others. The more of these basic resources available to the individual, the lower the suicide risk (Hatton, Valente, & Rink, 1977).

Living alone can be a higher risk situation. However, feelings of isolation and loneliness can be severe even for a person who lives with a group, and a person living alone may have a rewarding and satisfying support system available to her. The feeling of being isolated and detached seems to be the risk factor, rather than the actual living situation, although both should be noted.

Individuals who have suffered a recent, significant loss should be considered higher suicide risks. Such losses may take many forms; loss of job, status, loved one, physical health, or function of body parts. Even the loss of a pet can increase risk among certain individuals.

Substance Abuse Research is unequivocal in placing alcoholics and other substance abusers in a high-risk category (Fawcett et al., 1990; Murphy & Wetzel, 1990). It is clear from the research that the problems of suicide and substance abuse are closely linked. Abuse of alcohol and other substances place individuals at risk for suicide, especially if such abuse is associated with depression, social isolation, and other suicide risk factors.

One way in which alcohol and drug use increases suicide risk is by decreasing inhibition. People act more impulsively when they are in chemically altered states, and suicide is basically an impulsive act. No matter how much planning has preceded the suicide act, at the moment the pills are taken, the trigger is pulled, or the wrist is slit, some form of disinhibition has usually occurred. Alcohol and drug use may give people who are afraid to commit suicide the courage (or foolishness) required to carry out the plan.

Mental Disorders Most suicides are associated with a relatively small number of mental disorders or conditions. Patients with affective disorders and schizophrenia appear to be a special risk for suicide (Roy, 1989). Thought disorders such as a paranoid delusional system or auditory hallucinations that tell one to kill oneself or a loved one, especially when combined with depressed mood, put the sufferer at high risk (see chapter 10 of this text and Resnik, 1980). Individuals with psychotic depressive reactions are at especially high risk for suicide.

On the other hand, completed suicides are rarely associated with hysteria, antisocial personality, and various paraphilias, although suicide attempts in these groups are not uncommon (Robins, 1985). Even when a suicidal gesture appears to serve a manipulative purpose, as is frequently found with personality-disordered individuals, the gesture should be taken seriously. Moreover, all suicidal threats or attempts should be taken seriously. Even feigned suicide attempts may have fatal consequences.

For individuals who have been admitted to hospitals because of mental disorders, the period immediately following discharge is one of increased risk for suicide. This is particularly true of individuals who also:

1. Have tried suicide before
2. Suffer from a chronic mental disorder
3. Were admitted to the hospital recently
4. Live alone
5. Are unemployed
6. Are unmarried
7. Are vulnerable to depression (Roy, 1989).

Conducting a Thorough Suicide Assessment

Assessing Level of Depression

Because depression is implicated in many of the other risk factors, it is essential that you obtain a clear idea of the level of depression experienced by your client (see chapters 9 and 10). The first question to ask is simply how the client is feeling. Sad? Depressed? Helpless? Utterly hopeless? From the client's perspective, helplessness may indicate a feeling or belief that she is unable to make any changes necessary to feel better on her own. When she expresses

BOX 11-2

Answers and Explanations to the Suicide Quiz (from Box 11-1)

_T_ 1. Twenty-five to 50 percent of people who kill themselves have previously attempted to do so. [Previous suicide attempts constitute one of the better predictors of further attempts and possible suicide completion.]

_F_ 2. People who talk about suicide won't commit suicide. [People who eventually commit suicide often have tried to communicate their despair to others in a number of ways. All comments even vaguely associated with suicide or death, such as "Life just doesn't seem worthwhile anymore" or "I wish I were dead" should be considered attempts at communicating despair.]

_F_ 3. Suicide happens without warning. [Suicidal people usually leave clues or give warnings either verbally or through their behavior. For example, appearing depressed or apathetic is a potential clue that an individual is considering suicide.]

_T_ 4. If a parent of a child under five years of age commits suicide, the surviving child is many more times likely to grow up and commit suicide than a child who did not have that experience. [One research study showed that such children are nine times more likely to commit suicide when they grow up (Birtchnell, 1973).]

_T_ 5. Suicide attempters are more likely than other psychiatric patients to use substances in the twenty-four hours prior to admission to a hospital. [Ingestion of disinhibiting substances can help people "get up the nerve" to follow through on thoughts about suicide. The final act of attempting suicide, although perhaps preceded by detailed planning, requires strong uninhibited impulses (which are more likely to occur after ingestion of substances).]

_F_ 6. Patients under a doctor's care are not at risk of suicide. [Medical patients are often depressed because of their pain or prognosis. They may feel life isn't worth living anymore.]

_F_ 7. Life stress factors are good predictors of suicide. [This is false for two reasons. First, there are no "good" predictors of suicide. Second, many people with huge amounts of "life stress" are not the least bit suicidal.]

_T_ 8. More men commit suicide than women. [Most reports suggest men are about three times more likely to complete suicide than women. Women are about three times more likely to attempt suicide than men.]

_F_ 9. In the United States, suicide is more prominent among Protestants than Catholics. [There is some evidence that predominantly Catholic countries, such as Italy and Spain, have lower suicide rates than predominantly Protestant countries. However, in countries with heterogeneous religious compositions, the data are inconclusive.]

_F_ 10. A person who is very ill, perhaps even terminally ill, is not likely to commit suicide. [Many people who are terminally ill choose to terminate their own lives through suicide.]

_F_ 11. When a suicidal patient begins to improve, that's usually a sign that the "danger is over." [Sometimes, especially in depressed patients, improvement constitutes the time for greatest concern. Depressed patients may make the decision to commit suicide and consequently appear "improved." Other

(continued)

BOX 11-2 *Continued*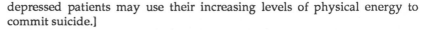

<table>
<tr><td></td><td></td><td>depressed patients may use their increasing levels of physical energy to commit suicide.]</td></tr>
<tr><td>F</td><td>12.</td><td>A great deal of regional variation in suicide can be accounted for by weather variables such as temperature and precipitation. [There is no conclusive evidence for this belief. Reports are also mixed on whether or not the moon is associated with suicidal behavior. Even when it appears that weather or lunar variables are associated with suicide, other variables can usually be found to be having an effect.]</td></tr>
<tr><td>T</td><td>13.</td><td>Increased standard of living is associated with higher rates of suicide and lower rates of homicide. [This statement has been supported by a number of studies. Doctors, lawyers, and children who appear to have the "best of everything" tend to commit suicide at higher rates than groups of people with "apparently" lesser quality of life (Pokorny, 1980).]</td></tr>
<tr><td>T</td><td>14.</td><td>The appearance of Halley's Comet is associated with historical increases in the number of suicides. [Strangely enough, this statement is true. Halley's Comet does not cause suicidal behavior, but the two phenomena are associated.]</td></tr>
<tr><td>T</td><td>15.</td><td>The most common means of suicide among women is a gun. [Contrary to popular belief, about 41 percent of female suicide victims use guns, while only about 25 percent use pills.]</td></tr>
</table>

helplessness, it may be an indirect request for help from the interviewer. She may believe that while she is unable to effect change in her life, you may be able to do so.

Perhaps even more extreme is the client who feels hopeless and believes no one can help and the future offers no hope of positive change. Depending on the client's personal style, hopelessness may be expressed in a variety of forms, such as "I don't see how things will ever be any different," or "I've felt like this for as long as I can remember and I'll probably always feel this way." You can use the client's ability to project into the future and make plans as a gauge of suicidal potential.

Believing the future is hopeless may be a more accurate indicator of suicide risk than overall level of depression (Beck, Brown, & Steer, 1989). As you might guess, suicide is less likely when a client believes there is hope for the future.

In addition to thoughts and feelings pertaining to hopelessness or helplessness, find out whether the client believes or feels himself to be worthless and whether he experiences excessive feelings of guilt. "Normal" sadness is less likely to include extreme, persistent, or recurrent thoughts and feelings of worthlessness or guilt.

If significant thoughts or feelings of hopelessness, helplessness, worthlessness, or guilt are present, determine the duration, frequency, and intensity of those thoughts and feelings. Is the mood disturbance of relatively recent onset, or is it of a longstanding nature? Do the thoughts and feelings come and go, or are they persistent and pervasive? Wollersheim (1985) suggests asking clients the following question to evaluate mood intensity: "Is it blue or black?"

Generally, suicide risk is probably higher in clients who have struggled with relatively intense depressive symptoms for an extended period without relief or hope for the future.

A common manifestation of depression is withdrawal from friends, family, and usual activities. Check if your client reports loss of interest and pleasure in activities that he used to do and enjoy. As noted previously, this is an important predictor of suicide in depressed clients (Fawcett et al., 1990). Listen for signs of emotional withdrawal from friends and family. At times, depressed persons are not fully aware of how withdrawn they are, and you may even need to obtain interviews with others who know the client if you have reason to believe you do not have the full picture.

Depression is often accompanied by a number of somatic changes, including sleep, appetite, and psychomotor change (marked slowing or nervous restlessness). In addition, sexual interest or drive is often greatly diminished. It is important to address these areas with regard to change. Have sleep patterns changed? Has weight been recently lost or gained? Are there any recent changes in communication patterns? In sexual activity? (See Hamilton, 1967.)

It is also important that you observe carefully the client's behavior during the interview. Psychomotor retardation may be apparent in overall slowed speech and increased pauses before responding. There may be little verbal input from the client or, in extreme cases, muteness. The client may exhibit slowed body movements or, conversely, may appear agitated and anxious, speak rapidly, pull on hair or clothing, rub hands together, or even pace. Agitation may also be evident in the client's report of feeling restless and feeling as if there is something he must do. Resnik (1980) notes that suicide risk is increased when depressed people begin to engage in active or energetic ways. This may be observed as anxiety, agitation, or anger, which may indicate energy and motivation for committing suicide.

You also need to assess cognitive changes in the client. Signs may include slowed thinking, loss of memory, and inability to concentrate. The client may have difficulty making decisions and solving problem. The inability to solve problems can lead to a kind of tunnel vision that prevents clients from seeing alternatives that could help ease the depression. Clients with extreme tunnel vision view suicide as the only available alternative to living with depression.

Exploring Suicidal Ideation

If you think you need to assess for suicide risk, do so by asking directly and calmly about your client's thoughts and feelings. Develop a standard question using words that you are comfortable with. Wollersheim (1974) provides the following example: "You certainly seem to feel extremely depressed. Feeling this miserable, have you found yourself thinking of suicide?" (p. 223). A common fear is that asking directly about suicide will put ideas in the person's head. As we've noted, there is *no* clinical evidence to suggest this occurs (Pipes & Davenport, 1990). Rather, most clients are relieved to have the opportunity to talk about suicidal thoughts. In addition, the invitation to share self-destructive thoughts reassures the client that the clinician is comfortable with the subject, in control of the situation, and capable of dealing with the problem (Wollersheim, 1974).

Most suicidal clients readily admit self-destructive thoughts when asked about them. However, some deny such thoughts in an attempt to reaffirm their self-control. If denial occurs, do not immediately drop the subject (sighing in relief). Make it easier for the person to admit such thoughts. Again we quote an illustration of a technique by Wollersheim:

> Well, I asked this question since almost all people at one time or another during their lives have thought about suicide. There is nothing abnormal about the thought. In fact it is very normal when one feels so down in the dumps. The thought itself is not harmful. However, if we find ourselves thinking about suicide rather intently or frequently, it is a cue that all is not well, and we should start making some efforts to make life more satisfactory. (1974, p. 223)

After a client admits to suicidal ideation, the duration, frequency, and intensity of suicidal thoughts should be explored. Exploring suicidal thoughts always leads to evaluating whether or not a client has a suicide plan.

Assessing Suicide Plans

Always ask if the client has threatened or attempted suicide in the past, or if close friends or family members have committed suicide. Such a history increases risks. Nearly three-fourths of those who ultimately commit suicide have a history of past attempts (Resnik, 1980). The greater the lethality of the last attempt, the higher the present risk.

Once rapport is established with an interviewer, most clients give details of any suicidal plans they have considered. Begin exploration of your client's plan with a paraphrase and a question such as "You've talked about how you sometimes think it would be better for everyone if you were dead. Have you planned how you would kill yourself if you decided to follow through on your thoughts?" Many clients will respond to such a question with reassurance that indeed they are not really contemplating a suicidal act. They may cite religion, fear, children, or some other reason not to commit suicide and note they simply think of it sometimes but would never follow through on such thoughts. In some cases, after hearing a client's reasons for living, the interviewer need not and should not further assess the client's suicidal plans but should move to the next area of inquiry, self-control. However, if a client identifies a potential suicide plan, further exploration of that plan is warranted.

When exploring and evaluating a client's suicide plan, assess the following four areas (Miller, 1985):

1. Specificity of the plan
2. Lethality of the method
3. Availability of the proposed method
4. Proximity of social or helping resources

Notice that these four areas of inquiry can be easily recalled with the acronym SLAP.

Specificity This refers to the details of a client's suicide plan. Has the person thought through all the details necessary to complete a suicide? The more specific the plan, the higher the risk. Some clients will clearly outline a particular method of suicide. Others will avoid the question. Still others will state something like, "Oh, I think about how things might be easier if I were dead, but I don't really have a plan." At this point it is up to your clinical judgment to determine how hard to push the client for specification of a plan. Again, we recommend following Wollersheim's (1974) advice in most cases by making "it easy for the client to answer in the affirmative if such is the case" (p. 223): "You know, most people who have thought about suicide have at least had passing thoughts about how they might do it. What kinds of thoughts have you had about how you would commit suicide if you decided to do so?"

Note that this interviewer statement is worded to accomplish two important objectives. First, the statement *reassures* the client that "most people" have thoughts about a suicidal plan. Second, the question is *open* in that it assumes the client has had such thoughts and inquires about them; the question is not closed in that it does not ask about whether or not a plan exists.

Lethality This refers to how quickly enactment of a client's plan could produce death. As one would assume, the greater the lethality, the higher the suicide risk. Lethality varies depending upon the way in which a particular method is used. If you believe your client is a very high suicide risk, you should inquire not simply as to your client's general method (e.g., firearms, toxic overdose, or razor blade), but also as to the way in which the method will be employed. For example, does your client plan to shoot herself in the stomach, temple, or mouth? Does she plan to use aspirin (depending upon her body weight, she may need over ninety five-grain tablets) or cyanide? Is her plan to slash her wrists or her throat with a razor blade? In each of these examples, the latter alternative is most lethal.

Availability This refers to how quickly a client could potentially implement a proposed plan. In other words, does the client have the means available for immediate implementation of the plan? If the client plans on overdosing with a particular medication, check whether that medication is available (but keep in mind that most people keep more than enough substances in their medicine cabinets in their homes to complete a suicide). If the client is considering committing suicide by driving a car off a cliff and has neither car nor cliff available, the immediate risk is lower than, for example, a person who plans to shoot herself and has a loaded gun in the bedroom. In most cases evaluating the availability of a suicide method is important in determining suicide risk and whether or not immediate intervention is necessary.

Proximity This refers to proximity of helping resources (i.e., other individuals who could intervene and rescue the client if an attempt is made). Does the client live with family or roommates? Does she live alone with no friends or neighbors nearby? Generally, the farther a client is from potential helping resources, the greater the suicide risk.

If you are working on an ongoing basis with a client, it is important to check in periodically with the client regarding her plan. Changes in the plan may act as important signals regarding progress or lack of progress in terms of suicide risk.

Assessing Client Self-Control

In assessing suicidal risk, Wollersheim (1974) has noted that considerable attention must be given to evaluating client conception of their own self-control. An individual who fears he may lose control and commit suicide is at high risk. Wollersheim (1974) suggests asking the following question: "Sometimes, have you been afraid that, in spite of yourself, in one of your really down periods, you might go ahead and commit suicide?" (p.224). If the client admits a fear of loss of control, the interviewer must take this revelation very seriously. It may be necessary to consider hospitalization or other changes so that external control is available for the client until the client feels more internal control.

It is important to explore thoroughly the issue of self-control. If a client has had suicidal thoughts in the past, ask what has kept her from losing control and committing suicide. This information may become a valuable therapeutic ally. What has worked in the past stands a chance of working again. For instance, you may find the client states something like the following:

C: "Yes, I often fear losing control late at night."

I: "Sounds like night is the roughest time."

C: "I hate midnight."

I: "So late at night, especially around midnight, you are sometimes afraid you will lose control and kill yourself. So far, something has kept you from doing it."

C: "Yeah. I think of the way my kids would feel when they couldn't get me to wake up in the morning. I just start bawling my head off at the thought. It always keeps me from really doing it."

When you have a client with this type of problem, of course, immediate supervision or consultation with peers is warranted. Although a brief verbal exchange should never be considered sufficient to make a determination that a client is safe on her own or that she needs hospitalization, it is important to note any strong mitigating factors, such as this client's love for her children, that will work against a loss of self-control.

In addition to the client's self-report of feeling in control or out of control, it is important to note any impulse-control problems in the client's behavioral history. For instance, if the client has a tendency toward explosive verbal outbursts or physical altercations, it may indicate a problem with impulse control. Also, clients who are emotionally overcontrolled most of the time but who on rare occasions completely lose control may be increased suicide risks.

Assessing Intent

Some clients are persistent and creative in their efforts to kill themselves. We have worked with clients who swallowed needles, razor blades, and virtually any dangerous substance they could locate (e.g., Drano and Campho Phenique). Some have run nude onto busy freeways or thrown themselves into large bodies of water in efforts to drown themselves. Others manage to hang themselves with pillowcases or slash their wrists with the top of soda bottles or cans. These clients may or may not have had specific plans to kill themselves. Instead, they were ready to take advantage of any means through which they could end their lives. It is an understatement to suggest that such clients intend to kill themselves; they are desperately seeking self-destruction.

The final area of suicide assessment is identifying a client's intent to kill oneself. Intent to kill oneself may be established through self-report, peer or family report, or behavioral observation. Essentially, assessing intent involves determining whether or not a client is talking or acting in ways that suggest he intends to kill himself.

Sometimes it is useful to ask clients to rate their mood on a scale of 1 to 10 (1 being the worst possible mood one could ever experience and 10 being euphoric). Similarly, it can be helpful to have clients rate their level of intent on a scale of 1 to 10 (1 being no intent and 10 being total intent). Generally speaking, intent should be rated by interviewers as absent, low, moderate, and high. Obviously, the greater the intent, the greater the suicide risk.

Crisis Intervention with Suicidal Clients

It is difficult to know how to best handle suicidal clients. The following guidelines, although not foolproof, provide you with basic ideas about how to handle yourself and your client during a suicide crisis.

Listening and Being Empathic

The first rule of working with suicidal clients is to listen closely to their thoughts and feelings. Often suicidal clients feel isolated from others, and therefore it is imperative that you establish an empathic connection with them. They may never have openly discussed their depressive or suicidal thoughts and feelings. Consequently, you need to openly align with them, letting them know that you hear accurately how miserable and desperate they feel (Shneidman, 1980).

Avoid expressions of shock or surprise when clients begin to discuss suicide. Deal with their thoughts and feelings in a matter-of-fact manner; this suggests to them that you've dealt with such issues previously, and it reassures them, to some degree, that their experiences are not all that unusual. In some situations you may want to be openly reassuring and supportive. Some of Wollersheim's (1974) suggestions are appropriate in this regard because in some situations the deviant response (i.e., feeling suicidal) is, in fact, a natural response:

"You've told me about some of the difficult experiences you've had recently, losing your wife, your job, and your health problems . . . and . . . given all that has happened it makes some sense that you'd give some thought to killing yourself and ending your discomfort. Most people in a situation like yours would think about whether or not life is still worth living."

Establishing a Therapeutic Relationship

As you make efforts to empathize with your client, you also should work on establishing a therapeutic relationship. You are a professional and as such it is your job to side with life. Continue to be empathic, but also let your client know your professional stance:

> "You know, right now it probably doesn't feel like life is worth much to you, but I want to let you know that things can and probably will get much better for you. It's a fact that just about everyone who gets depressed also gets over it and then feels much better. And you can accelerate the 'getting better' process by involving yourself in therapy."

Research indicates that people who are depressed or in a mood characterized by psychological or emotional discomfort have difficulty remembering positive events or previous experiences in which they felt positive emotions (Blaney, 1986; Clark & Teasdale, 1982, Eich, 1989). Consequently, it is important to encourage clients to focus on positive events and past positive emotional experiences, but interviewers must also remain empathic with the fact that it is simply very difficult for most depressed and suicidal clients to recall anything positive.

Finally, when it comes to establishing a therapeutic relationship with suicidal clients, it is important to be aware of the fact that they may be experiencing cognitive or attentional dysfunctions that make it difficult for them to attend to what you are saying. For that reason, Wollersheim (1974) recommends that suicide assessors speak slowly and clearly and that they occasionally repeat key messages when working with clients who are depressed and suicidal.

Identifying Alternatives to Suicide

> The primary thought disorder in suicide is that of a pathological narrowing of the mind's focus, called constriction, which takes the form of seeing only two choices; either something painfully unsatisfactory or cessation. (Shneidman, 1984, pp. 320-321)

It is a fact that suicide is a viable alternative to life. It is fruitless to attempt to debate with clients about whether or not suicide is a philosophically appropriate option. People commit suicide every day, and if a client wants to commit suicide badly enough, he will probably find a way to do it. Instead of arguing with your clients about whether or not they *should* commit suicide, help them identify options in addition to suicide.

Usually suicidal clients suffer from a form of mental constriction because of which they are unable to identify other viable options in their lives. As Shneidman (1980, p. 310) suggests, help your clients "widen" their view of life options. They need to take off their mental blinders and see that suicide is not the only alternative.

Suicidal clients should also be encouraged to examine the question, "Why commit suicide now?" Talk to your clients about the fact that there is no rush. An individual can always commit suicide later, after other life options have been explored. In fact, because suicide is a permanent choice, all other options should be explored first. The key here is that if you get your clients reinvolved with life, they often reap natural rewards and gratifications that eventually reduce the desire to commit suicide and thereby end life. When one's life becomes gratifying and worthwhile, the motivation to end it all must decrease.

Shneidman (1980) writes of an example wherein he goes through a list of alternatives with a pregnant and suicidal teenager in an effort to remove her blinders. This is a practical and concrete approach that can be used with clients to enhance the working relationship and at the same time open their minds to more constructive alternatives. Shneidman (1980) recommends using a pencil and paper to brainstorm alternative actions with regard to a specific life dilemma. Finally, after all alternatives are listed, the client is asked to rank the alternatives in order of preference. Of course, there is always the possibility that your client will decide that suicide is the best choice (at which point you have obtained some very important assessment information). On the other hand, it is surprising how often suicidal clients discover other, more preferable options through Shneidman's method.

Establishing Suicide-Prevention Contracts

Many writers and clinicians recommend establishing suicide-prevention contracts (Mahoney, 1990; Pipes & Davenport, 1990; Wollersheim, 1974). Although most clinicians we know use verbal suicide-prevention contracts, contracts may be formally written out as well. The typical contract is a verbal agreement between client and therapist (or interviewer), sometimes sealed with a handshake. The agreement ordinarily sounds something like:

> *I:* "You've said that sometimes you feel an urge to kill yourself. The possibility of you taking your own life during an impulsive moment concerns me. Can you promise me that if the urge to kill yourself wells up inside you, and you're afraid you're going to lose control and kill yourself, you'll call me first? We can talk things over and hopefully you'll be able to regain control."

> *C:* "Okay. Yeah, I can call you if I start to feel out of control."

Before reading on, stop and reread the previous suicide-prevention contract statement. What is wrong with this type of verbal agreement?

Several significant problems are associated with traditional suicide-prevention contracts. First, although as a professional helper you may feel you are completely committed to your clients, you may not want to deal with client crises at any time, night or day. Second, you may not be able to respond to your client immediately. For example, you may not be home, or you may be at home dealing with a smaller crisis of your own. Therefore, if you enter into a suicide contract similar to the one described above, be sure to provide your client with alternative telephone numbers (e.g., the local suicide hotline) in case you're unavailable when the suicidal urges occur. Third, what if your client simply calls you to "sign off"? For example: "Doc, I was calling 'cause you said to call if I felt out of control. Well, I just wanted to say good-bye; I'm gonna blow my head off."

Instead of the traditional "call me if you feel out of control" contract, Mahoney (1990) recommends making an agreement with clients that they meet with you face to face before following through with suicide impulses. Although this approach has several advantages, it also may be difficult for severely suicidal clients to honestly agree to such a contract. In order to avoid having clients feel pressured into establishing a suicide-prevention contract with you, give them an opportunity to decline your contract offer (e.g., "I only want you to agree to this contract if you really believe you can follow through with it."). In addition, when establishing any type of suicide contract with clients, be sure to acknowledge that you cannot always be available to them. Therefore, you should also provide them with numbers of local suicide hotlines in case they cannot reach you during their time of urgency.

Suicide-prevention contracts (even contracts that specify only telephone contact) probably decrease suicide risk in most cases because they constitute a lifeline between client and interviewer. Consequently, to be most effective, interviewers should establish a solid therapeutic relationship before entering into a suicide-prevention contract. In most cases a single interview is an adequate time period for establishing the type of relationship necessary to make a suicide-prevention contract effective. If it does not seem to you that you are relating well enough to a particular client to establish a suicide contract, it may be a sign that the client is severely suicidal and that more immediate intervention is warranted.

Suicide-prevention contracts also help evaluators assess client self-control and intent. If clients are willing to agree to a suicide-prevention contract, then they are probably in some control and have only low to moderate intent. Clients with low self-control or high intent usually will not agree to a suicide contract.

Becoming Directive and Responsible

When intervening with potentially suicidal clients, interviewers sometimes must become exceptionally directive and responsible (Shneidman, 1980).

When clients are unwilling or unable to protect their own well-being, it becomes the interviewer's responsibility to do so. This may involve directly telling the client what to do, where to go, who to call, and so forth. It also may involve prescriptive therapeutic interventions, such as urging the client to get involved in potentially rewarding activities—daily exercise, consistent recreational activity, church activities, or whatever seems therapeutic based on the individual client's needs.

Clients who are assessed as severely or extremely suicidal (see page 262) may require hospitalization. If you have such a client, be positive and direct regarding the need for and potential benefit of hospitalization. Clients may have stereotyped views of what life is like inside of a psychiatric hospital. Statements similar to some of the following may be helpful.

- "I wonder how you feel (or what you think) about the possibility of staying in a hospital for a while, until you feel safer and more in control?"
- "I think being in the hospital may be just the right thing for you. You can get away from the pressures of your daily life. You can rest and work on feeling better. And the staff at the hospital is great. They'll be there to talk with you, but they'll also leave you alone and let you rest."
- "Some people feel uncomfortable about the possibility of staying in a hospital for a while. In your case I think you should give it a try and see if it's helpful. If it isn't helpful, you can always check out in a week or so. My opinion is that life can be better for you, but that you need to take some steps to help make that happen. Going into the hospital is one of those steps . . . a chance to focus on yourself and how you can begin to feel life is worth living again."

Making Decisions about Hospitalization and Referral

When using interview methods to conduct a suicide assessment, most professionals follow procedures similar to those that have been described in this chapter. Once the assessment has been completed, there is still the question of how to proceed with the client's professional care. Unfortunately, there are no simple formulas to guide the interviewer in decisions about suicidal clients. Table 11-1 offers guidelines to help make the assessment and decision-making processes clearer.

During a suicide assessment, most interviewers are faced with the question, "What should I do?" Suicide is one issue that can propel interviewers into action. When working with suicidal clients, interviewers are very likely to rely on directive interviewing responses (e.g., questions, advice, and explanations). As a result, interviewers tend to feel heightened levels of responsibility for their clients, and they feel the pressure of making decisions that may determine whether a person lives or dies.

The first question to be addressed in the decision-making process is, How suicidal is the client? Suicidality can be measured along a continuum from nonexistent to extreme:

TABLE 11-1 Checklist of Suicide Assessment Issues

_____ Identify common risk factors associated with suicide that are characteristic of your client (e.g., sex, age, physical health).

_____ Evaluate for depression and associated risk factors within depressed populations (i.e., next three checklist items).

_____ Evaluate for panic attacks.

_____ Evaluate for general psychic anxiety.

_____ Evaluate for lack of interest or pleasure in usually pleasurable activities.

_____ Evaluate for alcohol abuse increase during affective episode.

_____ Evaluate for diminished concentration.

_____ Evaluate for global insomnia.

_____ Evaluate for feelings of hopelessness.

_____ Identify the frequency, duration, and intensity of suicidal ideation.

_____ Evaluate the specificity and lethality of the suicide plan, the availability of the means of suicide, and the proximity of resources that can prevent suicide.

_____ Evaluate client level of self-control by asking the client about his self-control and by exploring the client's history of impulsive behavior.

_____ Assess level of suicidal intent as absent, low, moderate, or high.

1. Nonexistent: No suicidal ideation or plans exist.

2. Mild: Suicidal ideation but no specific or concrete plans exist. Few risk factors are present.

3. Moderate: Suicidal ideation and a general plan exist. Self-control is intact; client knows several "reasons to live," and client does not "intend to" kill himself. Some risk factors are present.

4. Severe: Suicide ideation is frequent and intense. Plan is specific and lethal, means are available, and nearby helping resources are few. Self-control is questionable, but the client does not really "want" to kill himself; intent appears absent. Many risk factors may be present.

5. Extreme: Same description as Severe, except that client expresses a clear intent to kill himself as soon as the opportunity presents itself. Many risk factors are usually present.

Clients who present with mild to moderate suicide potential usually can be managed on an outpatient basis. Obviously, the more frequent and intense the ideation and the more clear the plan (assess using SLAP), the closer the client should be monitored. We recommend making verbal suicide-prevention contracts with clients who exhibit mild to moderate suicide potential. We also recommend discussing suicide as one of many alternatives. However, we are much less directive with and take much less responsibility for mild to moderately suicidal clients than for severely to extremely suicidal clients.

If moderately suicidal clients fit into several important high-risk categories, we sometimes treat them as if they were severely suicidal. For example: A fifty-five-year-old depressed male presents with a consistent suicide ideation and a vague plan. This client is socially isolated and has increased alcohol use since the onset of his depression. Depending upon a number of clinical issues, this client might be a good candidate for psychiatric hospitalization (a strategy usually employed with severely or extremely suicidal clients). He would especially be treated as high risk if he had made a previous suicide attempt.

Severely and extremely suicidal clients warrant swift and directive intervention. Such clients should not be left alone while you consider your intervention options. Instead, you should inform them in a supportive but directive manner that it is your professional responsibility to take actions needed to ensure their safety. Such actions may include contacting the police or a designated county or municipal mental health professional. If you believe a severely or extremely suicidal client should be escorted to a psychiatric facility, you should never attempt to do so on your own. Suicidal clients have jumped from moving vehicles, attempted to drown themselves in rivers, and thrown themselves into freeway traffic, in order to avoid hospitalization and accomplish their goal of suicide. Regardless of whether they succeed during such an attempt, the attempt itself will be unduly traumatic to both client and interviewer.

There are several reasons why hospitalization may not be the best option for moderately or severely suicidal clients (although it is probably always the best option for extremely suicidal clients). For some clients hospitalization itself is traumatic. They experience deflated self-esteem and regression to lower levels of functioning and become cut off from more socially acceptable support networks. Severely suicidal clients who are employed and have adequate social support networks may be maintained effectively without hospitalization. In such cases clinicians may greatly increase contact with clients, perhaps even meeting them for brief sessions on a five-times-weekly basis.

Regardless of how suicidal a client is, interviewers and therapists should consistently check with clients to determine whether or not suicidal status has changed. Do not assume that because your client was only mildly suicidal yesterday, she is still only mildly suicidal today.

Professional Issues

When you work with suicidal clients, it is very important that you be a competent and caring professional who lives up to professional standards of practice. Meeting professional standards will make your practice more effective and will help protect you if one of your clients actually completes a suicide (Moris, 1990).

Many important professional issues are associated with suicide assessment. Some of these issues are personal, while others emphasize professional or legal issues. It is sometimes difficult to disentangle the personal from the professional-legal. These issues are discussed briefly below.

Can You Work with Suicidal Clients?
Some interviewers are not well-suited to working with suicidal clients. If you are such an interviewer, it is good to know your limits.

Depressed and suicidal clients are often angry and hostile toward those who try to help them. Yet it remains the interviewer's responsibility to maintain rapport and not to become too irritated, even with hostile clients. Interviewers need to avoid taking the comments of suicidal clients personally.

If you are yourself prone to depression and suicide, it is wise to avoid working with suicidal clients consistently. Working with such clients may "push your emotional buttons" and cause you to become depressed and suicidal.

Some people strongly believe that suicide is a viable life choice and that clients should not be prevented from committing suicide if they truly want to (Szasz, 1986). Szasz states:

> All this points toward the desirability of according suicide the status of a basic human right (in its strict, political-philosophical sense). I do not mean that killing oneself is always good or praiseworthy; I mean only that the power of the state should not be legitimately invoked or deployed to prohibit or prevent persons from killing themselves. (p. 811)

On the other hand, Shneidman (1984) believes strongly that because of the psychological and emotional state of the suicidal person, suicide should not be considered a right: "Suicide is not a 'right' anymore than is the 'right to belch.' If the individual feels forced to do it he will do it" (p. 322).

If you have strong philosophical beliefs either for or against suicide, they may impede your ability to be maximally objective and helpful when you work with suicidal clients. If such is the case, you should consider referring suicidal clients to other professionals who can work more effectively with them.

Consultation

Consultation with peers and supervisors serves a dual purpose for professionals working with suicidal clients. It provides interviewers with much-needed professional support. Dealing with suicidal clients is difficult and stressful and help from other professionals should be welcomed. If only for the sake of preserving their own health and sanity, suicide assessors should not work in isolation. Consultation also provides interviewers with feedback regarding the appropriate standards of practice in each individual case. When it comes to defending your actions (or lack thereof) during a postsuicide trial, it will be expected that you have functioned in the *usual* and *customary* manner with regard to professional standards. Consultation is one way to ensure you are functioning in a professionally competent manner.

Documentation

Professional interviewers should always document the nature of their contact with clients (Soisson, VandeCreek, & Knapp, 1987). It is especially important when working with suicidal clients to document the bases of your clinical decisions. For example, if you are working with a severely or extremely suicidal client and decide against hospitalization, you should outline exactly why you made that particular decision. In such a case, you might be justified not hospitalizing your client if a suicide-prevention contract has been established and your client has good social support resources (e.g., family or employment).

When you work with a suicidal client, you should keep documentation to show that you:

1. Conducted a thorough suicide assessment.
2. Obtained adequate historical information.
3. Obtained records regarding previous treatment.
4. Asked directly about suicidal thoughts and impulses.
5. Consulted with one or more professionals.
6. Discussed limits of confidentiality with the client.
7. Implemented suicide interventions.
8. Gave resources (e.g., telephone numbers) to the client.

The legal bottom line with regard to documentation is that if an event was not documented, it did not happen.

Dealing with Completed Suicides

In the unfortunate event that one of your clients completes a suicide, you should be aware of several personal and legal issues.

First, you should seek professional and personal support. Sometimes therapists need psychotherapy or counseling to deal with their feelings of grief and guilt. In other cases postsuicide discussion with supportive colleagues is sufficient. Some professionals conduct what has been referred to as "psychological autopsies" in an effort to identify factors that contributed to the suicide. Psychological autopsies are especially helpful for professionals who regularly work with suicidal clients; autopsies may help them prevent suicides in future situations (Kaye & Soreff, 1991).

Second, consult with an attorney immediately. You need to know the nature of your legal situation and how to best protect yourself (Kottler & Brown, 1992).

Third, although your attorney may suggest otherwise, you probably should give the family of your deceased client full access to you. They may want to meet with you personally or simply discuss the case over the telephone. If you refuse to discuss the situation with a client's family, you risk their anger; angry families are more likely to prosecute you than are families who feel you have been open and fair with them (Moris, 1990).

Fourth, realize that anything you say to a deceased client's family can be used against you. Therefore, you should continue to consult with your attorney regarding what you can discuss openly.

Fifth, your attitude toward the deceased client's family may be more important than what you disclose about your client's case. Avoid saying, "My attorney recommended that I not answer that question." Make efforts to be open about your own sadness regarding the client's death, but avoid talking about your guilt (e.g., don't say, "Oh, I only wish I had decided to hospitalize him after our last session.").

Chapter Summary

Suicide is a significant social problem and is theoretically a preventable cause of death. There are many myths regarding suicide; this may be related to the fact that so many risk factors are associated with suicidal behavior. Some of the more prominent risk factors include depression, thoughts and feelings of hopelessness, age, sex, race, marital status, employment status, physical health, substance abuse, history of previous suicide attempt, and presence of a mental disorder. This chapter is designed to dispel suicide myths and facilitate competent suicide assessment.

Conducting a suicide assessment involves several important steps. First, as an interviewer you should learn the factors commonly associated with increased suicide risk. Although such factors are not infallible as indicators, they may help you make the difficult decisions associated with suicidal clients. Second, you should explore the extent of the client's depression. Third, you should evaluate the frequency, duration, and intensity of the client's suicidal thoughts (suicide ideation). Fourth, you should clarify whether or not the client has a suicide plan. Fifth, if appropriate, you should evaluate the client's suicide plan in terms of specificity of the plan, lethality and availability of the means, and proximity of supportive resources—or SLAP. Sixth, you should assess client self-control by asking about it directly, identifying reasons for living, and exploring the client's history of impulsive behavior.

When working with suicidal clients, it is important that you establish rapport and a therapeutic relationship through effective listening strategies. Supportive empathy is especially crucial. Suicidal clients may not have informed anyone previously of their suicidal thoughts and wishes. Let them know you hear their pain and misery, but at the same time inform them that there is good reason to be hopeful; most depressed and suicidal clients improve and begin to feel life is worth living again.

Avoid arguing with clients about whether or not suicide is a viable life option. Instead, focus on widening the client's view of personal options by emphasizing that suicide is only one of many life options. Reason that because suicide is a permanent choice, all other options should be explored first. Try to reinvolve clients in potentially reinforcing life activities.

Many interviewers establish suicide-prevention contracts with suicidal clients. Traditional suicide-prevention contracts are verbal or written agreements between client and interviewer that require the client to call the interviewer if the client believes he is going to lose control and attempt suicide. Mahoney (1990) recommends requiring in the agreement that the client commit to a face-to-face session before attempting suicide. Client willingness to establish such a contract usually indicates that client self-control is adequate and suicide intent is low.

Sometimes interviewers must become very directive and responsible when working with suicidal clients. They may need to recommend specific healthy activities or to urge hospitalization.

Deciding whether or not a client's suicidal impulses warrant immediate hospitalization is difficult and complex. A client's level of suicide risk can be rated to help facilitate decision making, but there is no foolproof formula available to help interviewers decide how to most effectively manage each suicidal case. The ratings of suicidality are nonexistent, mild, moderate, severe, and extreme. Clients who are mildly or moderately suicidal can normally be managed in an outpatient setting. Severely and extremely suicidal clients usually require hospitalization.

Depressed and suicidal clients can be extremely difficult to work with. Sometimes they are angry and hostile toward their counselors. If you have problems working with such clients, you should refer them to other professionals. If you have strong philosophical beliefs about suicide, they may interfere with your effectiveness with suicidal clients, and you may need to refer such clients elsewhere.

Interviewers should always know and adhere to professional standards when working with suicidal clients. Whenever possible, interviewers should consult with other professionals about their suicidal clients. All professional decisions should be clearly and concisely documented. In the unfortunate event of a client actually committing suicide, interviewers are advised to follow several key steps.

Suggested Readings

Bennett, B. E., Bryant, B. K., VandenBos, G. R., & Greenwood, A. (1990). *Professional liability and risk management.* Washington, D.C.: American Psychological Association. This text provides excellent guidelines for therapists who want to avoid professional liability in this age of frequent litigation.

Patterson, W. M., Dohn, H. H., Bird, J., & Patterson, G. A. (1983). Evaluation of suicidal patients: The SAD PERSONS scale. *Psychosomatics, 24,* 343–349. This is a useful article that provides an acronym to help clinicians recall suicide predictor variables.

Roy, A. (1989). Suicide. In H. Kaplan and B. Sadock (Eds.), *Comprehensive textbook of psychiatry* (5th ed.). Baltimore: Williams & Wilkins. This is an extensive chapter covering many dimensions of suicide.

Sterling-Smith, R. (1974). A medical toxicology index: An evaluation of commonly used suicidal drugs. In A. T. Beck, H. L. P. Resnik, & D. J. Lettieri, Eds., *The prediction of suicide.* Bowie, MD: Charles Press. This index provides a list of thirty drugs commonly used in suicide attempts. It is very useful if you are working with depressed clients who have access to various medications.

Szasz, T. S. (1986). The case against suicide prevention. *American Psychologist, 41,* 806–812. In this article Szasz outlines his provocative belief that coercive suicide-prevention efforts violate individual human rights.

Wollersheim, J. P. (1974). The assessment of suicide potential via interview methods. *Psychotherapy: Theory, Research and Practice, 11,* 222–225. Wollersheim's article focuses on assessing suicidal clients exclusively through interview procedures.

12

FACILITATING CLIENT *AND* INTERVIEWER DEVELOPMENT

What Is Development?

Client Development
    Listening
    Intentional Treatment Planning

Interviewer Development
    Questions to Ask Yourself
    Using Logic and Intuition
    Setting Personal Goals

Chapter Summary

Suggested Readings

We shall not cease from exploration
And the end of all our exploring
Will be to arrive where we started
And know the place for the first time.
          —T. S. ELIOT

What Is Development?

Just before author John Sommers-Flanagan was scheduled to give his usual lecture on developmental psychology to an introductory psychology class, he telephoned Leonard Burns, a colleague with extensive experience in the area, and asked him for something profound to tell the students about development. Len's reply was, "Tell them *things change with time.*" To be honest, John had hoped for something a little more verbose or at least funny to kick off his usual discussion of Piaget, Erickson, Ainsworth and the rest of the big names in developmental psychology. At first John didn't think much of his colleague's remark. The class, too, was relatively unimpressed. Hoping to impress the students with his scholarship and name dropping, John prefaced the quotation with the story of how he had asked an esteemed colleague for some profound words. Instead he observed a kind of "so what" look on their faces. Maybe he had overprepared them for the quote; but then again, he hadn't been all that impressed with it either.

Not until over a year later did John finally understand the significance of the colleague's comment, "Things change with time," and the reason why that class (and several classes since) had responded so unenthusiastically. Development is constant for living organisms. It is so commonplace, so ubiquitous, that we hardly notice the changes. And we don't want to move patiently through time, slowly adding to our knowledge, slowly maturing, slowly growing and, we hope getting better at what we do. We want instant results, sudden and visible changes, and giant steps toward being good, wise, and professional. Although this "I-want-change-now" attitude dominates Western culture, unfortunately, that just isn't how it works. As Len said, things change with time. We the authors would add that they change with effort, experience, patience, and tenacity, and that all too often, things change more slowly than we would like. This is especially true when it comes to developing a complex skill such as therapeutic interviewing.

One of our supervisors used to say, "Life is therapeutic" (Land, 1986). Unfortunately, life can be traumatic and antitherapeutic as well. War experiences, incest, and broken relationships all serve potentially to inhibit our developmental progress. Life experiences can powerfully facilitate or impede developmental progress, depending partly on the experience itself and partly on how we view and handle the experience.

Two factors fuel the developmental process: maturation and learning. Maturation refers to the constant developmental changes occurring within the body as a result of aging (rather than learning, injury, illness, or some other life experience). In other words, maturation involves change that would occur anyway, regardless of our particular experiences. In contrast, learning refers to the relatively permanent changes in our thoughts, feelings, and behaviors that occur as direct results of experience.

Theoretically, counseling and psychotherapy have no effect on maturation. On the other hand, a single clinical or therapeutic interview is a client experience that may powerfully affect learning. A single interview can produce relatively permanent and significant changes in a client's life. Therapeutic interviews do not change who the client *is*, but they can change who the client *is becoming*. Similarly, this textbook and the course-related experiences associated with it may help move you forward in the process of becoming a professional therapeutic interviewer.

Client Development

The general goal of therapeutic interviewing is to facilitate positive client development. This involves performing adequate assessment and evaluation, listening empathically, and obtaining a sense of what each client needs and wants in terms of personal growth. In the words of Fromm-Reichman (1950), "the patient needs an experience, not an explanation" (quoted in Korchin, 1976, p. 284). Part of the professional interviewer's role is to provide clients with *experiences*—if at all possible, therapeutic experiences.

Listening
It seems clear that most, if not all, clients benefit from the experience of having an empathic person listen closely to them as they talk about their lives. This is the least we can provide our clients, regardless of their developmental level (although some theorists have suggested that nondirective listening and empathic responding is the most important thing we can provide to our clients; Rogers, 1957; Strupp and Binder, 1984).

Beyond listening, therapeutic interviewing requires client assessment and technical counseling or psychotherapeutic interventions. Assessment involves not only evaluating a client's problem, but also an analyzing a client's personality or developmental status. We need to know where a client is in order to facilitate progress along life's journey. Similarly, to develop as interviewers, we need to know where we are, and where we're going.

Intentional Treatment Planning
An in-depth discussion of how to develop client treatment plans is beyond the scope of this book. Establishing treatment plans requires a theoretical foundation and practical knowledge regarding client and therapist capabilities. Treatment should not proceed in a haphazard and spontaneous manner (although some spontaneity in terms of treatment implementation is sometimes warranted). The following outline may be useful for formulating client treatment plans.

1. Identify the problem or problems you and the client would like to focus on during treatment. Characterize problems in terms of client development (i.e., clients seek to change or modify a particular pattern of thinking, feeling, or behaving).
   A. Identify the problems jointly. Doing so enhances the therapeutic alliance.

      B. Identify each problem as concretely and specifically as possible. This will make it easier to evaluate client progress.

      C. Seek to understand and help clients to understand their problems in developmental terms.

2. Establish short-term and long-term goals with respect to the identified problems.

      A. Formulate short-term goals that are clearly achievable (perhaps in days or hours). Achievable goals will help give clients a sense of immediate success and thereby enhance their motivation.

      B. Define long-term goals clearly. Long-term goals should be intrinsically connected with treatment termination.

3. Select appropriate methods of change.

      A. In general, use more supportive (e.g., behavioral or cognitive) methods with clients at lower developmental levels and more expressive (e.g., psychoanalytic, person-centered, feminist, and gestalt) methods with clients at higher developmental levels (see Ivey, 1991, and Luborsky, 1984, for information on evaluating client developmental levels).

      B. Consider other issues when selecting methods of change, such as what clients can afford in terms of time and money, what methods clients choose or are most comfortable with, and what kind of problems clients present with.

4. Identify methods of measuring client progress. One method will always be client self-report; others may include standardized assessment, peer reports, and more creative means of determining progress.

Whenever possible, client treatment plans should be intentional, concrete, and practical. They should be jointly discussed and established with clients in order to facilitate treatment alliance.

In some cases, however, it is best *not* to provide counseling or psychological treatment. Some clients lack the motivation or resources required to initiate, follow through with, or benefit from treatment (Seligman, 1986, 1990; Weiner, 1975). Frances, Clarkin, and Perry (1984) claim that clients who are highly resistant, who seek counseling in order to strengthen a disability claim, or who improve on their own are unlikely to benefit from psychological treatment. Perhaps the most important question to consider when initiating treatment (and it is a question not thoroughly addressed by this book) is whether or not the client is likely to benefit from or willing to participate in the therapeutic process.

Interviewer Development

As we have discussed throughout this text, becoming an effective therapeutic interviewer is a dynamic developmental process. Because experience enhances developmental processes through learning, we strongly recommend personal and professional experimentation to help you become a better therapeutic interviewer. In other words, gather experiences; work with different types of supervisors and clients; seek exposure to a variety of cultures, races, ages, and gender-related issues; broaden your therapeutic horizons.

We suggest that you keep a professional journal of all interviewing, therapy, testing, and supervisory experiences you have. Of course, do not include identifying data regarding clients, but rather record their problems areas, how you responded, what resulted, what supervisory and consultive guidance you were given, and what you learned. Recording your experiences offers many benefits. A few are listed below:

1. You will have a record of the kinds of professional experiences you've had (good material for your vita).
2. As an expert witness testifying in court some day, you will be able to tell the court exactly what your level of experience is and the number of relevant cases with which you have been involved.
3. You will have a record of your professional development.
4. You can discern patterns in your work and in choices you make and thereby identify gaps you want to address as time goes by.

Questions to Ask Yourself

The following list of questions (complete with our comments) is provided to stimulate your development as a professional interviewer.

Should I Implement Some of the Procedures I Might Choose to Use with Clients into My Own Life?   We believe that, generally speaking, before implementing therapeutic techniques with clients, we should experience them ourselves. For example, if you want to help clients relax more completely, you should experiment with relaxation procedures yourself. You may want to practice progressive relaxation, meditation, mental imagery, autogenic training, or other therapeutic procedures before suggesting them to a client. However, be sure to avoid the trap of believing that what works for you should work for your clients. Although you may enjoy and grow from meditation experiences, your clients may not.

What Types of Clients do I Want to (or Should I) Work With? You may have a special talent that enables you to work well with a particular type of client. Explore your special talents by working with a wide range of individuals. Your professional journal will be invaluable in this area, helping you sort out your personal reactions, your professional successes, and what parts of your professional and personal self are in greatest need of training or remediation. Don't be afraid to try working with people who seem a bit threatening. You may surprise yourself, rise to the challenge, and begin enjoying your work with a particular type of client. Author John Sommers-Flanagan's experience with angry adolescents has been more rewarding than he ever would have imagined (in fact, his affinity for working with such clients still surprises him). Of course, you should obtain professional supervision when working with new client populations or new types of client problems.

What Theoretical Orientation Best Fits Me? Choosing a theoretical orientation is closely related to development of one's professional identity. Consequently, choosing a theoretical orientation can produce reactions within would-be interviewers similar to reactions that occur during the adolescent identity crisis. Some interviewers will experience constant or consistent identity diffusion or confusion. Others will "foreclose" on a particular theoretical orientation without experiencing any confusion, quickly committing to that orientation at the suggestion of an authority figure. Others will experience a strong theoretical identity crisis and actively explore a number of perspectives in an effort to find a stable and desirable theoretical identity. Our main advice with regard to theoretical orientation is to avoid premature foreclosure (Marcia, 1966; Shaffer, 1989).

When author Rita Sommers-Flanagan decided to go to graduate school, she believed she was a "true-blue behaviorist." It took about two weeks for her to realize she didn't even know what a behaviorist was. When, years later, she felt she *could* roughly describe what one was, she recognized that she was not, primarily, a behaviorist after all. We do not recommend that students choose a theoretical orientation early on. Rather, you should try different theories and techniques. Note which ones seem to be consistent with your world view, your way of being with clients. Note which make sense to you and seem defensible as an explanation of human nature and how people change. Always be ready to modify, change, and grow. Many contemporary psychotherapists model openness and theoretical diversity (Cottone, 1992; Goldfried, 1990; Wollersheim, 1985).

On the other hand, we do not recommend sloppy eclecticism. It is acceptable to take ideas from a variety of sources, but you should know the roots of the ideas and understand each technique or belief in the context of the theory it represents. This is easier said than done. Years of study and good supervision are required to understand the premises of and begin to apply techniques based on psychoanalytic, behavioral, person-centered, cognitive, feminist, or behavioral theory. Still, we recommend in-depth exploration of theoretical orientations as the best option with regard to long-term professional development. This does not mean you cannot begin to be an effective interviewer and therapist before you fully understand the major theories. Our recommendations are simply that you know a theory well before using its premises and techniques and that you continue to grow and develop in this area throughout your career.

Should I Obtain Personal Counseling or Psychotherapy? Research on this issue has come to mixed conclusions (Clark, 1986; Greenberg & Staller, 1981; MacDevitt, 1987). There is evidence suggesting that obtaining personal psychotherapy during training is extremely helpful for some interviewers. There is also evidence that in some cases participation in psychotherapy stirs up personal issues within the therapist that can adversely affect interviewing performance (Greenberg & Staller, 1981).

Psychotherapy might be useful for the psychotherapist or counselor in training for several reasons. First, therapy can help you become more aware of your personal issues and deal with them more effectively when they emerge within you as the interviewer. This is the primary psychoanalytic rationale for obtaining psychotherapy. Second, being in the client role can help you develop greater empathy for your own clients. There is no substitute for actually experiencing what it is like to be a client. Third, on at least some occasions, everyone has problems in living. It is hypocritical to expect clients to seek professional help for their problems if you neglect to do so when problems arise in your own life. Obtaining therapy is a behavioral statement that you have faith in the profession.

Our bottom-line opinion on the question of whether therapists or counselors in training should receive personal counseling is yes. If you feel otherwise, we challenge you to explore your reasoning in your professional journal or with a supervisor or therapist.

Using Logic and Intuition

Although we believe the right brain/left brain dichotomy has been overused as an explanation for the variety of ways of thinking and behaving, it does provide a useful analogue for discussing the use of logic and intuition (Allen, 1983; Gazzaniga, 1983). The right brain purportedly operates more holistically than sequentially. When a person senses that some action is the right thing to do but has no logical explanation for why, this sense is said to be intuitive and to be associated with holistic, right-brain activity. "Trusting your gut," allowing your unconscious to integrate pieces of a situation into a sense of the big picture, and using art or music or meditation to move a client in therapy are all manifestations of therapeutic intuition. Intuition is sometimes said to represent the *art* of interviewing or of psychotherapy, and some individuals seem gifted with intuitive insight (Bugental, 1987). Others report having their intuitive skills grow by exposing themselves to therapy, meditation, art, music, journal writing, introspection, and a variety of other right-brain-based experiences.

The left brain theoretically represents and processes the sequential, rational, and logical issues relevant to life and therapy (Allen, 1983). Left-brain thinking might be considered the *science* of interviewing or psychotherapy. The scientific approach emphasizes measurement of therapeutic progress and acts, to a degree, as the test to which we must eventually put our intuitive work. Left-brain thinking asks questions like, How can I measure whether or not what I'm doing is effective? What is the likelihood of harming a client with this procedure? What are the efficacy data on this technique? Am I implementing this procedure properly? How can I maximize my effectiveness? Is this truly an intuitive stroke of genius or is it countertransference or indigestion on my part? Why? What are the scientifically identified signs of transference, rapport, and expertness? What are the facts in psychiatry, psychology, counseling, and social work?

Too much of either logic or intuition can be detrimental to good interviewing. However, we believe there is no such thing as too much education or too much dedication to continued personal growth. It is indefensible to let intuition run rampant. Intuition should be supported by experience, education, and supervision. Ultimately, it needs to stand the test of tangible, logical data. On the other hand, many brilliant interviewers cannot fully explain how they know what they know. They have a rich, deep intuitive side that guides them as they work with people. The difference between their work and "rampant intuition" is that they employ self-discipline and self-control to constantly put their intuitive insights to the test in terms of the results they yield. This balance is difficult to achieve, but it is an ideal worth striving toward.

Setting Personal Goals

If the statement that things change with time is true, then change is inevitable. We cannot *not* change. However, we have some control over the directions of those changes. No, you cannot become a superb therapeutic interviewer, complete with a wall of credentials, overnight. Yes, you can become better and better at what you do. Setting goals can facilitate personal and professional development regardless of your career aspirations.

Goal setting can be integrated into your professional journal. Perhaps on a yearly basis, identify an area or two in which you would like to grow. State your long-term goals clearly. Then identify intermediate objectives (short-term goals) that will move you toward your long-range goal. Set up a timetable. List the necessary resources and the possible ways to obtain them. Then begin, step by step, to move toward your goal. Not only will this system ensure that you continue to grow in positive ways, it will also help alleviate burnout, which is at least partly related to the feeling that one has reached a dead-end. Setting and pursuing goals is one way to take care of yourself as a person and professional. We sincerely wish you all the best as you proceed along your professional path.

Chapter Summary

Development occurs constantly. It is a process involving biological maturation and experiential learning. Clinical interviewers seek to enhance their clients' development by providing clients with therapeutic experiences. These experiences entail interviewers taking on several tasks, not the least of which is to listen empathically. Specific therapeutic interventions should be initiated only after client problems and developmental status have been assessed.

A simple outline for intentional treatment planning includes the steps of identifying specific client problems and developmental status, formulating of short- and long-term goals, selecting appropriate therapeutic change methods, and identifying methods of measuring client progress.

The process of becoming a competent therapeutic interviewer is dynamic and developmental. Gathering personal and professional experiences can help facilitate positive professional development. Interviewers in training should keep professional journals to track their professional experiences. In addition, interviewers can facilitate their own development by practicing therapeutic change procedures on themselves, obtaining personal counseling or psychotherapy, actively exploring various theoretical orientations, and experimenting with different clinical populations to find out with which they would most like to work.

Professional therapeutic interviewers remain open to new ways of working with clients. In this respect, both logic and intuition are used as ways of evaluating and applying therapeutic methods. Logic and rational thinking are very important in the science of specifying and evaluating treatment methods. Interviewers should use clinical intuition in combination with rational evaluation to sharpen their application of therapeutic techniques. Therapeutic interviewers can facilitate their own personal and professional development by setting specific short- and long-term goals in much the same ways they set such goals for their clients.

Suggested Readings

Bugental, J. F. T. (1987). *The art of the psychotherapist.* New York: W. W. Norton. This books focuses on the intuitive and artistic side of being a psychotherapist.

Ivey, A. E. (1991). *Developmental strategies for helpers.* Pacific Grove, CA: Brooks/Cole. Ivey's most recent book focuses on methods therapists can use to facilitate client development. The information on evaluating client developmental levels and applying appropriate treatment methods is especially useful.

Luborsky, L. (1984). *Principles of psychoanalytic psychotherapy: A manual for supportive-expressive treatment.* New York: Basic Books. This book focuses on identifying the differences between supportive and expressive approaches to psychotherapy. It provides important information regarding how to choose treatment techniques.

Seligman, L. (1990). *Selecting effective treatments.* San Francisco: Jossey-Bass. This book goes into great detail regarding the diagnosis and treatment-planning process from a counseling perspective.

Thorpe, S. A. (1987). An approach to treatment planning. *Psychotherapy, 24,* 729–735. This article describes a three-dimensional approach to treatment planning.

REFERENCES

Abt, I. R., & Stuart, L. E. (Eds.). (1982). *The newer therapies: A sourcebook.* New York: Van Nostrand Reinhold.

Adler, A. (1958). *What life should mean to you.* New York: Capricorn.

Ainsworth, M. D. S. (1984). Attachment. In N. S. Endler & J. McV. Hunt (Eds.), *Personality and the behavior disorders* (rev. ed.). New York: Wiley.

Ainsworth, M. D. S. (1989). Attachments beyond infancy. *American Psychologist, 44,* 709–716.

Alexander, J. A. (1990). *Functional family therapy.* Paper presented at continuing education workshop sponsored by Rivendell Hospitals of America, Butte, MT.

Allen, M. (1983). Models of hemispheric specialization. *Psychological Bulletin, 93,* 73–104.

American Psychiatric Association. (1987). *Diagnostic and statistical manual of mental disorders* (3rd ed., revised). Washington, DC: Author.

American Psychological Association. (1990). Ethical principles of psychologists (amended June 2, 1989). *American Psychologist, 45,* 390–395.

Arkoff, A. (Ed.). (1980). *Psychology and personal growth* (2nd ed.). Boston: Allyn & Bacon.

Bach, R. (1977). *Illusions.* New York: Delacort.

Balleweg, B. J. (1990). The interviewing team: An exercise for teaching assessment and conceptualization skills. *Teaching of Psychology, 17,* 241–242.

Banaka, W. H. (1971). *Training in-depth interviewing.* New York: Harper & Row.

Bandler, R., & Grinder, J. (1975). *The structure of magic I: A book about language and therapy.* Palo Alto, CA: Science and Behavior Books.

Bandler, R., & Grinder, J. (1979). *Frogs into princes.* Moab, UT: Real People Press.

Bandura, A. (1969). *Principles of behavior modification.* New York: Holt, Rinehart & Winston.

Barlow, D. H., & Cerny, J. A. (1988). *The psychological treatment of panic.* New York: Guilford.

Basow, S. A. (1980). *Sex role stereotypes: Traditions and alternatives.* Monterey, CA: Brooks/Cole.

Beck, A. T. (1976). *Cognitive therapy and the emotional disorders.* New York: International Universities Press.

Beck, A. T., Brown, G., & Steer, R. A. (1989). Prediction of eventual suicide in psychiatric inpatients by clinical ratings of hopelessness. *Journal of Consulting and Clinical Psychology, 57*, 309–310.

Beck, A. T., Rush, A. H., Shaw, B. F., & Emery, G. (1979). *Cognitive therapy of depression.* New York: Guilford.

Beitman, B. D. (1983). Categories of countertransference. *Journal of Operational Psychiatry, 14*, 82–90.

Bem, D., & Allen, A. (1974). On predicting some of the people some of the time: The search for cross-situational consistencies in behavior. *Psychological Review, 81*, 506–520.

Benjamin, A. (1981). *The helping interview.* (3rd ed.). Boston: Houghton-Mifflin.

Bennett, B. E., Bryant, B. K., VandenBos, G. R., & Greenwood, A. (1990). *Professional liability and risk management.* Washington, D.C.: American Psychological Association.

Bennett, C. C. (1984). "Know thyself." *Professional Psychology, 15*, 271–283.

Birdwhistell, M. L. (1952). *Introduction to kinesis: An annotation system for analysis of body motion and gesture.* Louisville, KY: University of Louisville Press.

Birdwhistell, M. L. (1970). *Kinesics and context.* Philadelphia: University of Pennsylvania Press.

Birtchnell, J. (1973). The use of psychiatric case register to study social and familial aspects of mental illness. *Social Science and Medicine, 7*, 145–153.

Blaney, P. H. (1986). Affect and memory: A review. *Psychological Bulletin, 99*, 229–246.

Bornstein, P. H. (1982). Personal communication.

Bornstein, P. H., & Bornstein, M. T. (1986). *Marital therapy: A behavioral-communications approach.* New York: Pergamon.

Bornstein, R. F. (1985). Personal communication.

Borysenko, J. (1986). *Minding the body, mending the mind.* New York: Simon & Schuster.

Bowlby, J. (1969). *Attachment & loss: Vol I Attachment.* London: Hogarth.

Bowlby, J. (1988). *A secure base.* New York: Basic Books.

Boyer, D. (1988). *In and out of street life: A reader on interventions with street youth.* Portland, OR: Tri-county Youth Services Consortium.

Brammer, L. M. (1979). *The helping relationship* (2nd ed.). Englewood Cliffs, NJ: Prentice-Hall.

Brockman, W. P. (1980). *Empathy revisited: The effect of representational system matching on certain counseling process and outcome variables.* Unpublished doctoral dissertation, College of William and Mary, Williamsburg, VA.

Brodsky, A. M. (1982). Sex, race, and class issues in psychotherapy research. In J. H. Harvey & M. M. Parks (Eds.), *The Master Lecture Series: Vol. I. Psychotherapy research and behavior change.* Washington, DC: American Psychological Association.

Brody, C. M. (Ed.). (1984). *Women therapists working with women: New theory and process of feminist therapy.* New York: Springer.

Brown, J. H., Henteleff, P., Barakat, S., & Rowe, C. J. (1986). Is it normal for terminally ill patients to desire death? *American Journal of Psychiatry, 143,* 208–210.

Brown, L., & Brodsky, A. M. (1992). The future of feminist therapy. *Psychotherapy, 29,* 51–57.

Bugental, J. F. T. (1987). *The art of the psychotherapist.* New York: W. W. Norton.

Buie, D. H. (1981). Empathy: Its nature and limitations. *Journal of the American Psychoanalytic Association, 29,* 281–307.

Burns, G. L. (1988). Personal communication.

Burns, G. L. (1990). Affective-cognitive-behavioral assessment: The integration of personality and behavioral assessment. In G. H. Eifert & I. M. Evans (Eds.), *Unifying behavior therapy: Contributions of paradigmatic behaviorism.* New York: Springer.

Capra, F. (1975). *The tao of physics.* New York: Random House.

Carkhuff, R. R. (1987). *The art of helping* (6th ed.). Amherst, MA: Human Resource Development Press.

Carver, C. S., & Scheier, M. F. (1978). Self-focusing effects of dispositional self-consciousness, mirror presence, and audience presence. *Journal of Personality and Social Psychology, 36,* 324–332.

Charlesworth, E. A., & Nathan, R. G. (1982). *Stress management: A comprehensive guide to wellness.* New York: Ballantine Books.

Clark, E. M., & Teasdale, J. D. (1982). Diurnal variation in clinical depression and accessibility of memories of positive and negative experiences. *Journal of Abnormal Psychology, 91,* 87–95.

Clark, M. M. (1986). Personal therapy: A review of empirical research. *Professional Psychology: Research and Practice, 17,* 541–543.

Clucas, T. J. (1990). Personal communication.

Corey, G. (1991). *Theory and practice of counseling and psychotherapy* (4th ed.). Monterey, CA: Brooks/Cole.

Cormier, W. H., & Cormier, L. S. (1985). *Interviewing strategies for helpers: Fundamental skills and cognitive behavioral interventions* (2nd ed.). Monterey, CA: Brooks/Cole.

Cormier, W. H., & Cormier, L. S. (1991). *Interviewing strategies for helpers: Fundamental skills and cognitive behavioral interventions* (3rd ed.). Monterey, CA: Brooks/Cole.

Corsini, R. (1989). *Current psychotherapies* (4th ed.). Itasca, IL: F. E. Peacock.

Cottone, R. R. (1992). *Theories and paradigms of counseling and psychotherapy.* Boston: Allyn & Bacon.

de Shazer, S. (1985). *Keys to solution in brief therapy.* New York: W. W. Norton.

DiBianco, J. T. (1979). The hemodialysis patient. In L. D. Hankoff & B. Einsidler (Eds.), *Suicide: Theory and clinical aspects.* Littleton, MA: PSG Publishing.

Dodson, F. (1987). How to discipline effectively. In E. Shiff (Ed.), *Experts advise parents.* New York: Dell.

Eagle, M. N. (1984). *Recent developments in psychoanalysis.* New York: McGraw-Hill.

Egan, G. (1985). *Exercises in helping skills: A training manual to accompany the skilled helper* (3rd ed.). Monterey, CA: Brooks/Cole.

Egan, G. (1986). *The skilled helper: Model, skills, and methods for effective helping* (3rd ed.). Pacific Grove, CA: Brooks/Cole.

Eich, E. (1989). Theoretical issues in state dependent memory. In H. L. Roediger & F. I. M. Craik (Eds.), *Varieties of memory and consciousness: Essays in honour of Endel Tulving.* Hillsdale, NJ: Erlbaum.

Eliot, T. S. (1943). *Four quartets.* New York: Harcourt, Brace, and Co., p. 39.

Elliott, R. (1988). Tests, abilities, race, and conflict. *Intelligence, 12,* 333–335.

Erdman, J. P., Klein, M. H., & Greist, J. H. (1985). Direct patient computer interviewing. *Journal of Consulting and Clinical Psychology, 53,* 760–773.

Erickson, M. H., Rossi, E., & Rossi, S. (1976). *Hypnotic realities.* New York: Irvington.

Evans, G., & Farberow, N. L. (1988). *The encyclopedia of suicide.* New York: Fact on File.

Fairbairn, R. (1952). *Object relations theory of the personality.* New York: Basic Books.

Fawcett, J., Scheftner, W. A., Fogg, L., Clark, D., Young, M. A., Hedeker, D., & Gibbons, R. (1990). Time-related predictors of suicide in major affective disorder. *American Journal of Psychiatry, 147,* 1189–1194.

Fenichel, O. (1945). *The psychoanalytic theory of neuroses.* New York: W. W. Norton.

Fenigstein, A. (1979). Self-consciousness, self-attention, and social interaction. *Journal of Personality and Social Psychology, 37,* 75–86.

Fenigstein, A., Scheier, M. F., & Buss, A. H. (1975). Public and private self-consciousness: Assessment and theory. *Journal of Consulting and Clinical Psychology, 43,* 522–527.

Fisher, S. (1973). *Body consciousness: You are what you feel.* Englewood Cliffs, NJ: Prentice-Hall.

Fitzgerald, L. F., & Nutt, R. (1986). The Division 17 principles concerning counseling/psychotherapy of women: Rationale and implementation. *Counseling Psychologist, 14,* 180–216.

Foley, R. & Sharf, B. F. (1981). The five interviewing techniques most frequently overlooked by primary care physicians. *Behavioral Medicine, 8,* 26–31.

Folman, R. Z. (1991). Therapist-patient sex: Attraction and boundary problems. *Psychotherapy, 28,* 168–173.

Folstein, M. F., Folstein, S. E., & McHugh, P. R. (1975). "Mini-mental state": A practical method for grading the cognitive state of patients for the clinician. *Journal of Psychiatric Research, 12,* 189–198.

Fong, M. L., & Cox, B. G. (1983). Trust as an underlying dynamic in the counseling process: How clients test trust. *Personal and Guidance Journal, 62,* 163–166.

Francis, A., Clarkin, J., & Perry, S. (1984). *Differential therapeutics in psychiatry.* New York: Brunner/Mazel.

Frank, J. D. (1973). *Persuasion and healing* (2nd ed.). Baltimore: John Hopkins University Press.

Frank, J. D. (1982). Therapeutic components shared by all psychotherapies. In J. H. Harvey & M. M. Parks (Eds.), *The Master Lecture Series: Vol. I. Psychotherapy research and behavior change* Washington, DC: American Psychological Association.

Frankl, V. E. (1960). Paradoxical intention: A logotherapeutic technique. *American Journal of Psychotherapy, 14,* 520–535.

Freud, A. (1946). *The ego and the mechanisms of defense.* (C. Baines, Trans.) New York: International Universities Press.

Freud, S. (1957). The future prospects of psycho-analytic therapy. In J. Strachey (Ed. and Trans.), *The standard edition of the complete psychological works of Sigmund Freud* (Vol. 11, pp. 141–151). London: Hogarth. (Original work published 1910)

Freud, S. (1958). Recommendations to physicians practicing psycho-analysis. In J. Strachey (Ed. and Trans.), *The standard edition of the complete psychological works of Sigmund Freud* (Vol. 12, pp. 111–120). London: Hogarth. (Original work published 1912)

Freud, S. (1955). Group psychology and the analysis of the ego. In J. Strachey (Ed. and Trans.), *The standard edition of the complete psychological works of Sigmund Freud* (Vol. 18, pp. 101–121). London: Hogarth. (Original work published 1921)

Freud, S. (1940/1949). *An outline of psychoanalysis.* New York: W. W. Norton.

Fromm-Reichman, F. (1950). *Principles of intensive psychotherapy.* Chicago: University of Chicago Press.

Gardner, H. (1983). *Frames of mind: The theory of multiple intelligences.* New York: Basic Books.

Gazda, G. M., Asbury, F. S., Balzer, F. J., Childers, W. C., & Walters, R. P. (1977). *Human relations development* (2nd ed.). Boston: Allyn & Bacon.

Gazda, G. M., Asbury, F. S., Balzer, F. J., Childers, W. C., & Walters, R. P. (1984). *Human relations development: A manual for educators* (3rd ed.). Boston: Allyn & Bacon.

Gazzaniga, M. S. (1983). Right hemisphere language following brain bisection: A 20-year perspective. *American Psychologist, 38,* 525–537.

George, R. L., & Cristiani, T. S. (1990). *Counseling: Theory and practice* (3rd ed.). Englewood Cliffs, NJ: Prentice-Hall.

Georgotas, A. (1985). Affective disorders: Pharmacotherapy. In H. I. Kaplan & B. F. Sadock (Eds.), *Comprehensive textbook of psychiatry* (4th ed.). Baltimore: Williams & Wilkins.

Gibbs, M. A. (1984). The therapist as imposter. In C. M. Brody (Ed.), *Women therapists working with women: New theory and process of feminist therapy.* New York: Springer.

Giffen, M. E., & Felsenthal, C. (1983). *A cry for help.* Garden City, NJ: Doubleday.

Gilligan, C. (1982). *In a different voice: Psychological theory and women's development.* Cambridge, MA: Harvard University Press.

Goldfried, M. (1990). Psychotherapy integration: A mid-life crisis for behavior therapy. Paper presented at the 24th annual meeting of the Association for the Advancement of Behavior Therapy, San Francisco.

Goldfried, M., & Davison, G. (1976). *Clinical behavior therapy*. New York: Holt, Rinehart & Winston.

Goldstein, A. P. (1980). Relationship-enhancement methods. In F. H. Kanfer & A. P. Goldstein (Eds.), *Helping people change*. New York: Pergamon.

Gough, H. G. (1957). *California Psychological Inventory manual*. Palo Alto, CA: Consulting Psychologists Press.

Gould, S. J. (1981). *The mismeasure of man*. New York: Norton.

Graves, J. R., & Robinson, J. D. (1976). Proxemic behavior as a function of inconsistent verbal and nonverbal messages. *Journal of Counseling Psychology, 23*, 333–338.

Greenberg, J. R., & Mitchell, S. A. (1983). *Object relations in psychoanalytic theory*. Cambridge, MA: Harvard University Press.

Greenberg, L. S., & Safran, J. D. (1987). *Emotion in psychotherapy: Affect, cognition, and the process of change*. New York: Guilford.

Greenberg, R. P., & Staller, J. (1981). Personal therapy for therapists. *American Journal of Psychiatry, 138*, 1467–1471.

Greenson, R. R. (1965). The working alliance and the transference neurosis. *Psychoanalytic Quarterly, 34*, 155–181.

Greenson, R. R. (1967). *The technique and practice of psychoanalysis* (Vol I). New York: International Universities Press.

Grinder, J., & Bandler, R. (1976). *The structure of magic II*. Palo Alto, CA: Science and Behavior Books.

Gunderson, J. G., Ronningstam, E., Bodkin, A. (1990). The diagnostic interview for narcissistic patients. *Archives of General Psychiatry, 47*, 676–680.

Gustafson, J. P. (1986). *The complex secret of brief psychotherapy*. New York: W. W. Norton.

Hadley, S. W., & Strupp, H. H. (1976). Contemporary views of negative effects in psychotherapy. *Archives of General Psychiatry, 33*, 1291–1302.

Haley, J. (1973). *Uncommon therapies: The psychiatric techniques of Milton Erickson*. San Francisco: Jossey-Bass.

Hall, C., & Lindzey, G. (1970). *Theories of personality*. New York: John Wiley & Sons.

Hall, E. T. (1966). *The hidden dimension*. Garden City, NJ: Doubleday.

Hamilton, M. (1967). A rating scale for depression. *Journal of Neurology, Neurosurgery, and Psychiatry, 23*, 56–62.

Hammer, A. (1983). Matching perceptual predicates: Effect on perceived empathy in a counseling analogue. *Journal of Counseling Psychology, 30*, 172–179.

Hanson, C. (1991). Personal communication.

Hatfield, E., & Walster, G. W. (1981). *A new look at love*. Reading, MA: Addison-Wesley.

Hathaway, S. R., & McKinley, J. C. (1943). *The Minnesota Multiphasic Personality Inventory*. Minneapolis: University of Minnesota Press.

Hatton, C. L., Valente, S. M., & Rink, A. (1977). Assessment of suicide risk. In C. L. Hatton, S. M. Valente, & A. Rink (Eds.), *Suicide: Assessment and intervention*. New York: Appleton-Century-Crofts.

Hayes, V. (1990). Personal communication.

Heinrich, R. K., Corbine, J. L., & Thomas, K. R. (1990). Counseling Native Americans. *Journal of Counseling and Development, 69,* 128–133.

Hersen, M., & Turner, S. M. (1985). *Diagnostic Interviewing.* New York: Plenum.

Hess, E. H. (1975). *The tell-tale eye.* New York: Van Nostrand Reinhold.

Hill, C. E., Helms, J. E., Tichenor, V., Spiegel, S. B., et al. (1988). Effects of therapist response modes in brief psychotherapy. *Journal of Counseling Psychology, 35,* 222–233.

Holinger, P. C., Offer, D., & Zola, M. A. (1988). A prediction model of suicide among youth. *Journal of Nervous and Mental Disease, 176,* 275–279.

Holt, R. R. (1969). *Assessing personality.* New York: Harcourt, Brace, & Jovanovich.

Horowitz, M., Marmar, C., Krupnick, J., Wilner, N., Kaltreider, N., & Wallerstein, R. (1984). *Personality styles and brief psychotherapy.* New York: Basic Books.

Hutchins, D. E., & Cole, C. G. (1986). *Helping relationships and strategies.* Monterey, CA: Brooks/Cole.

Huxley, A. (1932). *Brave new world.* New York: Harper & Row.

Ivey, A. E. (1988). *Intentional interviewing and counseling* (2nd ed.). Pacific Grove, CA: Brooks/Cole.

Ivey, A. E. (1991). *Developmental strategies for helpers.* Pacific Grove, CA: Brooks/Cole.

Izard, C. E. (1977). *Human emotions.* New York: Plenum.

Izard, C. E. (1982). *Measuring emotions in infants and children.* New York: Cambridge University Press.

Johnson, J., Weissman, M. M., & Klerman, G. L. (1990). Panic disorder, comorbidity, and suicide attempts. *Archives of General Psychiatry, 47,* 805–808.

Jones, E. E., & Thorne, A. (1987). Rediscovery of the subject: Intercultural approaches to clinical assessment. *Journal of Consulting and Clinical Psychology, 55,* 488–495.

Kaplan, H., & Saddock, B. (1989). *Comprehensive textbook of psychiatry* (5th ed.). Baltimore: Williams & Wilkins.

Kaye, N. S., & Soreff, S. M. (1991). The psychiatrist's role, responses, and responsibilities when a patient commits suicide. *American Journal of Psychiatry, 78,* 739–743.

Kazdin, A. E. (1979). Fictions, factions, and functions of behavior therapy. *Behavior Therapy, 10,* 629–656.

Kelly, G. A. (1955). *The psychology of personal constructs* (2 vols.). New York: W. W. Norton.

Kendall, P. C., & Bemis, K. M. (1983). Thought and action in psychotherapy: The cognitive-behavioral approaches. In M. Hersen, A. E. Kazdin, & A. S. Bellack (Eds.), *The clinical psychology handbook.* New York: Pergamon.

Kernberg, O. F. (1976). *Object relations theory and clinical psychoanalysis.* New York: Jason Aronson.

Kihlstrom, J. F. (1985). Hypnosis. *Annual Review of Psychology, 36,* 385–418.

Knapp, M. L. (1972). *Nonverbal communication in human interaction.* New York: Holt, Rinehart & Winston.

Knapp, M. L. (1978). *Nonverbal communication in human interaction* (2nd ed.). New York: Holt, Rinehart & Winston.

Kohut, H. (1972). *The analysis of the self.* New York: International Universities Press.

Kohut, H. (1977). *The restoration of the self.* New York: International Universities Press.

Kohut, H. (1984). *How does analysis cure?* London: University of Chicago Press.

Korchin, S. J. (1976). *Modern clinical psychology.* New York: Basic Books.

Korchin, S. J., & Sands, S. H. (1982). Principles common to all psychotherapies. In C. E. Walker (Ed.), *Handbook of clinical psychology.* Homewood, IL: Dow Jones-Irwin.

Kottler, J. A., & Brown, R. W. (1992). *Introduction of therapeutic counseling.* Pacific Grove: Brooks/Cole.

Krumboltz, J. D., & Thoresen, C. E. (Eds.). (1976). *Counseling methods.* New York: Holt, Rinehart & Winston.

Kurdek, L., & Smith, J. P. (1987). Partner monogamy in married, heterosexual, cohabitating, gay, and lesbian couples. *Journal of Sex Research, 23,* 212–232.

Laing, R. D. (1982). *The voice of experience.* New York: Pantheon Books.

Lambert, M. J., & Arnold, R. C. (1987). Research and the supervisory process. *Professional psychology: Research and practice, 18,* 217–224.

Land, J. (1986). Personal communication.

Langs, R. (1973). *The technique of psychoanalytic psychotherapy.* New York: Jason Aronson.

Langs, R. (1986). *Unconscious communication and the technique of psychotherapy.* Paper presented at continuing education seminar, Syracuse, NY.

Lansky, M. R. (1986). Marital therapy for narcissistic disorders. In N. S. Jacobson & A. S. Gurman (Eds.), *Clinical handbook of marital therapy.* New York: Guilford.

Lazarus, A. A. (1976). *Multimodal behavior therapy.* New York: Springer.

Lazarus, A. A. (1981). *The practice of multimodal therapy.* New York: McGraw-Hill.

Lazarus, A. A. (1992). The multi-modal approach to the treatment of minor depression. *American Journal of Psychotherapy, 46,* 50–57.

Lazarus, A. A., Beutler, L. E., & Norcross, J. C. (1992). The future of technical eclecticism. *Psychotherapy, 29,* 11–20.

Leary, T. (1957). *Interpersonal diagnosis of personality.* New York: The Ronald Press.

Le Guin, U. K. (1969). *The left hand of darkness.* New York: Ace Books.

Lennon, S. J., & Davis, L. L. (1990). Categorization in first impressions. *Journal of Psychology, 123,* 439–446.

Lerner, M. S., & Clum, G. A. (1990). Treatment of suicide ideators: A problem-solving approach. *Behavior Therapy, 21,* 403–411.

LeVine, S., & LeVine, R. A. (1985). Age, gender, and the demographic transition: The life course in agrarian societies. In A. S. Rossi (Ed.), *Gender and the life course.* New York: Aldine.

Levitt, E. A. (1964). The relationship between abilities to express emotional meanings vocally and facially. In J. R. Davis (Ed.), *The communication of emotional meaning.* New York: McGraw-Hill.

Luborsky, L. (1984). *Principles of psychoanalytic psychotherapy: A manual for supportive-expressive treatment.* New York: Basic Books.

Luborsky, L., Singer, B., & Luborsky, L. (1975). Comparative studies of psychotherapies. *Archives of General Psychiatry, 32,* 995–1008.

MacDevitt, J. W. (1987). Therapists' personal therapy and professional self-awareness. *Psychotherapy, 24,* 693–703.

Maholick, L. T., & Turner, D. W. (1979). Termination: That difficult farewell. *American Journal of Psychotherapy, 33,* 583–591.

Mahoney, M. J. (1990). Developmental psychotherapy. Workshop presented at the 24th annual meeting of the Association for the Advancement of Behavior Therapy, San Francisco.

Mahoney, M. J. (1991). *Human change processes.* New York: Basic Books.

Mallinckrodt, B. (1991). Client's representation of childhood emotional bonds with parents, social support, and formation of the working alliance. *Journal of Counseling Psychology, 38,* 401–409.

Marcia, J. E. (1966). Development and validation of ego identity status. *Journal of Personality and Social Psychology, 3,* 551–558.

Margulies, A. (1984). Toward empathy: The uses of wonder. *American Journal of Psychiatry, 141,* 1025–1033.

Marks, I. M. (1981). *Care and cure of neuroses.* New York: Wiley.

Maslow, A. H. (1970). *Motivation and personality* (2nd ed.). New York: Harper & Row.

Maurer, R. E., & Tindall, J. H. (1983). Effect of postural congruence on client's perception of counselor empathy. *Journal of Counseling Psychology, 30,* 158–163.

May, R. (1967). *The art of counseling.* Nashville, TN: Parthenon.

Mayerson, N. (1984). Preparing clients for group therapy: A critical review and theoretical formulation. *Clinical Psychology Review, 4,* 191–213.

McCarthy, P. R., & Foa, E. B. (1990). Obsessive-compulsive disorder. In M. E. Thase, B. A. Edelstein, & M. Hersen, (Eds.), *Handbook of outpatient treatment of adults: Nonpsychotic mental disorders.* New York: Plenum.

McIntosh, J. L. (1991). Epidemiology of suicide in the United States. In A. A. Leenaars (Ed.), *Life-span perspectives of suicide: Time-lines in the suicide process* (pp. 55–69). New York: Plenum.

Meador, B., & Rogers, C. R. (1984). Person-centered therapy. In R. J. Corsini (Ed.), *Current psychotherapies.* Itasca, IL: Peacock.

Means, J. R. (1981). Personal communication.

Means, J. R. (1990). Personal communication.

Meier, S. T. (1989). *The elements of counseling.* Belmont, CA: Wadsworth.

Meier, S. T. (1991). Personal communication.

Meissner, W. W. (1991). *What is effective in psychoanalytic therapy?: The move from interpretation to relation.* New Jersey: Jason Aronson.

Mezzich, J. E., & Shea, S. C. (1990). Interviewing and diagnosis. In M. E. Thase, B. A. Edelstein, & M. Hersen (Eds.), *Handbook of outpatient treatment of adults: Nonpsychotic mental disorders*. New York: Plenum.

Miles, C. P. (1977). Conditions predisposing to suicide: A review. *The Journal of Nervous and Mental Disease, 164*, 231–246.

Miller, J. B. (1986). *Toward a new psychology of women* (2nd ed.). Boston: Beacon Press.

Miller, J. P. (1979). *Suicide after sixty: The final alternative*. New York: Springer.

Miller, M. (1985). *Information Center: Training workshop manual*. San Diego: The Information Center.

Miller, P. H. (1983). *Theories of developmental psychology*. San Francisco: W. H. Freeman and Co.

Mischel, W. (1968). *Personality and assessment*. New York: Wiley.

Moras, K., & Strupp, H. H. (1982). Pretherapy interpersonal relations, patients' alliance and outcome in brief therapy. *Archives of General Psychiatry, 39*, 405–409.

Moris, R. (1990). *Forensic suicidology*. Paper presented at the meeting of the American Psychological Association, Boston.

Morshead, L. L. (1990). *Psychotherapists' responses to anger manifested by female clients*. Paper presented at the meeting of the American Psychological Association, Boston.

Mosak, H. H. (1989). Adlerian psychotherapy. In R. J. Corsini & D. Wedding (Eds.). *Current psychotherapies* (4th ed.). Itasca: F. E. Peacock.

Moursund, J. (1990). *The process of counseling and therapy* (2nd ed.). Englewood Cliffs, NJ: Prentice-Hall.

Murphy, G. E., & Wetzel, R. D. (1990). The lifetime risk of suicide in alcoholism. *Archives of General Psychiatry, 47*, 383–392.

Murphy, K. R., & Davidshofer, C. O. (1988). *Psychological testing*. Englewood Cliffs, NJ: Prentice-Hall.

Myers, D. G. (1989). *Psychology* (2nd ed.). New York: Worth.

Nutt, R. L., Hampton, B. R., Folks, B., & Johnson, R. J. (1990). *Applying feminist principles to supervision*. Paper presented at the meeting of the American Psychological Association, Boston.

Okun, B. F. (1987). *Effective helping: Interviewing and counseling techniques* (3rd ed.). Monterey, CA: Brooks/Cole.

Orlinsky, D., & Howard, K. (1978). The relation of process to outcome in psychotherapy. In S. Garfield & A. Bergin (Eds.), *Handbook of psychotherapy and behavior change: An empirical analysis*. New York: Wiley.

Othmer, E., & Othmer, S. C. (1989). *The clinical interview using DSM-III-R*. Washington, DC: American Psychiatric Press.

Parrot, L. (1992). Earliest recollections and birth order: Two Adlerian exercises. *Teaching of Psychology, 19*, 40–42.

Patterson, W. M., Dohn, H. H., Bird, J., & Patterson, G. A. (1983). Evaluation of suicidal patients: The SAD PERSONS scale. *Psychosomatics, 24*, 343–349.

Peck, M. S. (1978). *The road less travelled*. New York: Simon & Schuster.

Pederson, P. B. (1988). *A handbook for developing multicultural awareness.* Alexandria, VA: American Association for Counseling and Development.

Pederson, P. B. (Ed.). (1991). Special issue: Multiculturalism as a fourth force in counseling. *Journal of Counseling and Development, 70,* 1–250.

Pennebaker, J. W., Keicolt-Glaser, J. K., & Glaser, R. (1988). Disclosure of traumas and immune function: Health implications for psychotherapy. *Journal of Consulting and Clinical Psychology, 56,* 239–245.

Pennebaker, J. W., & O'Heeron, R. C. (1984). Confiding in others and illness rate among spouses of suicide and accidental death victims. *Journal of Abnormal Psychology, 93,* 473–476.

Phares, E. J. (1988). *Clinical psychology* (3rd ed.). Chicago: The Dorsey Press.

Pietrofesa, J. J., Hoffman, A., & Splete, H. H. (1984). *Counseling: An introduction* (2nd ed.) Boston: Houghton-Mifflin.

Pietsch, P. (1972, May). 'Shuffle brain.' *Harper's Magazine.*

Pipes, R. B., & Davenport, D. S. (1990). *Introduction to psychotherapy: Common clinical wisdom.* Englewood Cliffs, NJ: Prentice-Hall.

Plutchik, R. (1980). A language for the emotions. *Psychology Today, 13,* 68–78.

Poe, E. A. (1985). Silence: A fable. In *Works of Edgar Allan Poe.* New York: Avenel Books.

Pope, K. S. (1990). Therapist-patient sex as sex abuse: Six scientific, professional and practical dilemmas in addressing victimization and rehabilitation. *Professional Psychology: Research and Practice, 21,* 227–239.

Prochaska, J. O. (1984). *Systems of psychotherapy: A transtheoretical approach.* Chicago: The Dorsey Press.

Resnik, H. L. P. (1980). Suicide. In H. I. Kaplan and B. J. Sadock (Eds.), *Comprehensive textbook of psychiatry* (3rd ed.). Baltimore: Williams & Wilkins.

Retzlauff, P., Gibertini, M., Scolatti, M., Laughna, S., & Sommers, J. (1986). The Personality Adjective Inventory: Construction, reliability, and validity. *Educational and Psychological Measurement, 46,* 963–971.

Riskind, J. H., Beck, A. T., Brown, G., & Steer, R. A. (1987). Taking the measure of anxiety and depression: Validity of the reconstructed Hamilton Scales. *Journal of Nervous and Mental Disease, 175,* 474–479.

Robbins, S. B., & Jolkovski, M. P. (1987). Managing countertransference feelings: An interactional model using awareness of feeling and theoretical framework. *Journal of Counseling Psychology, 34,* 276–282.

Robins, E. (1985). Psychiatric emergencies. In H. I. Kaplan and B. J. Sadock (Eds.), *Comprehensive textbook of psychiatry* (3rd ed.). Baltimore: Williams & Wilkins.

Robinson, F. (1950). *Principles and procedures in student counseling.* New York: Harper & Row.

Rodolfa, E. R., Kraft, W. A., & Reilley, R. R. (1988). Stressors of professionals and trainees at APA-approved counseling and VA medical center internship sites. *Professional Psychologist: Research and Practice, 19,* 43–49.

Rogers, C. R. (1942). *Counseling and psychotherapy.* Boston: Houghton-Mifflin.

Rogers, C. R. (1951). *Client-centered therapy.* Boston: Houghton-Mifflin.

Rogers, C. R. (1957). The necessary and sufficient conditions of therapeutic personality change. *Journal of Consulting Psychology, 21*, 95–103.

Rogers, C. R. (1958). The characteristics of a helping relationship. *Personnel and Guidance Journal, 37*, 6–16.

Rogers, C. R. (1961). *On becoming a person.* Boston: Houghton-Mifflin.

Rogers, C. R. (1972). *Carl Rogers on counseling, a personal perspective at 75 [Film].* Corona Del Mar, CA: Psychological and Educational Films.

Rosenthal, R. H., & Akiskal, H. S. (1985). Mental status examination. In M. Hersen & S. M. Turner (Eds.), *Diagnostic interviewing.* New York: Plenum.

Roy, A. (1989). Suicide. In H. Kaplan and B. Sadock (Eds.), *Comprehensive textbook of psychiatry* (5th ed.). Baltimore: Williams & Wilkins.

Saint-Exupery, A. de. (1971). *The little prince.* New York: Harcourt, Brace, & Jovanovich.

Salinger, J. D. (1945). *The catcher in the rye.* Boston: Little, Brown.

Sattler, J. M. (1988). *Assessment of children.* San Diego: Jerome M. Sattler.

Schact, T. E., Binder, J. L., & Strupp, H. H. (1984). The dynamic focus. In H. H. Strupp and J. L. Binder, *Psychotherapy in a new key.* New York: Basic Books.

Scheflin, A. E., & Scheflin, A. (1972). *Body language and social order.* Englewood Cliffs, NJ: Prentice-Hall.

Seay, T. A. (1978). *Systematic eclectic therapy.* Jonesboro, TN: Pilgrimage Press.

Seligman, L. (1986). *Diagnosis and treatment planning in counseling.* New York: Human Sciences Press.

Seligman, L. (1990). *Selecting effective treatments.* San Francisco: Jossey-Bass.

Shaffer, D. R. (1989). *Developmental psychology: Childhood and adolescence* (2nd ed.). Pacific Grove, CA: Brooks/Cole.

Sharpley, C. F. (1984). Predicate matching in NLP: A review of research on the preferred representational system. *Journal of Counseling Psychology, 31*, 238–248.

Shea, S. C. (1988). *Psychiatric interviewing: The art of understanding.* Philadelphia: W. B. Saunders.

Shneidman, E. S. (1980). Psychotherapy with suicidal patients. In T. B. Karasu and L. Bellak (Eds.), *Specialized techniques in individual psychotherapy.* New York: Brunner/Mazel.

Shneidman, E. S. (1984). Aphorisms of suicide and some implications for psychotherapy. *American Journal of Psychotherapy, 38*, 319–328.

Siassi, I. (1984). Psychiatric interview and mental status examination. In G. Goldstein & M. Hersen (Eds.), *Handbook of psychological assessment.* New York: Pergamon.

Siegel, B. (1986). *Love, medicine, and miracles.* New York: Harper & Row.

Sifneos, P. E. (1987). *Short-term dynamic psychotherapy.* New York: Plenum.

Silverman, C. (1968). The epidemiology of depression—a review. *American Journal of Psychiatry, 124*, 883–891.

Skinner, B. F. (1971). *Beyond freedom and dignity.* New York: Alfred A. Knopf.

Sloane, R. B., Staples, F., Cristol, A., Yorkston, N., & Whipple, K. (1975). *Psychotherapy versus behavior therapy.* Cambridge, MA: Harvard University Press.

Smith, M. L., Glass, G. V., & Miller, T. I. (1980). *The benefits of psychotherapy.* Baltimore: Johns Hopkins University Press.

Smith-Hanen, S. S. (1977). Effects of nonverbal behaviors on judged levels of counselor warmth and empathy. *Journal of Counseling Psychology, 24,* 87–91.

Snyder, M. (1974). Self-monitoring of expressive behavior. *Journal of Personality and Social Psychology, 30,* 526–537.

Soisson, E. L., VandeCreek, L., & Knapp, S. (1987). Thorough record keeping: A good defense in a litigious era. *Professional Psychology: Research & Practice, 18,* 498–502.

Sommers, J. (1986). *Psychiatric and familial sabotage in a case of obsessive-compulsive disorder.* Paper presented at the meeting of the Western Psychological Association, Seattle.

Sommers-Flanagan, J. (1990). *Common fears of beginning interviewers.* Unpublished manuscript. Portland, OR.

Sommers-Flanagan, J., & Means, J. R. (1987). Thou shalt not ask questions: An approach to teaching interviewing skills. *Teaching of Psychology, 14,* 164–166.

Sommers-Flanagan, J., & Sommers-Flanagan, R. (1989). A categorization of pitfalls common to beginning Interviewers. *The Journal of Training and Practice in Professional Psychology, 3,* 58–71.

Sonne, J. L., & Pope, K. S. (1991). Treating victims of therapist-patient sexual involvement. *Psychotherapy, 28,* 174–187.

Spitzform, M. (1982). Personal communication.

Spooner, S. E., & Stone, S. C. (1977). Maintenance of specific counseling skills over time. *Journal of Counseling Psychology, 24,* 66–71.

Staats, A. W. (1990). Paradigmatic behavior therapy: A unified framework for theory, research, and practice. In G. H. Eifert & I. M. Evans (Eds.), *Unifying behavior therapy: Contributions of paradigmatic behaviorism.* New York: Springer.

Sterling-Smith, R. (1974). A medical toxicology index: An evaluation of commonly used suicidal drugs. In A. T. Beck, H. L. P. Resnik, & D. J. Lettieri (Eds.), *The prediction of suicide.* Bowie, MD: Charles Press.

Sternberg, R. J. (1985). *Beyond IQ: A triarchic theory of human intelligence.* New York: Cambridge University Press.

Sternberg, R. J., & Wagner, R. K. (Eds.). (1986). *Practical intelligence: Origins of competence in the everyday world.* New York: Cambridge University Press.

Strong, S. R. (1968). Counseling: An interpersonal influence process. *Journal of Counseling Psychology, 15,* 215–224.

Strong, B., & DeVault, C. (1989). *The marriage and family experience* (4th ed.). St. Paul, MN: West.

Strub, R. L., & Black, F. W. (1977). *The mental status examination in neurology.* Philadelphia: F. A. Davis.

Strupp, H. H. (1955). The effect of the psychotherapist's personal analysis upon his techniques. *Journal of Consulting Psychology, 19,* 197–204.

Strupp, H. H. (1978). The therapist's theoretical orientation: An overrated variable. *Psychotherapy, 15,* 314–317.

Strupp, H. H. (1983). Psychoanalytic psychotherapy. In M. Hersen, A. E. Kazdin, & A. S. Bellack (Eds.), *The clinical psychology handbook.* New York: Pergamon.

Strupp, H. H., & Binder, J. L. (1984). *Psychotherapy in a new key.* New York: Basic Books.

Strupp, H. H., Hadley, S. W., & Gomes-Schwartz, B. (1977). *Psychotherapy for better or worse: The problem of negative effects.* New York: Jason Aronson.

Strupp, H. H., & Hadley, S. W. (1979). Specific vs. nonspecific factors in psychotherapy: A controlled study of outcome. *Archives of General Psychiatry, 36,* 1125–1136.

Sudak, H. S., Ford, A. B., & Rushforth, N. B. (1984). Adolescent suicide: An overview. *American Journal of Psychotherapy, 38,* 350–363.

Sue, D. W., Arredondo, P., & McDavis, R. J. (1992). Multicultural counseling competencies and standards: A call to the profession. *Journal of Counseling and Development, 70,* 477–486.

Sue, D. W., & Sue, S. (1987). Cultural factors in the clinical assessment of Asian-Americans. *Journal of Consulting and Clinical Psychology, 55,* 479–487.

Sue, D. W., & Sue, D. (1990). *Counseling the culturally different* (2nd ed.). Somerset, NJ: Wiley & Sons.

Sullivan, H. S. (1953). *The interpersonal theory of psychiatry.* New York: W. W. Norton.

Sullivan, H. S. (1970). *The psychiatric interview.* New York: W. W. Norton.

Szasz, T. S. (1961). *The myth of mental illness.* New York: Hoeber-Harper.

Szasz, T. S. (1970). *The manufacture of madness: A cooperative study of the inquisition and the mental health movement.* New York: McGraw-Hill.

Szasz, T. S. (1986). The case against suicide prevention. *American Psychologist, 41,* 806–812.

Teyber, E. (1988). *Interpersonal process in psychotherapy: A guide for clinical training.* Chicago: The Dorsey Press.

Thoresen, C. E., & Mahoney, M. J. (1974). *Behavioral self-control.* New York: Holt, Rinehart & Winston.

Thorpe, S. A. (1987). An approach to treatment planning. *Psychotherapy, 24,,* 729–735.

Tracey, T., Hays, K. A., Malone, J., & Herman, B. (1988). Changes in counselor response as a function of experience. *Journal of Counseling Psychology, 35,* 119–126.

Tuckman, J., & Youngman, W. F. (1968). Assessment of suicidal risk in attempted suicide. In H. L. P. Resnik (Ed.), *Suicidal behaviors.* Boston: Little, Brown.

Ullmann, L. P., & Krasner, L. (1965). *Case studies in behavior modification.* New York: Holt, Rinehart & Winston.

Vacc, N. A., Wittmer, J., & DeVaney, S. B. (1988). *Experiencing and counseling multicultural and diverse populations.* Muncie, IN: Accelerated Development.

Van Wagoner, S. L., Gelso, C. J., Hayes, J. A., & Diemer, R. A. (1991). Countertransference and the reputedly excellent therapist. *Psychotherapy, 28,* 411–421.

Wakefield, J. C. (1992). The concept of mental disorder: On the boundary between biological facts and social values. *American Psychologist, 47*, 373–388.

Walters, R. P. (1980). *Amity: Friendship in action: Part I. Basic friendship skills.* Boulder, CO: Christian Helpers.

Watkins, C. E., & Terrell, F. (1988). Mistrust level and its effects on counseling expectations in Black client-White counselor relationships: An analogue study. *Journal of Counseling Psychology, 35*, 194–197.

Watkins, J. G., (1987). *Hypnotherapeutic technique: The practice of clinical hypnosis.* (Vol. 1). New York: Irvington.

Watkins, J. G. (1978). *The therapeutic self.* New York: Human Sciences Press.

Watzlawick, P., Weakland, J., & Fisch, R. (1974). *Change: Principles of problem formation and problem resolution.* New York: Norton.

Webster's ninth new collegiate dictionary. (1985). Springfield, MA: Merriam-Webster.

Wechsler, D. (1958). *The measurement and appraisal of adult intelligence.* (4th ed.). Baltimore: Williams & Wilkins.

Wechsler, D. (1975). Intelligence defined and undefined. *American Psychologist, 30*, 135–139.

Wechsler, D., & Stone, C. P. (1945). *Wechsler memory scale manual.* New York: The Psychological Corporation.

Weinberg, G. (1984). *The heart of psychotherapy: A journey into the mind and office of the therapist at work.* New York: St. Martin's.

Weiner, I. B. (1975). *Principles of psychotherapy.* New York: Wiley.

Weiss, A. R. (1986). Teaching counseling and psychotherapy skills without access to a clinical population: The short interview method. *Teaching of Psychology, 13*, 145–147.

Westefeld, J. S., & Furr, S. R. (1987). Suicide and depression among college students. *Professional Psychology: Research and Practice, 18*, 119–123.

Westermeyer, J. (1987). Cultural factors in clinical assessment. *Journal of Consulting and Clinical Psychology, 55*, 471–478.

Wolberg, L. R. (1988). *The technique of psychotherapy* (4th ed., Parts 1 & 2). New York: Grune & Stratton.

Wolff, S. (1989). Personal communication.

Wollersheim, J. P. (1974). The assessment of suicide potential via interview methods. *Psychotherapy: Theory, research, and practice, 11*, 222–225.

Wollersheim, J. P. (1985). Personal communication.

World Health Organization. (1978)). *International classification of diseases.* Geneva: Author.

Yalom, I. D. (1985). *The theory and practice of group psychotherapy* (3rd ed.). New York: Basic Books.

Zaro, J. S., Barach, R., Nedelman, D. J., & Dreiblatt, I. S. (1977). *A guide for beginning psychotherapists.* New York: Cambridge University Press.

Zuckerman, M. (1990). Some dubious premises in research and theory on racial differences: Scientific, social, and ethical issues. *American Psychologist, 45*, 1297–1303.

NAME INDEX

Abt, I. R., 34
Adler, A., 201, 202
Ainsworth, M. D. S., 138, 270
Akiskal, H. S., 240
Alexander, J. A., 148
Allen, A., 207
Allen, M., 275
American Psychological Association, 46, 47
Arkoff, A., 32
Arnold, R. C., 3, 11
Arrendo, P., 7, 65
Asbury, F. S., 53, 117

Bach, R., 33
Balleweg, B. J., 8
Balzer, F. J., 53, 117
Banaka, W. H., 55
Bandler, R., 73, 84
Bandura, A., 133
Barach, R., 212, 216
Barlow, D. H., 7, 98
Basow, S. A., 24
Beck, A. T., 5, 6, 7, 110, 208, 216, 247, 252, 267
Beitman, B. D., 131, 132, 133
Bem, D., 207
Bemis, K. M., 5
Benjamin, A., 34, 35, 37, 38, 39, 49, 69, 84, 93, 100, 101, 108, 149, 157, 186, 190, 216
Bennett, C. C., 24, 28, 32, 267
Beutler, L. E., 7
Binder, J. L., 2, 5, 6, 18, 19, 53, 209, 210, 211, 271
Bird, J., 267
Birdwhistell, M. L., 53, 54, 251
Black, F. W., 218, 242

Blaney, P. H., 258
Bodkin, A., 216
Bornstein, M. T., 216
Bornstein, P. H., 9, 216
Bornstein, R. F., 131
Borysenko, J., 26, 32, 89
Bowlby, J., 138
Boyer, D., 19
Brammer, L. M., 75
Brockman, W. P., 73
Brodsky, A. M., 64, 141
Brody, C. M., 65, 114, 118
Brown, G., 216, 247, 252
Brown, J. H., 249
Brown, L., 141
Brown, R. W., 265
Bryant, B. K., 267
Bugental, J. F. T., 275, 277
Buie, D. H., 121, 123
Burns, G. L., 208
Buss, A. H., 23

Capra, F., 218
Carkhuff, R. R., 81, 121
Carver, C. S., 23
Cerny, J. A., 7, 98
Charlesworth, E. A., 26, 32
Childers, W. C., 53, 117
Clark, D., 247, 249, 253
Clark, E. M., 258
Clark, M. M., 22, 27, 274
Clarkin, J., 272
Clucas, T. J., 45
Cole, C. G., 57, 84, 96, 100, 183, 184
Corbine, J. L., 8
Corey, G., 3, 11, 114, 212
Cormier, L. S., 51, 53, 57, 58, 65, 92, 96, 100, 110, 139, 140, 183, 190, 196

Cormier, W. H., 51, 53, 57, 58, 65, 92, 96, 100, 110, 139, 140, 183, 190, 196
Corsini, R., 5, 11
Cottone, R. R., 274
Cox, B. G., 141, 145
Cristiani, T. S., 87, 96
Cristol, A., 5

Davenport, D. S., 38, 39, 44, 47, 53, 113, 132, 248, 253, 259
Davidshofer, C. O., 166
Davis & Lennon, 42
Davis, L. L., 42
Davison, G., 3, 5, 53, 125, 129, 133, 139
de Shazer, S., 89
DeVaney, S. B., 8, 59, 65
DeVault, C., 104
DiBianco, J. T., 249
Diemer, R. A., 132
Dodson, F., 104
Dohn, H. H., 267
Dreiblatt, I. S., 212, 216

Eagle, M. N., 134
Edelstein, B. A., 179
Egan, G., 53, 65, 81, 87, 92, 96, 102, 124
Eich, E., 258
Eliot, T. S., 269
Elliott, R., 236
Ellis, A. E., 6
Emery, G., 7
Erdman, J. P., 207
Erickson, M. H., 100
Evans, I. M., 248

Fairbairn, R., 134
Farberow, N. L., 248
Fawcett, J., 247, 249, 253
Felsenthal, C., 247
Fenichel, O., 88, 89, 129
Fenigstein, A., 23, 25
Fisch, R., 89
Fisher, S., 21
Fitzgerald, L. F., 145
Foa, E. B., 105
Fogg, L., 247, 249, 253
Foley, R., 149, 150, 173, 179
Folks, B., 142
Folman, R. Z., 118
Folstein, M. F., 234, 242

Folstein, S. E., 234, 242
Fong, M. L., 141, 145
Ford, A. B., 247, 248
Francis, A., 7
Frank, J. D., 15
Frankl, V. E., 136
Freud, A., 88
Freud, S., 4, 5, 123, 127, 129, 132

Gardner, H., 236
Gazda, G. M., 53, 110, 117
Gazzaniga, M. S., 275
Gelso, C. J., 132
George, R. L., 96
Georgotas, A., 247
Gibbons, R., 247, 249, 253
Gibbs, M. A., 69, 84
Gibertini, M., 26
Giffen, M. E., 247
Gilligan, C., 59, 65
Glaser, R., 200
Glass, G. V., 5
Goldfried, M., 3, 5, 7, 53, 125, 129, 133, 139, 197, 208, 274
Goldstein, A. P., 139
Gough, H. G., 26
Gould, S. J., 236
Graves, J. R., 58
Greenberg, J. R., 134
Greenberg, L. S., 89, 200
Greenberg, R. P., 22, 27, 274, 275
Greenson, R. R., 89, 110, 124, 145
Greenwood, C. W., 267
Greist, J. H., 207
Grinder, J., 73, 84
Gunderson, J. G., 216
Gustafson, J. P., 18, 126, 216

Hadley, S. W., 3, 14, 18, 119
Haley, J., 101
Hall, C., 11, 54
Hall, E. T., 53
Hamilton, M., 253
Hammer, A., 73
Hampton, B. R., 142
Hanson, C., 121
Harvey, J. H., 64
Hatfield, E., 103
Hathaway, S. R., 26
Hatton, C. L., 249

Hayes, V., 44, 132
Hays, K. A., 148
Hedeker, D., 247, 249, 253
Heinrich, R. K., 8
Helms, J. E., 120
Henteleff, P., 249
Herman, B., 148
Hersen, M., 20, 216
Hess, E. H., 54
Hill, C. E., 120
Holinger, P. C., 247
Holt, R. R., 42
Horowitz, M., 141
Howard, K., 97
Hutchins, D. E., 57, 84, 96, 100, 183, 184
Huxley, A., 244

Ivey, A. E., 52, 53, 54, 61, 90, 95, 96, 149, 159, 160, 272, 277
Izard, C. E., 57, 81

Johnson, R. J., 142, 245
Jolkovski, M. P., 131
Jones, E. E., 28

Kaltreider, N., 141
Kaplan, H., 11
Kaye, N. S., 265
Kazdin, A. E., 5
Keicolt-Glaser, J. K., 200
Kelly, G. A., 207
Kendall, P. C., 5
Kernberg, O. F., 134
Kihlstrom, L. L., 100
Klein, M. H., 207
Klerman, G. L., 245
Knapp, M. L., 54, 57
Knapp, S., 264
Kohut, H., 121, 125, 134
Korchin, S. J., 15, 16, 271
Kottler, J. A., 265
Kraft, W. A., 47
Krasner, L., 208
Krumboltz, J. D., 124
Krupnick, J., 141
Kurdek, L., 103

Laing, R. D., 217
Lambert, M. J., 3, 11
Land, J., 270

Langs, R., 34
Lansky, M. R., 125
Laughna, S., 26
Lazarus, A. A., 7, 196, 197, 216
Le Guin, U. K., 148
Leary, T., 208, 215
Lennon, S. J., 42
Lettieri, D. J., 267
LeVine, R. A., 65
Levine, S., 65
Levitt, E. A., 56, 57
Lindzey, G., 11
Luborsky, L., 3, 4, 5, 6, 18, 68, 71, 75, 97, 116, 120, 155, 209, 272, 277

MacDevitt, J. W., 22, 274
Maholick, L. T., 174
Mahoney, M. J., 5, 17, 197, 259, 260, 266
Malone, J., 148
Marcia, J. E., 274
Margulies, A., 123
Marks, I. M., 34
Marmar, C., 141
Maslow, A. H., 24, 25
Maurer, R. E., 55
Mayerson, N., 97
McCarthy, P. R., 105
McDavis, R. J., 7, 65
McHugh, P. R., 234, 242
McIntosh, J. L., 247
McKinley, J. C., 26
Meador, B., 72, 75, 84
Means, J. R., 6, 8, 9, 10, 93, 217
Meichenbaum, D., 110
Meier, S. T., 6, 56, 68, 71, 90, 102, 184, 189
Meissner, W. W., 5, 129
Mezzich, J. E., 8, 179, 181
Miles, C. P., 246
Miller, J. B., 59, 65, 125
Miller, J. P., 247, 248
Miller, M., 254
Miller, P. H., 11
Miller, T. I., 5
Mischel, W., 208
Mitchell, S. A., 134
Moras, K., 119
Moris, R., 263, 265
Morshead, L. L., 24
Mosak, H. H., 202
Moursund, J., 100, 149, 191

Murphy, G. E., 245, 249
Murphy, K. R., 166
Myers, D. G., 56, 134

Nathan, R. G., 26, 32
Nedelman, D. J., 212, 216
Norcross, J. C., 7
Nutt, R. L., 142, 145

Offer, D., 247
O'Heeron, R. C., 200
Okun, B. F., 90, 96
Orlinsky, D., 97
Othmer, E., 3, 113, 114, 120, 121, 125, 139, 140, 145, 150, 220, 223, 234, 242
Othmer, S. C., 3, 113, 114, 120, 121, 125, 139, 140, 145, 150, 220, 223, 234, 242

Parks, M. M., 64
Parrot, L., 202
Patterson, G. A., 267
Patterson, W. M., 267
Peck, M. S., 117, 118
Pederson, P. B., 65
Pennebaker, J. W., 200
Perls, F., 6
Perry, S., 272
Phares, E. J., 3, 13
Pietrofesa, J. J., 122
Pietsch, P., 85
Pipes, R. B., 38, 39, 44, 47, 53, 113, 132, 245, 253, 259
Plutchik, R., 57
Poe, E. A., 67
Pokorny, G., 252
Pope, K. S., 118
Prochaska, J. O., 7

Reilley, R. R., 47
Resnik, H. L. P., 247, 248, 249, 253, 254
Retzlauff, P., 26
Rink, A., 249, 250
Riskind, J. H., 216
Robbins, S. B., 131
Robins, E., 250
Robinson, F., 58, 69
Rodolfa, E. R., 47
Rogers, C. R., 4, 6, 8, 19, 25, 72, 74, 75, 77, 84, 101, 110, 112, 114, 115, 116, 117, 119, 121, 123, 124, 144, 145, 271

Ronningstam, E., 216
Rosenthal, R. H., 240
Rossi, E., 100
Rossi, S., 100
Rowe, C. J., 249
Roy, A., 246, 250, 267
Rush, A. H., 7
Rushforth, N. B., 247, 248

Saddock, B., 11
Safran, J. D., 89, 200
Saint Exupery, A. de., 182
Salinger, J. D., 51
Sands, S. H., 15
Sattler, J. M., 236
Schact, T. E., 209
Schaffer, T. 274
Scheflin, A., 65
Scheflin, A. E., 65
Scheier, M. F., 23
Scolatti, M., 26
Seay, T. A., 196
Seligman, L., 96, 272, 277
Sharf, B. F., 149, 150, 173, 179
Sharpley, C. F., 73, 74
Shaw, B. F., 7
Shea, S. C., 8, 39, 53, 149, 150, 158, 159, 160, 164, 170, 172, 177, 179, 181, 186, 193
Shneidman, E. S., 244, 248, 257, 258, 259, 260, 264
Siassi, I., 218
Siegel, B., 26, 44
Sifneos, P. E., 211
Silverman, C., 246
Singer, B., 5
Skinner, B. F., 34
Sloane, R. B., 5
Smith-Hanen, S. S., 59
Smith, J. P., 103
Smith, M. L., 5
Snyder, M., 56, 57
Soisson, E. L., 264
Sommers-Flanagan, J., 6, 8, 10, 69, 93, 124
Sommers-Flanagan, R., 124
Sommers, J., 26, 228
Sonne, J. L., 118
Soreff, S. M., 265
Spiegel, S. B., 120
Spitzform, M., 172

Spooner, S. E., 92
Staats, A. W., 208
Staller, J., 22, 27, 274, 275
Staples, F., 5
Steer, R. A., 216, 247, 252
Sterling-Smith, R., 267
Sternberg, R. J., 236
Stone, C. P., 234
Stone, S. C., 92
Strong, B., 104
Strong, S. R., 42, 139, 141
Strub, R. L., 218, 242
Strupp, H. H., 2, 3, 5, 6, 14, 18, 19, 22, 53, 110, 119, 135, 138, 209, 210, 211, 271
Stuart, L. E., 34,
Sudak, H. S., 247, 24
Sue, D. W., 7, 28, 65
Sue, S., 28
Sullivan, H. S., 127, 129
Szasz, T. S., 3, 264, 267

Teasdale, J. D., 258
Terrell, F., 7
Teyber, E., 209, 216
Thase, M. E., 179
Thomas, K. R., 8
Thoresen, C. E., 124, 197
Thorne, A., 28
Thorpe, S. A., 277
Tichenor, V., 120
Tindall, J. H., 55
Tracey, T., 148
Tuckman, J., 248
Turner, D. W., 174
Turner, S. M., 20, 216

Ullmann, L. P., 208

Vacc, N. A., 8, 59, 65
Valente, S. M., 249

VandeCreek, L., 264
VandenBos, G. R., 267
Van Wagoner, S. L., 132

Wagner, R. K., 236
Wakefield, J. C., 3
Wallerstein, R., 141
Walster, G. W., 103
Walters, R. P., 53, 54, 117
Watkins, C. E., 7
Watkins, J. G., 9, 101, 121
Watzlawick, P., 89
Wcakland, J., 89
Wechsler, D., 234, 235
Weinberg, G., 113
Weiner, I. B., 87, 88, 89, 110, 128, 129, 132, 136, 272
Weiss, A. R., 8, 10
Weissman, M. M., 245
Westermeyer, J., 7
Wetzel, R. D., 245, 249
Whipple, K., 5
Wilde, O., 1
Wilner, N., 141
Wittmer, J., 8, 59, 65
Wolberg, B., 6, 113, 191, 192
Wolff, S., 15
Wollersheim, J. P., 43, 252, 253, 254, 255, 256, 257, 258, 259, 267, 274

Yalom, I. D., 23, 91, 103, 110
Yorkston, N., 5
Young, M. A., 247, 249, 253
Youngman, W. F., 248

Zaro, J. S., 212, 216
Zola, M. A., 247
Zuckerman, M., 27, 32

SUBJECT INDEX

Abstract thinking, 236–237
Abuse:
  alcohol and drug, 207, 220, 247, 249, 262
  child, 105, 107, 128, 156
  physical, 105, 128, 190, 193, 196
  of power and authority, 105
  of questions, 92, 93, 182, 183, 216
  sexual, 118, 141, 193, 196, 201, 212
  substance, 249
Acceptance, 119
Accurate empathy, 4, 87, 111, 115, 121–124, 127, 145
Active listening, 3, 14, 31–32, 84
Advanced empathy, 87
Advice, 17, 69, 80, 85, 95, 97, 100–103, 105–106, 109, 110, 141, 183
Affect:
  and the BASIC ID, 196–197
  defined, 221
  descriptors of, 223
  and memory, 203
  and mood, 217, 219, 221, 223
  and speech content, 223
Agreement-disagreement, 85, 103–104
  alternatives to, 104
  potential effects of, 103–104, 106
  primary intent/effect, 106
Appearance, 217, 219–220
  of clients, 219–220
  of interviewers, 41–42
  as a manifestation of client mental state, 219–220
Approval-disapproval, 85, 105–108
  primary intent/effect, 106
Armchair diagnosis, 38
Assessment:
  ABC model of, 197

BASIC ID model of, 196–197
  inadequate, 18
  suicide, 243–267
Attending behavior, 51–59, 61–62, 67, 71, 80
  negative, 51, 53, 58–59
  positive, 51, 53, 59
  skill-building activities for, 55, 67
Attitude:
  of client toward interviewer, 217, 220–222
  defined, 220
  descriptors of client, 222
Attractiveness, 111, 140–141
Audiotaping, 33, 40, 41
Awareness (see Self-awareness)

BASIC ID, 196–197
Body language, 53–55
  and mirroring, 54–55
  positive, 54
Body phase (of the interview), 147, 163–170
  checklist for, 170
  and information gathering, 164–165
Brief nondirective interviews, 67, 80, 93

Clarification, 67, 74–76, 80
  forms of, 74–75
  guidelines for use, 75–76
  purpose of, 74, 80
Client(s):
  affect and mood, 221, 223
  appearance of, 219–220
  attitude toward the examiner (interviewer), 217, 220–222
  background and personal history of, 199–207

Client(s): (continued)
  common fears of, 111, 113–115
  common problems of, 15, 193
  current functioning of, 211–212
  development, 269, 271–272
  expectations, 156–157
  goals of, 212
  interpersonal style of, 207–211
  memory and intelligence of, 232–238
  opening statements of, 160–163
  orientation and consciousness of,
    230–232
  perceptual disturbances of, 228–230
  registration forms for, 212–213
  rehearsed opening statements of, 160
  reliability, judgment, and insight of,
    236–239
  speech and thought of, 223–228
  symptom analysis of, 194–196
Clinical judgment, 165–166
  sources of, 165–166
Closing phase (of the interview), 147,
    170–174
  checklist for, 173
  guiding and empowering clients
    during, 173
  instilling hope during, 172–173
  reassuring and supporting clients
    during, 171–172
  summarizing crucial themes during,
    172
  tying up loose ends during,174
Common client problems:
  conceptualizing, 193, 196–199
  prioritizing, 193–194
Confidentiality, 33, 45–47
  defined, 45
  as an ethical principle, 46
  informing clients about, 46–47
  legal and ethical limits of, 46–47
Confrontation, 85, 93–96
  as a directive listening response, 93–96
  firm, 94–95
  gentle, 94
  measuring the effectiveness of, 95
  primary intent/effect, 96
Congruence
  and Carl Rogers, 4, 111, 115–117
  and physical touch, 116, 118
  implications of, 116, 118–119

problems associated with, 117–118
  tempering of, 117–118
Core conditions (according to C. Rogers),
    111–112, 115–127
Countertransference, 111, 130–133
  coping with, 133
  as an impediment to psychotherapy,
    132
  and interviewer unconscious process,
    132
  and transference, 131
Crisis intervention with suicidal clients,
    243, 257–263
Cultural issues, 7, 27, 51, 54, 59–60
  and differences in attending skills, 51,
    54, 59–60
  and eye contact, 54
Cultural self-awareness, 7, 27–28

Delusions, 226–227
Depression:
  and memory, 233–234
  and suicide, 246–247, 250, 252–253
  symptoms of, 198
Desensitization:
  and objective self-awareness, 25–26
  and silence, 81–82
Development:
  client, 269, 271–272
  interviewer, 269, 272–276
  what is, 270–271
Developmental self-awareness, 26–27
Diagnosis:
  armchair, 38
  criteria for dysthymia, 198
  and DSM-III-R, 166–167, 198
  learning procedures of, 3, 4, 86,
    166–168, 170
  procedures, 166–168, 170, 198
  syndromes, 197–199
Directive action responses:
  agreement-disagreement, 103–104,
    106
  approval-disapproval, 105–108
  explanation (providing information),
    97–100, 106
  giving advice, 101–103, 106
  suggestion, 100–101, 106
  urging, 105–106
Directive historical leads, 201–207

Directive listening responses:
  confrontation, 93–96
  feeling validation, 90–92, 96
  interpretation, 87–90, 96
  interpretive reflection of feeling, 86–88,
    96
  questions, 92–93, 96
Documentation, 264–265

Emotional or psychological disorders,
  166–168, 170
Emotional expression, 57, 81–82
Empathy:
  advanced, 87
  asking the question of, 121–122
  and client ambivalence, 126–127
  and crisis intervention, 257–258
  defined, 121
  effects of, 124
  misguided attempts at, 124–126
  strategies, 123–124
  and various theoretical orientations, 5,
    125
Empowerment, 111, 143–144
Enhancing feeling capacity and
  vocabulary, 67
Ethical issues, 33, 45–47, 264–265
Expertness, 111, 139, 140
Explanation (providing information), 85,
  97–100, 106
  and cognitive behavioral therapists, 99
  as reassurance, 98–99
  as role induction, 97
  types of, 97–99
Eye contact, 53–54

Feedback, 51, 62–63
Feeling capacity and vocabulary, 81–82
Feeling validation, 85, 90–91, 96
Feminist issues, 69, 111, 118–119, 125,
  141–144
Free association, 4

Generating sensory-based and/or feeling
  words, 62, 82–83
Giving advice, 85, 101–106
Goals and objectives of this book, 18

Hallucinations:
  forms of, 228–230

questioning clients about, 229–230
Hierarchy of needs (Maslow), 24
Humor, 108

Identification, 111, 133–135
Individual differences, 60,
Insight:
  as an effect of interpretation, 85, 87–90,
    96
  in mental status examinations, 237–239
  measuring client, 237–239
Intake interviews:
  current functioning of client during,
    211–212
  evaluating client interpersonal style
    during, 207–211
  identifying and exploring client
    problems through, 192–199
  objectives of, 192
  obtaining historical information
    during, 199–207
Intelligence:
  defined, 235
  forms of, 236
  and memory, 217, 232–237
  questions used to assess, 237
Internalization:
  of bad objects, 134–135
  of good objects, 134–135
  and identification, 111, 133–135
Interpersonal:
  circumplex, 208–209
  styles, 208
Interpretation:
  and genetic material, 89
  primary intent/effect, 96
  psychoanalytic or classical, 88–89
  and reframing, 89–90
  trial, 210–211
  and the unprepared patient, 89
Interpretive reflection of feeling, 85–88, 96
Interviewer:
  development, 269, 272–276
  expectations and misconceptions, 28
  personal goals, 276
  response analysis, 107
  self-statement, 20
  use of logic and intuition, 275–276
Interviewer development activities:
  brief nondirective interviews, 80–81

Interviewer development activities:
(*continued*)
enhancing feeling capacity and
vocabulary, 81
gathering information with questions,
183, 188
generating sensory-based and/or
feeling words, 82
interviewer response analysis, 107
rubber band exercise, 55
silence desensitization, 81–82
Interviewer opening statement, 147
Interviewer response analysis, 107
Interviewing:
defined, 13–14
favorite phase, 169
Introduction phase (of the interview):
addressing clients during, 152–155
and base rates, 153–154
checklist for, 158
conversation and small talk, 152–153,
155–156
defined, 150
educating clients during, 156–158
initial face-to-face meeting, 152–154
standardized, 153–154
and telephone contact, 150–152

Judgment:
assessing client, 237–238
of clients, 237–238
clinical, 165–166

Leary's interpersonal circumplex,
208–209
Less-directive, 70
Listening skills, 13, 18, 271

Marital therapy (counseling):
and empathy, 125
interviewing approaches, 216
Maturation, 270–271
Memory:
confabulation of, 233
and intelligence, 217, 232–235
methods of measuring client, 233–235
and pseudodementia, 234
types of, 232–235
Mental status examination:
a generic approach to, 219–239

what is a, 218–219
when to use, 240
Mental status report, 239
Mirroring, 55
Mood:
and affect, 217, 219, 221, 223
descriptors of, 223
Mutuality, 111, 142, 143

Negative attending behavior(s), 51, 53,
56, 58–59, 61–62
and doodling, 61–62
excessive eye contact, 58
excessive head nods, 58
excessive mirroring, 58
excessive "uh-huhs," 58
Negative psychotherapy outcomes, 14,
17–18
Neurolinguistic programming (NLP), 73
Nondirective historical leads, 200–201
Nondirective listening responses:
attending behavior, 71, 80
clarification, 74–76, 80
nondirective reflection of feeling,
76–77, 80
paraphrase, 72–74, 80
silence, 67–69, 71–72, 80
summarization, 77–80
Nondirective reflection of feeling:
accuracy of, 77
and feeling validation, 90
intent/effect, 76, 80
Note-taking, 33, 38–40
informing clients of, 39
rules for, 39

Objective self-awareness, 13, 22–23, 25–26
Obsessions:
and compulsions, 227–228, 230
questioning clients about, 230
Opening phase (of the interview):
checklist for, 164
client statements, 160–163
interviewer's statement, 159–160
Orientation and consciousness:
descriptors of, 232
levels of, 231
questions directed toward client,
230–232
Other-awareness, 7

Paralinguistics, 55–57
Paraphrase (*see also* Reflection of content):
    generic, 73
    metaphorical, 74
    primary intent/effect, 72, 80
    sensory based, 73–74, 80
Parataxic distortion, 127
Payment for services, 16
Perceptual disturbances:
    hallucinations, 228–230
    illusions, 228–229
    questioning clients about, 229–230
Personal therapy, 274–275
Physical setting, 33
Premature advice, 102–103
Privacy, 34–35
Probe, 92
Problem conceptualization systems,
    196–199
Problem prioritization, 193–194
Professional:
    background and affiliation, 213
    relationships with clients, 15–17
    relationships, 15–17
    worth, 16
Professional issues, 243
    completed suicides, 265
    consultation, 264
    documentation, 264–265
    work with suicidal clients, 243, 263–264
Psychiatric interviewing, and empathy, 125
Psychodiagnostic interviewing, 218
Psychomotor activity, 217

Questions, 85, 92, 93, 96, 181–192
    and overuse, 92, 93
    benefits and liabilities of, 187–189
    classifying, 187–192
    closed, 184–185
    gathering information with, 188
    guidelines in using, 189–192
    indirect, 186
    open, 183–184
    primary intent/effect, 96
    projective, 186–187
    swing, 185–186
    types of, 183–187, 192

Rapport, 3, 111, 112, 113–115, 149
Rapprochement, 7

Reflection of content (*see also*
    Paraphrase), 67, 72, 73, 74, 80
Registration forms, 212, 213
Reliability, of client reports, 236–238
Resistance:
    managing, 137–138
    to medical intervention, 135
    recognizing, 136–137
    and the terrible twos, 136
Role induction:
    and the effectiveness of
        counseling/psychotherapy,
        97–98
    explanation and, 97–98
Room, 33–36

Seating arrangements, 33–38
Self-awareness:
    cultural, 7, 27, 28
    developmental, 26–27
    forms of, 23
    objective, 13, 22–23, 25–26
    physical, 23–24
    psychosocial, 24–26
Self-disclosure, 108
Self-presentation:
    and first impressions, 41–42
    grooming and attire, 41–42
    presenting credentials, 42–43
Sentence completion test for beginning
    interviewers, 29–30
Sex biases, 23–24
Silence:
    and client discomfort, 68–71
    guidelines for using, 71–72
    and interviewer discomfort, 68–71
Silence desensitization, 67, 81–82
Speech:
    describing client, 223–224
    rate and volume, 223–224
    and thought, 217, 223–224
Stereotypes, sexual (gender), 23–24
Stress management:
    for interviewers, 33, 47,48
    suggested readings, 49
Structural models, 147, 149–150
Suggestion:
    as compared with advice, 100, 101
    and hypnosis, 100, 101
    interview effect, 106

Suicide:
  alternatives to, 243, 258–259
  assessment, 243, 250–257
  and client self-control, 243, 256–257
  and depression, 243, 25–257
  hospitalization, 261–263
  ideation, 243, 253–254
  intent, 243, 257
  myths, 243, 246
  plans, 243, 254–256
  prediction, 244–245
  prevention contracts, 243, 259–260
  quiz, 245
  quiz answers, 251–252
  risk factors associated with, 243,
    246–250
  sad persons scale, 267
  SLAP, 254–256
  statistics, 243, 244–245
Summarization:
  difficulties associated with, 78–79
  guidelines for, 79
  primary intent/effect, 77, 80
Symptom analysis, 194–196

Termination phase (of the interview):
  checklist for, 176
  facing, 176–177
  guiding or controlling, 175–176
  significant client statements and
    actions during, 174
  watching the clock, 174
Textbook organization, 1, 9
Theoretical orientations:
  behavioral, 5, 70, 99–100, 111, 125, 129,
    133, 138–141, 196–197, 210
  cognitive, 5, 70, 99–100, 196–197, 210
  feminist, 69, 111, 118–119, 125, 141–144
  object relations, 134–135
  person-centered, 4–5, 70, 111, 118–119
  psychoanalytic, 70–71, 88, 100–101,
    111, 118–119, 125, 127–138, 207, 210
Therapeutic interviewing:
  defined, 13–14

guiding factors underlying, 20
Thought:
  content, 226–228
  process, 225–226
  and speech, 217, 223–224
Time:
  and client tardiness, 44
  ending sessions on, 45
  excuses for extending session length,
    45
  starting sessions on, 43–44
  when clients are early, 44
Total awareness interviewing, 1, 8, 9
Transference:
  and ambivalence, 129–130
  interpretation of, 129
  as an old map, 127–128
  and self-fulfilling prophecies, 128
Treatment planning, 218, 269, 271, 272
Trial interpretation, 210–211
Trust:
  defined, 141
  tests of, 141
Trustworthiness, 111, 141

Unconditional positive regard, 4, 111,
  119–121
  direct expressions of, 120
  how to express, 120–121
Urging, 85, 105, 106
  and crisis situations, 105
  primary intent/effect, 106

Verbal tracking, 53, 56
Videotaping, 33, 40–41
Vocal qualities (*see also* Paralinguistics),
  53, 55–56

Working alliance, 111, 124, 129, 138
  and attachment theory, 138
  as a predictor of psychotherapy
    response, 138
  and suicidal clients, 258